Placebo Effects

Placebo Effects

SECOND EDITION

Fabrizio Benedetti, MD
Professor of Neurophysiology and Human Physiology
Department of Neuroscience
University of Turin Medical School, Italy
National Institute of Neuroscience, Turin, Italy

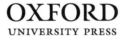

OXFORD
UNIVERSITY PRESS

OXFORD
UNIVERSITY PRESS

Great Clarendon Street, Oxford, OX2 6DP,
United Kingdom

Oxford University Press is a department of the University of Oxford.
It furthers the University's objective of excellence in research, scholarship,
and education by publishing worldwide. Oxford is a registered trade mark of
Oxford University Press in the UK and in certain other countries

First Edition published in 2009
Second Edition published in 2014

Impression: 1

Published in the United States of America by Oxford University Press
198 Madison Avenue, New York, NY 10016, United States of America

British Library Cataloguing in Publication Data
Data available

Library of Congress Control Number: 2014936312

ISBN 978-0-19-870508-6

Printed in Great Britain by
Clays Ltd, St Ives plc

Reviews of the First Edition

Benedetti is highly analytical in his approach and, at the same time, has the ability to explain complex matters so that they are easily understood. This book should be a must for all who struggle to make sense out of the intriguing phenomenon we call placebo. (*Pharmaceutical Press*)

Benedetti's book is a lucid and extensive review entrenched in the neuroscience of placebo research and heralding the importance of this area of study. (*PsycCRITIQUES*®)

. . . comprehensive and thoughtful volume . . . All physicians could learn much from this volume. (*New England Journal of Medicine*)

The breadth of topics addressed . . . make this book an important read for anyone in the medical field. (*Journal of the Neurological Sciences*)

For Claudia and Federica, with affection and love.

Preface to the Second Edition

There are at least three reasons why I decided to write a Second Edition of this book. First, the First Edition was well received by scientists, physicians, psychologists, sociologists, philosophers, and students. Indeed, there was the need for a book of this kind, in order to better describe what placebo effects are, how they work, and what their meaning is within the clinical context and more in general within the modern biomedical paradigm. Second, there has been a dramatic increase in placebo studies over the past 5–6 years, particularly by using a biological approach. This has originated a true science of placebo, whose study represents today a melting pot of concepts and ideas for neuroscience, ranging from a reductionist to a more integrative approach. Therefore, this Second Edition represents an update with the more recent findings over the past 5 years. The third reason why I present this new Edition is that many medical schools and psychology courses are using this book for teaching. I am particularly delighted that now students can learn something more about placebo effects while they are also learning medical and psychological skills and practice. Accordingly, I subdivided this Second Edition into five parts. The first is about some general principles, the second and third parts are a systematic description of placebo effects across different medical conditions, whereas the fourth part is about some clinical, ethical, and methodological considerations. I also decided to add a very short fifth part on some interesting issues outside the healing environment, such as physical and cognitive performance as well as some aspects investigated by social psychology. Hopefully, this fifth part will stimulate further research outside the strict biomedical field. Finally, I added several boxes, which I hope will be of interest to those readers who want to learn some more about some unfamiliar topics. I hope I was able to reach all of these goals.

Preface to the First Edition

The progress of modern medicine basically resides in the advancement of anatomy, physiology, molecular biology and, more in general, a better knowledge of how molecules, cells and tissues behave and interact with each other. Within this context, the modern physician has many effective tools in his hands to treat and prevent diseases, from pharmacology to genetic therapy and from physical intervention to surgery. Besides this materia medica, the patient's mind, emotions and beliefs also matter and play a central part in any therapy, as emphasized and investigated by different biomedical disciplines, like psychosomatics and psychoneuroimmunology.

With this book on placebo and placebo-related effects, I want to give scientific evidence to the old tenet that patients must be both cured and cared for. Curing the disease only is not always sufficient and care of the patient must often be careful and appropriate, as in many circumstances the patient's mind really matters. However, maybe paradoxically, anatomy, physiology, cells and molecules are all crucial to understand this psychological aspect of the therapy. In fact, today we know that placebo effects are mediated by many molecules in the brain which, in turn, may affect the course of a disease and the response to a treatment. Therefore, this is a biological book which emphasizes the importance of the psychological component of a therapy by using the same biological tools of the materia medica.

Many misunderstandings and misconceptions about the placebo effect have permeated the history of medicine. Perhaps, the most common resides in its very definition. The inappropriate use of the words "placebo effect" and "placebo response" has pervaded the medical literature for many years, and even today these terms are sometimes confused with other phenomena. In clinical trials, for example, several authors continue to wrongly coin the terms "placebo effect" or "placebo response" when they want to describe the therapeutic outcome in those groups of patients who received a placebo (an inert treatment). Indeed, the common and widespread use of "placebo effect" and "placebo response" refers to the outcome in placebo groups, without considering that many factors are responsible for the reduction of a symptom when patients take a placebo. Therefore, what most studies deal with when they talk about placebo effects and placebo responses is actually a complex set of phenomena that are responsible for the clinical improvement.

For example, when a group of patients takes a placebo and improves, this can be due to the spontaneous remission of the disease or symptom, to the effects of a co-intervention, to the biases of the patient who wants to please his doctor, or to a real neurobiological placebo response whereby a brain network anticipates a clinical benefit and acts on some physiological functions. Therefore, when describing the outcome in a placebo group, we must not talk about "the placebo effect," or "the placebo response," but rather about the improvement that occurs in the group of patients who received the placebo. Indeed, throughout this book I will use these definitions carefully, in order to clearly distinguish between real neurobiological placebo effects on the one hand, and improvements in placebo groups attributable to other factors on the other.

Throughout this book, it will appear clear that a real placebo effect is not spontaneous remission or the effect of a co-intervention, or the patients' biases. The placebo effect is a real psychobiological phenomenon whereby the brain is actively involved and anticipates a clinical benefit. Therefore, this book strives to make it clear that when we study the placebo, we are actually studying how the brain anticipates an event in the clinical setting.

Another common misunderstanding about the placebo effect is that there is only one placebo effect. Actually, there is not a single placebo effect but many (Benedetti 2008). The brain may anticipate a clinical benefit through different mechanisms, such as expectation of a reward or expectation that reduces anxiety, as well as classical conditioning, and this may occur in different systems and apparatuses of the body. Therefore, if the main mechanism of a given placebo effect is reward, one is actually studying reward mechanisms. Likewise, if the main mechanism is classical conditioning, one is actually studying Pavlovian conditioning. This is the principal reason why the title of this book refers to the plural (placebo effects).

In recent times, it has also emerged that the term placebo effect is too restrictive and should be extended to related phenomena which share similar mechanisms. Thus, as described throughout this book, besides classical placebo effects, today we can describe several placebo-related effects, the latter being characterized by the fact that no placebo is administered. In fact, by adopting a strict definition, the placebo effect follows the administration of a placebo. If no placebo is given, we cannot call it a placebo effect. I believe that these strict definitions help us in a number of ways. First, they remind us what a placebo and a placebo effect are exactly. Second, they underscore that it is not always necessary to administer a placebo to obtain a therapeutic effect, as sometimes the doctor's words and attitudes are enough. Third, these definitions remind us that the psychosocial context can produce therapeutic effects in a variety of ways, regardless of the administration of a placebo.

During the many courses I teach at my University, from Physiology to Neuroscience, from Pain Pathophysiology to Pain Management, and from Clinical Trials Methodology to the Patient–Provider Interaction, I strive to make the students aware of the placebo phenomenon. Unfortunately, what I have found thus far is only a very limited understanding and a very restricted usage of the word placebo. What students know about placebos and placebo effects, from those in the medical schools to those in the nursing schools and to those in more advanced courses (Neurology, Surgery, Anaesthesiology, and such like), is their use in double-blind clinical trials and its importance in Evidence-Based Medicine, whereby effective treatments must work better than placebos.

On the basis of these considerations, many years ago I started talking of placebos in more detail during my lessons to students and to doctors of any kind, until I took the decision to write this book. I soon realized the difficulty of teaching medical students, and even doctors, that placebo effects often play a part in treatment. Therefore, this book is directed at medical students, doctors of any kind, nurses, psychologists and psychotherapists, as well as to all those neuroscientists and biologists who are interested in understanding the biological link between a complex mental activity and the body. In other words, this book does not talk of the most known aspects of placebos and placebo effects, such as clinical trials methodology and designs, but rather it talks of what is less known about placebos—its psychobiological aspects and mechanisms.

In an interesting article that was published in 1972 in the *Lancet*, Blackwell et al. (1972) proposed an experiment to be performed in a class of medical students. With its intriguing title "Demonstration to medical students of placebo responses and non-drug factors" this article is a classic experiment in which medical students participate in a simulation of a clinical trial that tests the sedative effects of blue capsules (actually a placebo that the students believe to be a sedative) and the stimulant effects of pink capsules (a placebo believed to be a stimulant). I think demonstrations like this should be more common in medical schools.

The widespread use of the word placebo in the medical literature, and its use in many experimental procedures, is evidence of the importance of this phenomenon in modern biomedical sciences. If one considers the modern clinical approach of evidence-based medicine, which basically relies on the superiority of a treatment over a placebo, the central role of the placebo emerges even more. Thus the knowledge of placebo effects is essential in modern medicine, and the crucial questions to be answered are "where," "when" and "how" placebo effects work. I believe that these questions are worthy of intense scientific scrutiny, as they will lead to fundamental insights into human biology. And, in particular, I hope this book may at least partially answer some of these questions.

The plan of this book can be summarized as follows. Chapter 1 presents an historical overview about the emergence of the concept of placebo. It also describes where and how placebos are used in clinical trials and in routine medical practice, without going into too many methodological details. In Chapter 2 a more modern view of the placebo concept is presented, explaining the methodological drawbacks and pitfalls in its investigation as well as the general underlying mechanisms, according to both a psychological and a neuroscientific approach and conceptualization. Chapters 3 to 9 provide detailed analysis of placebo and placebo-related effects in different medical conditions. Chapter 3 is about pain, where most of our neurobiological understanding of the placebo effect comes from. Chapter 4 describes the placebo effect in neurological disorders, and Chapter 5 covers mental and behavioral disorders. A detailed account of the involvement of behavioral conditioning in the immune and endocrine system is given in Chapter 6. This is a mechanism that is particularly relevant to understanding the placebo phenomenon. In the following chapters it becomes clear that we know much less about placebo and placebo-related effects in cardiovascular and respiratory diseases (Chapter 7), gastrointestinal and genitourinary disorders (Chapter 8) and some special conditions like oncology, surgery and alternative and complementary therapies (Chapter 9). Chapter 10 discusses some important clinical and ethical implications and applications, particularly those that derive from recent advances in placebo research. Finally, Chapter 11 explores some methodological details, showing how some of the experiments described throughout the book were carried out in my laboratory.

At the beginning of each chapter there is a list of summary points, which are key learning points; and at the end of each chapter there is a list of points intended to stimulate further discussion and give an idea of possible future lines of research. I hope these points are of particular help to readers using this book as a textbook in medical schools or studying psychology courses.

References

Benedetti F (2008). Mechanisms of placebo and placebo-related effects across diseases and treatments. *Annual Review of Pharmacology and Toxicology,* **48**, 33–60.

Blackwell B, Bloomfield SS and Buncher CR (1972). Demonstration to medical students of placebo responses and non-drug factors. *Lancet,* **1**, 1279–82.

Acknowledgments

I started working on the placebo effect in 1994 and this topic has been for me a fascinating, challenging, and fertile field of research for many years. Despite the many travels and visits to foreign institutions, the University of Turin Medical School has been my professional home for all these years. Therefore, I want to thank all my colleagues from my home institution who helped and supported me in a number of ways.

In particular, I owe a great debt to Piergiorgio Strata who was for me one of the best advisers and friends, after being an excellent mentor when I was a medical student more than 30 years ago, as well as to Piergiorgio Montarolo, who was partially responsible for the acquisition of my technical skills and for my scientific growth.

Special thanks to all my collaborators who helped me in planning and doing the experiments, analyzing the data, and interpreting the results. They are: Luana Colloca, Martina Amanzio, Antonella Pollo, Sergio Vighetti, Elisa Carlino, Elisa Frisaldi, Bruno Bergamasco, Leonardo Lopiano, Michele Lanotte, Elena Torre, Giovanni Asteggiano, Innocenzo Rainero, and Giuliano Maggi. Many colleagues from around the world also helped in many ways, both directly and indirectly. For example, I will never forget the nice experience during the years 2002–2004 spent with the "Placebo Group," organized by Anne Harrington as part of the program of the Harvard University Mind–Brain–Behavior Initiative. This was one of the most exciting academic experiences I have ever had, thus I want to thank all members of that group for the excellent discussions and stimulating exchange of ideas: thanks to Anne Harrington, Dan Moerman, Howard Fields, Nick Humphrey, Jamie Pennebaker, and Ginger Hoffman.

Not to mention the many invitations I have had from Stephen Strauss and Linda Engel of the US National Institutes of Health during the years 2000–2004 to discuss and plan future projects and strategies for a better understanding of the placebo effect. Another more recent intellectual collaboration with Manfred Schedlowski and Paul Enck, who stimulated me to co-organize an exciting meeting on placebo and nocebo effects in Tutzing, Germany, in 2007 and in Tuebingen, Germany, in 2013, and with Damien Finniss, Don Price, Ron Kupers, and Serge Marchand, with whom I co-organized another placebo meeting in Copenhagen, further boosted my desire to publish this book. I also want to highlight the ongoing intellectual discussions with Ted Kaptchuk and Jian Kong, who are helping me to generate new ideas and hypotheses. I want to thank them all for this and I apologize if I forget someone.

Finally, my family was crucial for getting this book done—both my wife Claudia and my daughter Federica. My wife has contributed with her continuous, lovely support as well as in choosing, classifying, and organizing the figures and revising the references. My daughter has always kept me smiling and has drawn several figures with her skills acquired at the Italian Academy of Fine Arts.

Contents

List of Boxes

Part 1

General concepts and mechanisms

This first part is dedicated to the general concepts related to the placebo effect, from the evolution of the word placebo over the centuries (Chapter 1) to a more modern view and approach (Chapter 2). In addition, the general mechanisms that have been identified over the past years are described. Unfortunately, we do not know whether different medical conditions and therapeutic interventions share common mechanisms, or rather, whether there are mechanisms that are specific for different diseases. Therefore, in this first part the mechanisms will be described according to a mechanism-based classification of placebo effects, in contrast to the second and third parts, where a systematic approach to different diseases will be used. Moreover, this first part tries to put placebo effects within the broader context of the doctor–patient relationship (Chapter 3), a challenging enterprise that is aimed at understanding why and how medical care and placebo responses have emerged during evolution as a unique and special biological/social system.

Chapter 1

The traditional concept of placebo

Summary points

- The history of medicine is basically the history of placebos, as most medical interventions were nothing but placebos—that is, inert.

- Over the centuries doctors started using sham treatments to see whether the clinical improvement was attributable to the patient's imagination and/or spontaneous remission.

- Today placebos are widely used in clinical research to validate the efficacy of a therapy.

- Besides clinical research, doctors and nurses use placebos to please and placate anxious patients.

- The placebo effect is a good example of how a mental activity may affect several physiological functions; thus it is an excellent model for studying mind–body interactions.

- The nocebo effect, which is opposite to the placebo effect, is another good model for understanding mind–body interactions.

1.1 The origin of the placebo concept and methodology

1.1.1 Many bizarre ineffective therapies were developed over the past centuries

In their book *The Powerful Placebo: From Ancient Priest to Modern Physician*, Shapiro and Shapiro (1997a) assert that the history of medical treatment is essentially the history of the placebo effect (see also Shapiro and Shapiro, 1997b). Indeed, by considering the very definition of placebo as an ineffective treatment for the symptom or disorder being treated, most of the therapies that were developed over the past centuries were actually placebos. Starting from the very beginning of medical care, that is, the time when special care to a sick person was provided for the first time, which is likely to have emerged in early hominids (Evans, 2002), many bizarre treatments were developed that were aimed at both relieving symptoms, like pain, and curing diseases. Most, if not all, of these medicaments and procedures were based neither on a scientific rationale nor on the assessment of real efficacy, but rather they emerged from metaphysical beliefs, social influences, and scientific ignorance about anatomy and physiology related to that particular historical period.

Shapiro and Shapiro (1997a, 1997b) provide us with a neat account of the many medicaments and procedures available across different historical times and different cultures and societies. The eccentricity and oddity of these treatments are shown by the use of many bizarre concoctions made of a variety of ingredients, like moss from the skull of victims of violent death, frogs, worms, feathers, hair, horns, hoofs, ants, scorpions, viper flesh, crab eyes, bee glue, fox lung, spider webs, teeth, sexual organs, and so forth (see Box 1.1 for some examples). Some of the most famous and widespread of these concoctions were *theriac* and *mattioli*, which contained up to 230 substances. Some other substances, such as *bezoar* (believed to be a crystallized tear from the eye of a deer bitten by a snake) and *mandrake*, were used by physicians to treat virtually any kind of malady. The Emperor Huang Ti refers to more than 2000 drugs and 16,000 prescriptions that were used in China. Records from Sumerians, Babylonians, and Assyrians describe 265 remedies, and over 600 drugs were used in ancient India. A rough estimation of all the remedies available across the centuries comes to about 4785 drugs and 16,842 prescriptions—a massive and astonishing pharmacopoeia (Shapiro and Shapiro, 1997a, 1997b).

As emphasized by Shapiro and Shapiro (1997a, 1997b), besides substances and concoctions, several other procedures were used by physicians, such as purging, puking, cutting, blistering, bleeding, freezing, heating, sweating, and leeching, not to mention their attempts to perform surgical operations in which different organs were manipulated, cut, or removed. Most, if not all, of these drugs and procedures were ineffective, with only a few possible but unlikely speculative exceptions. For example, if the concoction contained opium, it was likely to show specific analgesic properties. Likewise, bleeding was likely to have specific effects in some circulatory diseases.

It should be noted, however, that one of the most intriguing aspects of pre-scientific medicine is not so much the existence of the myriad of bizarre ineffective medical interventions, but rather the belief that they were effective. These beliefs were often reinforced by the occurrence of real clinical improvements sometimes observed by physicians and experienced by patients. There are several explanations for these improvements. First and foremost, spontaneous remissions of symptoms and diseases often occurred, but they were misinterpreted as the beneficial effects of the medical treatments being used. Similarly, physicians often treated patients who were not ill but probably merely anxious, so that no real improvement actually took place. Last, but not least, some clinical improvements might have been due to the patient's expectations of clinical benefit and to changes in their emotional state (the true psychobiological placebo effect).

It should be noted that many bizarre and ineffective therapies persist today; they fall into the category of alternative and/or complementary medicine (see section 10.4). For example, today there are many concoctions, procedures, and even talismans that are as bizarre as those used centuries ago. There is the widespread belief among many people that these treatments are effective, even though they have not passed the rigorous tests of modern science. Therefore, the oddity, nonsense, eccentricity, and irrationality of many medicaments are not features of the past, because they pervade our society outside mainstream science. This is not only true for pharmacological agents or physical procedures, but also for psychological interventions. There are more than 400 psychotherapies available today for the treatment of a number of diseases and ailments

Box 1.1 Healing recipes in ancient Rome

The following are examples of healing recipes in ancient Rome in the second half of the second century and the first half of the third century after Christ, taken from the *Liber Medicinalis* by Quintus Serenus Sammonicus. Most of these treatments were likely to lack any therapeutic effect. If a positive outcome occurred, this was likely to be due to either the spontaneous remission of the ailment or the psychological effects of "imagination."

Therapies for earache and excruciating pain in other areas of the face

Instill juice of ash tree twigs and urine of young virgin into the painful ear, or otherwise lukewarm oil in which red worms from an old tree had been crushed. A mixture of boiled worms and fat from a hoarse-crying goose is effective as well. In some circumstances, amelioration occurs with ox bile blended with urine of a stinky sheep. For stabbing pain in the eyes, place the eye of a live shrimp as a talisman on the painful eye, cabbage, incense, wine, and milk of a parturient goat.

How to treat sterility and facilitate parturition

The woman must eat the vulva of a hare. Or she has to drink the drool dripping from the tender mouth of sheep while they are ruminating grazed grass in the sheepfold. To facilitate delivery, the woman must eat snails. A ring of droppings of black vulture can be applied to the vagina to relieve the pain of childbirth.

How to treat epileptic seizures

Pour bile of dark vulture in old wine, or drink blood from a swallow mixed with incense, lamb bile, honey. Ashes from weasel and swallow are effective as well. Otherwise, one can drink rainwater collected in a human skullcap in supine position. Good relief from seizures can also be achieved by picking up a pebble from a swallow nest and hanging it around the neck of the sufferer.

Therapy of delirium, and how to free the brain

Wrap the head of the sick person with lungs just explanted from a sheep. Do not forget to perform fumigations with dirty wool and nauseating odors. To prevent delirium, it is necessary to free the brain of healthy subjects. To do this, chew pyrethrum roots, grease the body with young elder, inhale ivy lymph, vinegar, and rue.

How to facilitate sleep

Albeit weird and bizarre, the following is an example of a possible effective treatment, because the recipe contains ingredients that are known to be hypnogenic, i.e., poppy and mandrake.

Dissolve the ashes of a sheet written with any word into lukewarm water and drink it. Grease the forehead with Pallade liquor with rose scent, together with poppy. Eat mandrake and the subcutaneous nodules of the thighs of a ram.

(Parloff, 1986; Moerman, 2002), but it is hard to believe that all of them are really effective (see section 6.5). Some psychological interventions that are bordering on magic still persist in Western and non-Western society, and people trust and use them, as they did centuries ago.

1.1.2 When doctors became aware of the ineffectiveness of many therapies

As the knowledge about anatomy and physiology of both animals and humans was growing over the centuries, the need for a scientific explanation of many medical treatments emerged among physicians and the scientific community. According to Kaptchuk (1998), an important historical period when scientific skepticism emerged about the efficacy of some medical remedies is approximately in the second half of the 1700s, and involved "mesmerism," "perkinism," and "homeopathy."

Mesmerism was introduced in the second half of the 1700s by Franz Anton Mesmer, who claimed to have discovered a healing fluid which he called "animal magnetism." In order to assess the very nature and the effectiveness of mesmerism, King Louis XVI appointed a commission headed by Benjamin Franklin. This commission performed what can be considered one of the first blind assessments and sham (placebo) interventions in the history of medicine (Kaptchuk, 1998). Some women were blindfolded and asked where the "mesmeric energy" was being applied. The commission observed that: "while the woman was permitted to see the operation, she placed her sensations precisely in the part towards which it was directed; that on the other hand, when she did not see the operation, she placed them at hazard, and in parts very distant from those which were the object of magnetism. It was natural to conclude that these sensations, real or pretended, were determined by the imagination" (Franklin et al., 1785, p. 30; Kaptchuk, 1998). In another series of experiments, real mesmerism was found to work as well as sham mesmerism. Thus the conclusion was that the mesmeric fluid had no existence and any effects were attributable to imagination.

It was during this same period that Elisha Perkins introduced "perkinism," a kind of healing method whereby two metal rods were supposed to conduct pathogenic fluid away from the body. John Haygarth decided to investigate the efficacy of perkinism by replacing the two metal rods with two sham wooden rods—perhaps representing one of the first sham (placebo) devices in the history of medicine. He found that both the metal and the wooden rods had the same probability of inducing clinical improvement (Haygarth, 1801; Kaptchuk, 1998), which indicates that the metal rods had no specific therapeutic effects.

In the first half of the 1800s, Armand Trousseau tested the efficacy of homeopathy, a novel therapeutic approach introduced by Samuel Hahnemann based on the belief that a disease can be cured by very small amounts of the same substances that cause it. Trousseau probably used the first inert substances (placebos) in the history of medicine for assessing the effectiveness of a medical treatment (Trousseau and Gouraud, 1834; Kaptchuk, 1998). In fact, he used bread pills and told the patients that they were a homeopathic treatment. What the investigators found was a positive effect of bread pills and they attributed this to the natural course of disease and to imagination.

Many experiments and assessments of this kind were performed in the following years, and they were refined more and more over time. What was emerging was the physicians' awareness that the outcome of many therapies was nothing more than spontaneous remission or imagination, and the need for carrying out rigorous trials in order to validate the efficacy of a medicament.

The word *placebo* is old (it is the Latin word for "I shall please"). It entered the medical lexicon to indicate sham treatments and inert substances (such as sugar pills and saline solutions) that physicians give deliberately to please or placate their anxious patients, but its use in clinical research emerged gradually over time to indicate a control group receiving a sham treatment (as was done with sham mesmerism, sham rods in perkinism, and sham homeopathy). Therefore, the word "sham" was replaced with the word "placebo," so that today we could use the terms placebo mesmerism, placebo rods in perkinism, and placebo homeopathy.

It should be pointed out that the awareness of the scientific community about the ineffectiveness of many treatments over the past years was not paralleled by awareness among many other people, including some physicians. As already discussed in section 1.1.1, many bizarre concoctions and procedures are still present in our modern society, and this is attributable to the fact that many people trust, and thus use, them. Needless to say, this is an important point in the context of this book: trust, beliefs, and expectations are crucial in placebo and placebo-related effects.

1.1.3 The traditional concept of placebo effect is a first source of confusion

To give a placebo to a group of patients means to give a sham medical treatment. Accordingly, the therapeutic outcome is called "placebo effect," which means the effect that follows the administration of the placebo. These definitions generated some confusion which, unfortunately, even pervades scientific literature today. As described in detail in Chapter 2, the very nature of this confusion resides in the fact that the improvements that may take place in patients who receive placebo may be due to many factors, for example, spontaneous remission or expectation of therapeutic benefit or other factors (Fig. 1.1). Most clinical investigators referred to the placebo effect as: any improvement that may occur in the placebo group, regardless of whether it is a spontaneous remission or a psychobiological phenomenon; whereas most psychologists referred to the placebo effect as: the psychological phenomenon that involves expectation and anticipation of clinical improvement (Kirsch, 1999). Some authors have tried to distinguish between the terms placebo effect (the global outcome in the placebo group) and placebo response (the psychobiological phenomenon) (Hoffman et al., 2005, see also section 2.2.1), but unfortunately this recommendation has not been followed in many clinical trials. It should therefore be realized that even today many authors wrongly equate the outcome seen in the group of patients who received the sham treatment with the placebo effect, or response, without considering that such an outcome can be due to the natural course of the disease, or to expectation, as well as to other factors (see Chapter 2).

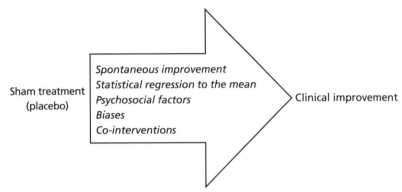

Fig. 1.1 The clinical improvement that occurs following administration of a placebo treatment is due to many factors and is often and mistakenly called a "placebo effect" or "placebo response." Actually, the real placebo effect is only the improvement that is attributable to psychosocial factors, for example, the expectation of therapeutic benefit. Therefore, the correct definition of the clinical improvement in this figure is "the improvement that takes place in the group of patients that received the placebo treatment."

This point has been well conceptualized by Ernst and Resch (1995) with the terms "true" and "perceived" placebo effects. The former represents the real psychobiological phenomenon, that is the target of the present book, and the latter is the sum of many factors (the natural course of the disease, statistical regression to the mean, unidentified parallel interventions, and such like) that have nothing to do with the psychological events taking place in the patient's brain. A review of the literature shows that most authors confuse the "perceived" with the "true" placebo effect and unfortunately this confusion is still present, even in more recent times in which more attention should be paid to both terminology and methodology (Ernst and Resch, 1995).

The main reason for this is that physicians, clinical investigators, and drug companies are mainly interested in demonstrating the superiority of a treatment compared to the placebo, regardless of the underlying mechanisms. In other words, they are not so much interested in knowing *why* an improvement occurs in the placebo group, but rather if the active treatment *works better* than the placebo. If one then considers the modern clinical approach of evidence-based medicine, which basically relies on the superiority of a treatment over a placebo, this point emerges even more. There is no need to know why placebos work, but rather there is an urgent need to know whether they are worse than active treatments.

It is not surprising, therefore, why the term placebo effect is still used in a very broad sense and with a very broad meaning. However, it will appear clear throughout this book that, by taking the recent neurobiological discoveries about real psychobiological placebo phenomena into consideration, the scientific community is becoming more and more aware that it is necessary to differentiate real placebo effects from other phenomena that are present in clinical trials, thus dissolving the traditional confusion about the placebo terminology.

1.2 **The placebo in clinical trials and medical practice**

1.2.1 **Placebos are the tenet of the randomized, double-blind, placebo-controlled trial design**

As the awareness of the possible influences of imagination and suggestion on thera-peutic outcome increased over time, physicians and clinician scientists introduced the blind assessment (real treatment versus sham treatment) into clinical medicine. For ex-ample, in the period 1911–1914, Bingel (1918) tested 937 patients for the effectiveness of diphtheria antitoxin. Patients were subdivided into those who received true diph-theria antitoxin serum and those who received sham treatment (normal horse serum), according to what could be called today a double-blind design. In fact, neither the patients nor the physicians knew the nature of the test serum.

Besides the concerns about the influence of suggestion on the outcome, it should be noted that many trials were aimed not so much at uncovering suggestion and imagina-tion, but rather at identifying the natural course of a disease. In other words, physicians used the blind assessment and the placebo administration in order to discriminate between specific therapeutic effects and spontaneous fluctuations of the disease. For example, in the Michigan tuberculosis trial in the period 1926–1931, the investigators administered sodium-gold-thiosulfate to some patients and distilled water to others, to compare the specific effects of the drug under test with the natural variations in the severity of the disease (Amberson et al., 1931). Likewise, in the 1930s, Evans and Hoyle (1933) were not concerned with suggestion and imagination, but rather with the natu-ral variations of the symptoms. They tested several drugs, like nitrates, narcotics, and digitalis, in the treatment of angina pectoris against a no-treatment group, and actually found no difference, thus indicating that the spontaneous fluctuations of angina pecto-ris played a key role in remissions and relapses.

Another important point that was crucial for the modern use of placebos in clinical trials was the emerging awareness that even physicians and clinical investigators were susceptible to suggestion, imagination, and biases. This led to the more and more wide-spread use of the double-blind design, in which neither the investigator nor the patient knew the nature of the tested therapy (it could be either real or sham). In fact, in many previous trials a single-blind design had been adopted, whereby only the patients were blind as to the treatment; the investigators still knew whether a real or sham treatment was being administered. For example, the Michigan tuberculosis trial by Amberson et al. (1931) was a single-blind trial. Randomization (that is, the random allocation of patients to real and sham groups) was also crucial, contributing to elimination of both uncertainty and variability in the outcome measures; this was seen in 1948 in the first randomized clinical trial in the history of medicine, performed with streptomycin in tuberculosis (Hill, 1990).

Today, in some clinical trials, active placebos are used. An active placebo is a com-pound that mimics the side effects of the active treatment under test. Thus, an active placebo is not inert. Active placebos are used whenever blinding is problematic, that is, when the patient easily realizes that an active treatment has been administered be-cause of its side effects. For example, if the active substance under test induces drow-siness and/or a dry mouth, it will be easy to guess which group the patient belongs to. To avoid the possibility of this "unblinding," the placebo group might receive, for example, a benzodiazepine, which also causes drowsiness. In this way, the subjects in the "active placebo" group are made to believe that the real treatment is being administered. Although many clinical trials use active placebos, some ethical aspects must be mentioned. For example, in some circumstances it is unethical to induce even minor side effects in the placebo group.

Clinical trials are conducted in phases. For example, with pharmacological agents, phase 1 trials try to determine dosing, to document how a drug is metabolized and excreted, and to identify acute side effects. In this phase, a small number of healthy volunteers (between 20 and 80) are usually involved. Phase 2 trials include more participants (100–300) who have the disease or condition that the medication could potentially treat. In phase 2, researchers seek to gather further safety data and preliminary evidence of the drug's beneficial effects (efficacy). If the phase 2 trials indicate that the pharmacological agent may be effective, and the risks are considered acceptable, given the observed efficacy and the severity of the disease, the drug moves on to phase 3. In phase 3 trials, the drug is studied in a much larger number of people with the disease (1000–3000). This phase further tests the medication's effectiveness, monitors side effects, and, in some cases, compares the medication's effects to a standard treatment (if one is already available). As more and more participants are tested over longer periods of time, even rare side effects can be revealed. Sometimes, phase 4 trials are conducted after a drug is already approved and on the market, in order to better understand the treatment's long-term risks, benefits, and optimal use, as well as to test the medication in special populations such as children.

Placebos are generally used in phase 2 and phase 3 clinical trials, as phase 1 is only aimed at assessing how a drug is metabolized and excreted. Of course, the placebo must be identical to and undistinguishable from the true medication. In some cases, it is considered unethical to use placebos, particularly if an effective treatment is available and when, in fact, withholding a treatment even for a short time would expose participants to unreasonable risks. For example, it would be unethical to give placebos to depressed patients who are at risk of suicide (see also section 11.1).

With all these elements in the hands of modern physicians and clinical investigators, the randomized, double-blind, placebo-controlled trial, the so-called RCT, represents the tenet of clinical research today for validating a therapy. It contains all the elements that are necessary to control for suggestion, imagination, and biases of both patient and investigator, and to control for other confounding factors such as the spontaneous fluctuations of diseases and symptoms. The concept of placebo, with its traditional meaning of sham treatment as evolved over the centuries, is at the very heart of the modern clinical experimental approach (Kaptchuk, 1998), and in more recent times it has also acquired a central role in evidence-based medicine, which relies on the superiority of a treatment over a placebo.

1.2.2 Placebos may be used with other experimental designs

The randomized, double-blind, placebo-controlled trial, in which patients who receive real treatment are compared with patients who receive sham treatment, has undergone several changes in more recent times in order to improve the experimental design as well as to try to resolve unanswered questions (Farrar, 2010; Enck et al., 2011; Enck and Klosterhalfen, 2013). The main purpose of different experimental protocols is to determine whether a given therapy is really effective in a particular clinical condition. This approach of the typical clinical trial has been called "pragmatic," as opposed to the "explanatory" approach whereby one of the main purposes is to elucidate the biological mechanisms underlying the symptom and/or the action of the treatment (Schwartz and Lellouch, 1967). Certainly, most clinical trials are pragmatic, as the main interest of both physicians and drug companies is to demonstrate the efficacy of the therapy under test.

The crossover design represents a kind of evolution of the classical clinical trial. In contrast to the randomized design, in which each patient receives a single treatment, in a crossover design each patient receives all the treatments. To do this, patients first receive the real treatment, then they are switched to the placebo treatment, or vice versa. Studying true and placebo treatment in the same person has obvious advantages, such as a reduction in the sample size required and a reduction of the variability in reporting symptoms (Louis et al., 1984). The reduction of variance in crossover designs leads to greater statistical power. However, the crossover approach has important limitations. One of these is the possibility of persistence of the effects of the first treatment. In fact, if the therapy-induced changes are not soon reversed when the therapy is withdrawn and replaced with the placebo, crossover designs are not appropriate. Another limitation has to do with the high dropout rates because of the increased length compared with randomized controlled studies. A further limitation is the rapidly changing underlying disease—the total duration of the crossover study should be short enough to avoid within-patient variations.

One of the main concerns with the crossover design is persistence of the effects of the first treatment, the so-called carryover effects. Of course, these carryover effects may be present when the first treatment is a pharmacological agent. In this case, both the persistence of drug metabolites and possible changes in the brain and/or other tissues may occur. Thus, when the drug is replaced with a placebo, particular attention must be paid to all these factors. However, if the first treatment is the placebo, some carryover psychological effects may occur as well. For example, if the subject does not respond to the placebo, this negative effect may influence the subsequent replacement of the placebo with the true treatment. This is due to the fact that the placebo effect is a learning phenomenon (see section 2.3.3).

Other designs have been developed that use placebo administration. For example, two-stage clinical trials are aimed at selecting either placebo nonresponders or good drug responders at a first stage, and then enrolling these patients in a second stage of the trial (Box 1.2). In other words, placebo responders can be identified in a first placebo run-in period, and then discarded from the second stage of the trial, thereby increasing the sensitivity of the trial when comparing placebo nonresponders with the real treatment.

It can be seen from this brief description of some clinical trial methodology that the main use of placebo has to do with control conditions. Therefore, most of this methodology is pragmatic, as it is aimed at enhancing the sensitivity of the trial in order to validate the effectiveness of the therapy under test. Certainly, the administration of placebos in these clinical trials is not aimed at investigating the placebo effect per se.

Box 1.2 Run-in and enriched clinical trials

In order to increase the sensitivity of a clinical trial, i.e., the difference between the active treatment group and the placebo group, some new designs have been developed over the past years. The main criticism against these designs is that they do not represent the real world, that is the general population. The following are two examples.

Placebo run-in

In the placebo run-in design, patients are given a placebo treatment for several days, then those who respond to the placebo and those who show poor adherence are discarded. The remaining patients, who are mainly represented by placebo nonresponders and good adherers, are randomized to active treatment and placebo (Fig. 1.2). In this way, the specific effect of the treatment under test is supposed to be better evidenced. The main question is: Is it correct to include in the randomization only the placebo nonresponders?

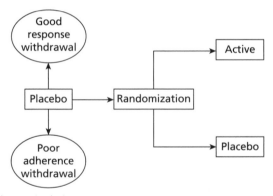

Fig. 1.2 Placebo run-in design.

Enriched enrollment with randomized withdrawal

According to this paradigm, patients are treated with the active treatment for several days, then those who do not respond and those who show severe adverse events are discarded. The remaining patients, who are represented by good responders to active treatment, are randomized to active treatment or placebo (Fig. 1.3). Therefore, the good response to the treatment under validation is supposed to be better evidenced compared to the placebo. The main question is: Is it correct to include in the randomization only the good active treatment responders?

Box 1.2 Run-in and enriched clinical trials (continued)

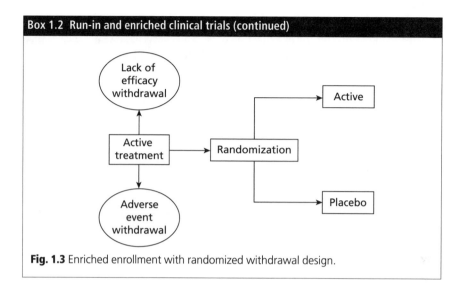

Fig. 1.3 Enriched enrollment with randomized withdrawal design.

In contrast to the designs described earlier, it is also possible to manipulate the information provided to the subjects and the timing of the treatment that is given (Enck et al., 2011). For example, the balanced placebo design has been developed for better understanding the role of suggestion in the therapeutic outcome. This design, formulated by Ross et al. (1962), refers to a methodology for studying many aspects of human behavior and drug effects, orthogonally manipulating instructions ("told drug" versus "told placebo") and drug administered ("received drug" versus "received placebo") (Fig. 1.4). It has been used in many conditions such as alcohol research (Marlatt et al., 1973; Rohsenow and Bachorowski, 1984; Wilson et al., 1985; Epps et al., 1998),

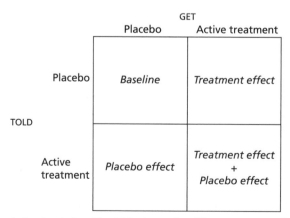

Fig. 1.4 Balanced placebo design. The table shows the different outcomes following different combinations of what the patients "get" and what they are "told," which allow investigators to identify the modulation of drug action by verbal suggestions.

smoking (Sutton, 1991), and amphetamine effects (Mitchell et al., 1996). This design is particularly interesting for the investigation of placebo effects because it indicates that verbally induced expectations can modulate the therapeutic outcome, both in the placebo group and in the active treatment group. For example, Flaten et al. (1999) showed that carisoprodol, a centrally acting muscle relaxant, resulted in different outcomes, either relaxant or stimulant, depending on the combination of verbal suggestion and drug administration (including the placebo). The balanced placebo design produces information that cannot be derived from conventional clinical trials. For example, it provides a baseline against which drug and placebo effects can be measured, and provides a direct assessment of the drug effect with the placebo component removed. The problem with the balanced placebo design is that it entails deception; thus it is ethically questionable (see Chapter 11).

In an attempt to overcome the limitations of the balanced placebo design, another strategy has been devised (Enck et al., 2011). In the balanced crossover design, subjects are divided into four groups, and all are told that they are participating in a conventional randomized, double-blinded, and placebo-controlled crossover trial, in which they will receive both the drug and the placebo at two different occasions, according to a randomized and double-blind order. However, only the groups "active treatment–placebo" and "placebo–active treatment" (Fig. 1.4) will be exposed to drug and placebo in a balanced way, i.e., half the subjects will receive the drug first and then the placebo, whereas the other half will receive first placebo and then the drug. In this case, the groups "active treatment–placebo" and "placebo–active treatment" represent the conventional drug trial assuming the additive model for drug and placebo response (that is, therapeutic outcome = drug effect + placebo effect). In group "active treatment–active treatment," the minimal value of both measures would represent the true drug response, and the difference between both would be the expectancy component of the drug response. In group "placebo–placebo," the maximum value should represent the true placebo response, and the difference between both values should be the expectancy component of the placebo response. Comparing these expectancy effects between groups "active–active" and "placebo–placebo" would allow us to test whether the expectancy component of the placebo response is equal under drug and placebo conditions (which is the assumption of the additive model). Although this approach is certainly interesting, it is quite complex in the setting of a clinical trial. In addition, the balanced crossover design has the important limitation of the possible interference of carryover and sequence effect, as in any crossover design.

Another possible manipulation is related to the timing of treatment administration. For example, if a drug can elicit its action at a predefined time point after ingestion, for example, through a coating technology, the comparison between drug and placebo, along with the manipulation of timing instructions and delay of drug release, might provide important information on both pharmacological and placebo responses (Enck et al., 2011).

1.2.3 Placebos are widely used in routine medical practice

Placebos are traditionally used in clinical practice to please or placate anxious and complaining patients. Indeed the word *placebo* ("I shall please") was introduced in the medical dictionary to mean an inert treatment that is given to patients more to please than to cure (de Craen et al., 1999; Wall, 1999). In contrast to clinical research, placebo administration in clinic entails deception. In fact, in a double-blind study the patients do know that they may receive either the real or the sham treatment, but in clinical practice physicians give placebos deceptively, by telling their patients that actually they are real drugs. In a typical situation, which is very common among physicians and nurses, a patient who complains of pain during the night in the ward is given by either the doctor or nurse an inert pill or a saline shot to placate further complaints. Of course the patient is told that the pill or the shot is a powerful painkiller. This is true not only with inpatients, but also with outpatients. For example, a common situation is when a patient goes to the doctor's office many times complaining of chronic pain and discomfort. In order to placate this anxious patient who visits the doctor repeatedly, the doctor may give a long-lasting placebo treatment, and reassurance that it will reduce any discomfort in the long run. Thus placebos can be given in both acute and chronic conditions, although it is not easy to know exactly how often such therapies are administered. Many doctors and nurses are reluctant to admit they have used and/or are using inert substances in routine clinical practice, as the use of placebos is often considered to be ethically questionable.

Some recent surveys, performed among medical personnel, indicate the widespread use of placebos in routine medical practice. For example, Berger (1999) surveyed resident physicians in the United States on the use of placebos, and found that 59% were familiar with the use of placebo in patient care; 50% of these had learned about their use from another physician. Physicians were more likely to consider placebo administration for suspected and factitious pain. In a similar survey in Denmark, Hrobjartsson and Norup (2003) found that 86% of general practitioners reported using placebos at least once, and 48% used them more than ten times within the last year. In this survey, the most important reason for using placebo interventions was to avoid a confrontation with the patient. About 30% of physicians believed in an effect of placebos on objective outcomes; 46% found their use ethically acceptable.

In another survey, performed in Israel by Nitzan and Lichtenberg (2004), 60% of physicians and nurses used placebos; among those users, 62% prescribed a placebo as often as once a month or more, and 68% deceived patients completely by telling them that they were receiving real medication. In addition, 94% reported that they found placebos generally or occasionally effective. In a subsequent survey among academic physicians in the United States, Sherman and Hickner (2007) found that 45% had used placebos in clinical practice; the most common reasons for using them were to calm the patient and as supplemental treatment. As many as 96% of them believed that placebos can have therapeutic effects, and 40% reported that placebo could benefit patients physiologically. Only 12% said that placebos should be prohibited in clinical practice.

More recent studies have investigated the use of placebos among physicians in more detail. For example, by considering the distinction between pure placebos (substances with no pharmacological effect, such as sugar pills and saline solutions) and impure placebos (substances with pharmacological effect but not for the condition being treated, such as antibiotics in viral infections), doctors have been found to rely more on impure placebos (Kermen et al., 2010; Fent et al., 2011; Louhiala, 2012; Howick et al., 2013). Interestingly, impure placebos are often not recognized as such by practitioners;

thus they remain at the fringe of many ethical debates and discussions concerning policy and regulation (Harris and Raz, 2012). Therefore, impure placebos used in clinical practice present unresolved ethical concerns so far, and information and education are necessary in order to make doctors and medical students understand what impure placebos are and which drugs are really effective in specific conditions (the typical cases are represented by the ineffectiveness of antibiotics in viral infections as well as the lack of efficacy of vitamins in a number of medical conditions).

1.2.4 Psychologists consider the placebo effect as an example of the power of mind

Not only have placebos been conceptualized in terms of methodology in clinical trials for the validation of different therapies, but they have also traditionally been taken as an example of the powerful interaction between mind and body. Clearly, this stems from the early studies (described in section 1.1.2) in which a sham treatment was compared with an active treatment such as mesmerism and perkinism. In these cases, the main conclusion was that imagination played a major role in the therapeutic outcome, thus underlining the important role of the mind in the modulation of a number of physiological functions. The seminal work by many authors, such as Shapiro and Shapiro (1997a, 1997b) and Brody (2000), contributed to the conceptualization of the placebo effect in terms of the mind–body interaction. Therefore, besides the traditional concept of placebo in clinical trial design and for validating different treatments, the placebo concept has permeated psychology literature for many years (for example, see White et al., 1985) and has, for example, played a key role in many aspects of psychotherapy (see section 6.5).

Within this context, starting from the early notion of the role of imagination in the therapeutic outcome, as occurred in the earliest clinical trials (section 1.1.2), several factors have been considered to be important in the placebo effect. For example, according to Ross and Buckalew (1985), many elements are at work during a placebo response, such as the relationship between the doctor and the patient, the patient's expectations and needs, the patient's personality and psychological state, the severity and discomfort of the symptoms, the type of verbal instructions given, the preparation characteristics, and the environmental milieu. Each of these factors can be manipulated in order to produce an optimal effect, although in the experimental setting it is not always easy to manipulate all these factors independently of each other.

The traditional importance of the mind–body interaction in the placebo effect clearly emerges in the definition by Brody (2000), who emphasizes the role of symbolic meaning, and defines the placebo effect as: a change in the body, or the body–mind unit, that occurs as a result of the symbolic significance which one attributes to an event or object in the healing environment. This definition is embedded in the notion that symbols induce expectations of an outcome, thus highlighting the crucial role of meaning and expectation. In other words, the therapeutic context has a meaning that induces expectations which, in turn, shape experience and behavior (Kirsch, 1999). In this sense, it is important to stress that the psychological conceptualization of the placebo has been very important in focusing our attention on what is really important (the meaning and meaning-induced expectations), and deflecting it from what is not (the inert pills and, in general, inert medical treatments) (Moerman, 2002; Moerman and Jonas, 2002). In fact, placebos have typically been identified as inert agents or procedures aimed at pleasing the patient rather than exerting a specific effect. However, if a placebo is inert, it cannot cause an effect, as something that is inert has no inherent properties that allow it to cause an effect. This paradox is highlighted in the many attempts to define placebo and the placebo effect, resulting in a degree of confusion and debate (Price et al., 2008). Therefore, whereas in the clinical trial setting the conceptualization of placebo focuses on distal, or external, factors—such as inert treatments, inert pills, and inert substances—in the context of psychology the concept of placebo focuses on proximal, or internal, factors—like expectations, beliefs, and mind–body relationship.

Nocebo phenomena, which are opposite to placebo phenomena, have also traditionally been recognized. In this case, the pathogenic effects of imagination and negative expectations and beliefs in tribal societies have been described in a number of ways, and taken as a good example of the power of the mind. For example, in some aboriginal people of Australia, pointing a bone at someone may induce negative outcomes; and in Latin America and Africa, someone believing that he is bewitched may result in a sort of "voodoo" death (Cannon, 1942). Although many of these phenomena are certainly anecdotal (Lewis, 1977), it is not surprising that Cannon (1942) explains them as a stress-induced activation of the sympathetic nervous system. Similar explanations were put forward by Lex (1974), who interprets some forms of voodoo death as the imbalance between the sympathetic and parasympathetic nervous system.

Within the traditional context of the mind–body unit, Hahn (1985, 1997) goes further by proposing a sociocultural model of illness and healing, whereby placebos and nocebos are fundamentally involved. By performing an anthropological analysis, he conceives the processes of sickness and healing as a complex interaction of human beings with their environment. For example, depression may derive from an intricate interaction of both internal and external factors, such as beliefs, values, and psychological coping devices, as well as society's rules, attitudes, and behaviors. At the heart of these social interactions are the pathogenic effects of nocebos and the therapeutic effects of placebos. In the first case, beliefs and expectations may sicken and kill, as in the extreme case of voodoo death, whereas in the second case, beliefs and expectations may reduce discomfort and may heal. Speculatively, Hahn (1985, p. 185) noted that:

> It is unlikely that belief in the healing power of large doses of arsenic would transform this chemical into a healing agent; yet I submit, though I will not attempt to prove it, that such a belief would retard its poisonous effects. Likewise, lack of faith in antibiotics may diminish the potency of these drugs, and faith or scepticism about pharmacologically inert materials or practices may shift the results in expected directions.

Nocebo phenomena, and the impact of negative expectations and imagination, are not limited to the past and to tribal societies. They are also present in Western societies and are described in many other sections of this book. For example, many side effects both in clinical trials and in clinical practice are psychological. Likewise, many health warnings, like those broadcasted by the media, may induce negative expectations and negative outcomes. Anticipatory nausea and vomiting in cancer chemotherapy, the emotional impact of negative diagnoses, and the distrust of both doctors and therapies are all examples of nocebo and nocebo-like phenomena in Western societies.

The merits of this psychosocial/anthropological approach, albeit mostly speculative in many cases, reside in the fact that it paved the way for the neuroscientific investigation of mind–body phenomena, such as placebo and placebo-related effects. Therefore, the psychological conceptualization of the placebo effect in terms of the mind–body relationship represents an important step in the transition from the placebo concept as a methodological approach in clinical trials design to neuroscientific investigation of the placebo effect as a psychobiological phenomenon. Starting from the first biological investigations of the placebo effect, for example, in the early 1960s in animals (Herrnstein, 1962) and in the late 1970s in humans (Levine et al., 1978), today placebo research is a complex field of investigation which spans psychology to psychophysiology, pharmacology to neurophysiology, and cellular and molecular analysis to modern neuroimaging techniques.

1.3 **Points for further discussion**

1 It should be stressed that there is a clear-cut difference between the two definitions "placebo effect, or response" (the psychobiological phenomenon) and "improvement in the group of patients who received the placebo" (the global improvement, which also encompasses spontaneous remission). Unfortunately, many clinical trialists today still call the outcome in the placebo group the "placebo effect, or response."

2 Complex clinical trial designs, such as the balanced placebo design, need to be evaluated carefully in order to better understand their usefulness across different medical conditions.

3 It would be interesting to undertake surveys in several countries to compare the use of placebo in routine medical practice among different cultures and societies.

4 Placebo effects need to be included within the context of those models that study the mind–body interaction. In particular, it would be useful to consider the placebo effect as an experimental approach to analyze how a complex mental activity interacts with the neuronal circuitry of the brain.

References

Amberson JB, McMahon BT and Pinner M (1931). A clinical trial of sanocrysin in pulmonary tuberculosis. *American Reviews of Tuberculosis*, **24**, 401–35.

Berger JT (1999). Placebo medication use in patient care: a survey of medical interns. *West Journal of Medicine*, **170**, 93–6.

Bingel A (1918). Über Behandlung der Diphtherie mit gewöhnlichem Pferdeserum. *Deutsches Archiv für Klinische Medizin*, **125**, 284–332.

Brody H (2000). *The placebo response*. Harper Collins, New York.

Cannon WB (1942). Voodoo death. *American Anthropologist*, **44**, 169–81.

de Craen AJ, Kaptchuk TJ, Tijssen JG and Kleijne J (1999). Placebos and placebo effects in medicine: historical overview. *Journal of the Royal Society Medicine*, **92**, 511–15.

Enck P and Klosterhalfen S (2013). The placebo response in clinical trials—the current state of play. *Complementary Therapies in Medicine*, **21**, 98–101.

Enck P, Klosterhalfen S and Zipfel S (2011). Novel study designs to investigate the placebo response. *BMC Medical Research Methodology*, **11**, 90.

Epps J, Monk C, Savage S and Marlatt GA (1998). Improving credibility of instruction in the balanced placebo design: a misattribution manipulation. *Addictive Behaviors*, **23**, 426–35.

Ernst E and Resch KL (1995). Concept of true and perceived placebo effects. *British Medical Journal*, **311**, 551–3.

Evans D (2002). Pain, evolution, and the placebo response. *Behavioral and Brain Sciences*, **25**, 459–60.

Evans W and Hoyle C (1933). The comparative value of drugs used in the continuous treatment of angina pectoris. *Quarterly Journal of Medicine*, **26**, 311–38.

Farrar JT (2010). Advances in clinical research methodology for pain clinical trials. *Nature Medicine*, **16**, 1284–93.

Fent R, Rosemann T, Fässler M, Senn O and Huber CA (2011). The use of pure and impure placebo interventions in primary care—a qualitative approach. *BMC Family Practice*, **12**, 11.

Flaten MA, Simonsen T and Olsen H (1999). Drug-related information generates placebo and nocebo responses that modify the drug response. *Psychosomatic Medicine*, **61**, 250–5.

Franklin B, Majault, Le Roy et al. (1785). *Report of Dr. Benjamin Franklin, and other commissioners, charged by the King of France, with the examination of animal magnetism, as now practiced in Paris.* Translated by W. Godwin. J. Johnson, London. Available at: https://archive.org/details/56721030R.nlm.nih.gov.

Hahn RA (1985). A sociocultural model of illness and healing. In L White, B Tursky and GE Schwartz, eds. *Placebo: theory, research, and mechanisms*, pp. 167–95. Guilford, New York.

Hahn RA (1997). The nocebo phenomenon: scope and foundations. In A Harrington, ed. *The placebo effect: an interdisciplinary exploration*, pp. 56–76. Harvard University Press, Cambridge, MA.

Harris CS and Raz A (2012). Deliberate use of placebos in clinical practice: what we really know. *Journal of Medical Ethics*, **38**, 406–7.

Haygarth J (1801). *Of the imagination, as a cause and as a cure of disorders of the body; exemplified by fictitious tractors and epidemical convulsions.* R. Cruttwell, Bath.

Herrnstein RJ (1962). Placebo effect in the rat. *Science*, **138**, 677–8.

Hill AB (1990). Suspended judgement: memories of the British streptomycin trial in tuberculosis. The first randomized clinical trial. *Controlled Clinical Trials*, **11**, 77–9.

Hoffman GA, Harrington A and Fields HL (2005). Pain and the placebo: what we have learned. *Perspectives Biology and Medicine*, **48**, 248–65.

Howick J, Bishop FL, Heneghan C et al. (2013). Placebo use in the United Kingdom: results from a national survey of primary care practitioners. *PLoS One*, **8**, e58247.

Hrobjartsson A and Norup M (2003). The use of placebo interventions in medical practice—a national questionnaire survey of Danish clinicians. *Evaluation and the Health Professions*, **26**, 153–65.

Kaptchuk TJ (1998). Intentional ignorance: a history of blind assessment and placebo controls in medicine. *Bulletin of the History of Medicine*, **72**, 389–433.

Kermen R, Hickner J, Brody H and Hasham I (2010). Family physicians believe the placebo effect is therapeutic but often use real drugs as placebos. *Family Medicine*, **42**, 636–42.

Kirsch I (ed.) (1999). *How expectancies shape experience.* American Psychological Association, Washington, DC.

Levine JD, Gordon NC and Fields HL (1978). The mechanisms of placebo analgesia. *Lancet,* **2,** 654–7.

Lewis G (1977). Fear of sorcery and the problem of death by suggestion. In J Blacking, ed. *The anthropology of the body,* pp. 111–44. Academic Press, New York.

Lex BW (1974). Voodoo death: new thoughts on an old explanation. *American Anthropologist,* **76,** 818–23.

Louhiala P (2012). What do we really know about the deliberate use of placebos in clinical practice? *Journal of Medical Ethics,* **38,** 403–5.

Louis TA, Lavori PW, Bailar JC 3rd and Polansky M (1984). Crossover and self-controlled designs in clinical research. *New England Journal of Medicine,* **310,** 24–31.

Marlatt GA, Demming B and Reid JB (1973). Loss of control drinking in alcoholics: an experimental analogue. *Journal of Abnormal Psychology,* **81,** 223–41.

Mitchell SH, Laurent CL and de Wit H (1996). Interaction of expectancy and the pharmacological effects of d-amphetamine: subjective effects and self-administration. *Psychopharmacology,* **125,** 371–8.

Moerman DE (2002). *Meaning, medicine and the placebo effect.* Cambridge University Press, Cambridge.

Moerman DE and Jonas WB (2002). Deconstructing the placebo effect and finding the meaning response. *Annals of Internal Medicine,* **136,** 471–6.

Nitzan U and Lichtenberg P (2004). Questionnaire survey on use of placebo. *British Medical Journal,* **329,** 944–6.

Parloff MB (1986). Frank's "common elements" in psychotherapy: non-specific factors and placebos. *American Journal of Orthopsychiatry,* **56,** 521–30.

Price DD, Finniss DG and Benedetti F (2008). A comprehensive review of the placebo effect: recent advances and current thought. *Annual Review of Psychology,* **59,** 565–90.

Rohsenow DJ and Bachorowski J (1984). Effects of alcohol and expectancies on verbal aggression in men and women. *Journal of Abnormal Psychology,* **93,** 418–32.

Ross S and Buckalew LW (1985). Placebo agentry: assessment of drug and placebo effects. In L White, B Tursky and GE Schwartz, eds. *Placebo: theory, research, and mechanisms,* pp. 67–82. Guilford, New York.

Ross S, Krugman AD, Lyerly SB and Clyde DJ (1962). Drugs and placebos: a model design. *Psychological Reports,* **10,** 383–92.

Schwartz D and Lellouch J (1967). Explanatory and pragmatic attitudes in therapeutic trials. *Journal of Chronic Diseases,* **20,** 637–48.

Shapiro AK and Shapiro E (1997a). *The powerful placebo: from ancient priest to modern physician.* Johns Hopkins University Press, Baltimore, MD.

Shapiro AK and Shapiro E (1997b). The placebo: is it much ado about nothing? In A Harrington, ed. *The placebo effect: an interdisciplinary exploration,* pp. 12–36. Harvard University Press, Cambridge, MA.

Sherman R and Hickner J (2007). Academic physicians use placebos in clinical practice and believe in the mind-body connection. *Journal of General Internal Medicine,* **23,** 7–10.

Sutton SR (1991). Great expectations: some suggestions for applying the balanced placebo design to nicotine and smoking. *British Journal Addiction,* **86,** 659–62.

Trousseau A and Gouraud H (1834). Repertoire clinique: experiences homéopathique tentées à l'Hotél-Dieu de Paris. *Journal des Connaissances Médico-Chirurgicales*, **8**, 338–41.

Wall PD (1999).The placebo and the placebo response. In PD Wall and R Melzack, eds. *The textbook of pain*, pp. 1297–308. Churchill Livingstone, Edinburgh.

White L, Tursky B and Schwartz GE eds (1985). *Placebo: theory, research, and mechanisms*. Guilford, New York.

Wilson GT, Niaura RS and Adler JL (1985). Alcohol: selective attention and sexual arousal in men. *Journal of Studies on Alcohol*, **46**, 107–15.

Chapter 2

A modern view of placebo and placebo-related effects

Summary points

- By definition, the placebo effect is the effect that follows the administration of an inert treatment (the placebo), whereas in a placebo-related effect no placebo is given.

- The placebo effect, or placebo response, is a psychobiological phenomenon that must not be confounded by other phenomena, such as spontaneous remission and statistical regression to the mean.

- The nocebo effect, or nocebo response, is a negative placebo effect, which goes in the opposite direction of the placebo effect.

- There are many placebo effects with different biological mechanisms and in different systems and apparatuses, which are triggered by the psychosocial context around the patient and the therapy. This psychosocial context constitutes the ritual of the therapeutic act.

- Expectation of a future outcome plays a central role, and may act through different mechanisms, such as modulation of anxiety and activation of reward circuits.

- Learning plays a crucial role and powerful placebo effects may be induced through a conditioning procedure. Through conditioning, it is also possible to elicit placebo responses in animals.

- Modern interpretations of classical conditioning suggest that many conditioned placebo responses are consciously mediated by complex cognitive factors.

- Other mechanisms related to personality traits and genetic variants have also been identified, and these may be associated with good or poor placebo responsiveness.

- Placebo and placebo-related effects may be related to other self-regulatory processes and may have emerged during evolution as a defense mechanism of the body.

2.1 **What they are not**

2.1.1 **Many phenomena are mistakenly taken for placebo effects**

As already mentioned in Chapter 1, a first and important source of confusion about the placebo effect is in its definition. By looking through the online resource PubMed and searching for the word "placebo," approximately 170,000 papers can be found, and the word placebo is often associated with the terms "effect" or "response." Most of these papers, particularly those involving clinical trials, use these words inappropriately or in a very broad and confusing sense. In fact, if we followed the definition of most clinical trial studies, the placebo response and/or effect would be: the outcome that is found in those groups of patients who receive a placebo (the inert treatment). It is very common to find titles of studies like "High rate of placebo responses in clinical trials on . . ." or "Analysis of the placebo response in clinical trials on. . . ." Going through these papers, you soon realize that most of the studies analyze the time course of some symptoms in placebo groups. As a point of fact, the reduction of a symptom in the group that received a placebo can be due to many causes that have nothing to do with the real placebo effect, or response (Kienle and Kiene, 1997; Benedetti and Colloca, 2004), as shown in Fig. 1.1 and described in detail in Table 2.1.

Spontaneous remission, habituation, patient and/or observer bias, the effects of unidentified co-interventions, and many other factors are all phenomena that are sometimes taken for placebo effects (Table 2.1). In other words, if a clinical improvement occurs in the group of patients who received the placebo, most studies describe this effect as "placebo effect" or "placebo response," regardless of whether the improvement is attributable to a spontaneous reduction of symptom severity or to a real psychobiological placebo effect in which the brain anticipates the benefit.

As this is the most common source of misunderstanding about the placebo effect, we should abandon the terms "placebo effect" and "placebo response" when describing the outcome of a placebo group in a clinical trial, and should replace them with words like "improvement in the group that received the placebo." In this way, we make it clear that those patients who took the placebo did improve, although the cause of the improvement is unknown. It might be due to a spontaneous regression of a symptom, to a real active involvement of the brain in anticipating the outcome, or it might represent a biased report of the patient who wants to please the doctor.

2.1.2 **Spontaneous remission is frequently and erroneously defined as placebo effect**

Most chronic conditions show a spontaneous variation in symptom intensity that is known as natural history (Fields and Levine, 1984). If someone takes a placebo just before his symptom starts decreasing, he may believe that the placebo is effective, although that decrease would have occurred anyway. Clearly, this is not a placebo effect but a misinterpretation of the cause–effect relationship, due to a spontaneous remission of the symptom.

Spontaneous fluctuations and remissions of symptoms are probably the most common source of confusion about placebo effects. For example, in his classic work on the

Table 2.1 Factors that can cause the false impression of placebo effect. Reprinted from *Journal of Clinical Epidemiology*, 50(12), Gunver S Kienle and Helmut Kiene, *The Powerful Placebo Effect: Fact or Fiction?* pp. 1311–1318, Copyright (1997), with permission from Elsevier

Natural course of a disease
Spontaneous improvement
Fluctuation of symptoms
Regression to the mean
Habituation
Additional treatment
Observer bias
Conditional switching of treatment
Scaling bias
Poor definition of drug efficacy
Irrelevant response variables
Subsiding toxic effect of previous medication
Patient bias
Answer of politeness and experimental subordination
Conditioned answers
Neurotic or psychotic misjudgment
No placebo given at all
Psychotherapy
Psychosomatic phenomena
Voodoo medicine
Uncritical reporting of anecdotes
Misquotation
False assumption of toxic placebo effects created by
Everyday symptoms
Misquotation
Persistence of symptoms

power of placebos, Beecher (1955) was likely to interpret the improvement of common cold after 6 days as a placebo effect following administration of a placebo. He did not consider that many patients with the common cold get better spontaneously within 6 days (Diehl, 1953). Similarly, in two studies (Keats and Beecher, 1950; Keats et al., 1951) in which the reduction of postoperative pain was claimed to be a placebo effect by Beecher (1955), subsequent analysis showed that it was actually the spontaneous decline of postoperative pain (Kienle and Kiene, 1997).

In this book, it will become clear that many clinical trials claiming high placebo responses do not consider spontaneous remission as an important contributing factor in symptom reduction. For example, in the genitourinary apparatus (see Chapter 9), although placebo groups have been analyzed in some detail, no definitive conclusion can be drawn because spontaneous remission cannot be ruled out. The only way to rule out spontaneous fluctuations is to use an untreated group as a control. With a no-treatment group it is possible to assess the natural course, or natural history, of the disease; comparison between a placebo group and a natural history (no-treatment) group allows us to identify the component of the symptom that is subject to spontaneous fluctuations.

Figure 2.1 is an example of spontaneous fluctuation of pain, the so-called natural history of pain. If a placebo, or an otherwise ineffective treatment, is administered at

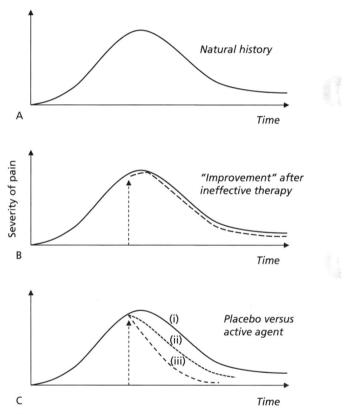

Fig. 2.1 Graph (A) shows the natural fluctuation of pain in a given painful condition; (B) shows an ineffective therapy (dashed line) administered at the time indicated by the arrow, compared to natural history (solid line). If it is not known that a remission in severity might occur without treatment, then any remission will be mistakenly attributed to that treatment. In (C) the natural history of pain intensity (i) is compared with that following placebo administration (ii) and active therapy (iii). The analgesia attributable to the active therapy is represented by the difference between (ii) and (iii), whereas the analgesia attributable to the placebo therapy is represented by the difference between (i) and (ii). Reprinted from *Trends in Neurosciences*, 7 (8), Howard L. Fields and Jon D. Levine, Placebo analgesia—a role for endorphins?, pp. 271–273, Copyright (1984), with permission from Elsevier.

Random numbers			Selection ≥ 0.70	
Series 1	Series 2		Series 1	Series 2
0.71	0.21		**0.71**	0.21
0.11	0.31			
0.70	0.74		**0.70**	0.74
0.23	0.28			
0.49	0.12			
0.26	0.63			
0.35	0.18			
0.63	0.15			
0.25	0.90			
0.55	0.34			
0.95	0.84		**0.95**	0.84
0.09	0.57			
0.92	0.55		**0.92**	0.55
0.32	0.11			
0.86	0.32		**0.86**	0.32
0.59	0.03			
0.02	0.63			
0.96	0.18		**0.96**	0.18
0.36	0.57			
0.68	0.30			
0.04	0.51			
0.63	0.83			
0.80	0.34		**0.80**	0.34
0.05	0.54			
0.55	0.57			
0.93	0.52		**0.93**	0.52
0.61	0.61			
0.72	0.95		**0.72**	0.95
0.24	0.25			
0.14	0.51			

A   m = 0.49   m = 0.45   m = 0.84   m = 0.52

          p = N.S.   p < 0.04

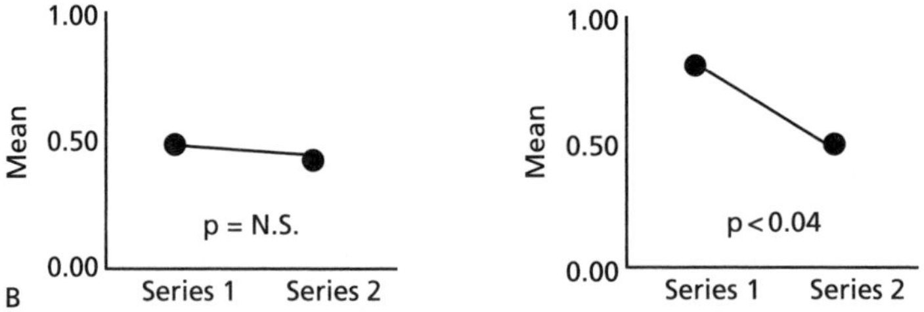

Fig. 2.2 Selection bias may be introduced by factors such as the severity of symptoms, the selection of the diagnostic test, or the definition of the baseline. Every selection gives a model with regression to the mean. In (A) regression to the mean is illustrated by two random series of numbers with values between 0.00 and 1.00. The means of both sets of figures are given, and the statistical difference between the means is not significant (p = N.S.). The figures in bold have values ≥ 0.70. These selected figures were analyzed again on the right side; now their means show a significant difference (p < 0.04). In (B)

the time indicated by the arrow, the reduction in pain can be mistakenly attributed to the placebo, or the ineffective treatment. In other words, pain would have subsided anyway, regardless of placebo administration. To avoid this mistake, the natural history is compared with a placebo treatment *and* an active treatment. The difference between the natural history and the placebo treatment represents the placebo component of the therapy, whereas the difference between the placebo treatment and the active treatment represents the specific component of the therapy. Therefore, it is important to realize that a real placebo effect has nothing to do with the natural history of a symptom, although, as previously mentioned, many clinical trials fail to underscore this difference.

2.1.3 **Regression to the mean is common in clinical trials**

Spontaneous improvement can be considered a special case of regression to the mean, whereby there is a tendency for extreme values to move closer to the mean after repeated measurements. Indeed, regression to the mean is a statistical phenomenon that assumes individual people tend to have extreme values of a physiological parameter (e.g., glucose levels) when enrolled in a clinical trial, and that these extreme values tend to be lower at a second measurement (Davis, 2002). In such cases, the improvement cannot be attributed to any intervention they might have undergone. One very important factor in this phenomenon is the selection criteria used for inclusion in a clinical trial. Figure 2.2 shows an example with random numbers. It is sufficient to randomly generate numbers from 0.00 to 1.00 in order to obtain a model of regression to the mean (Ruck and Sylven, 2006), which indicates that regression to the mean is not a biological phenomenon but rather a mathematical model. It can be seen that there is no difference between the means of the first and second series of numbers. However, if a selection is done, in this case values ≥ 0.70, the sample regresses to the mean with statistical significance. Therefore, every selection bias gives a model with regression to the mean. If these random numbers are replaced with a physiological parameter, such as the plasma level of glucose, the selection of glucose levels above a given value (e.g., ≥ 500 mg/100 mL) would produce similar results, giving the impression of improvement at the second measurement.

When assessing the possibility that an improvement is due to regression to the mean, rather than to a real placebo effect, adequate variables must be carefully selected. For example, in a trial of cholestyramine versus placebo (for the management of high levels of cholesterol), patients were selected on the basis of high plasma levels of cholesterol (Lipid Research Clinics Program, 1984). One of the known side effects of cholestyramine is constipation, and 3% of patients were found to have constipation before the treatment. After 1 year of treatment, 39% of those who received cholestyramine had

Fig. 2.2 (continued) the means for both sets of data are represented graphically. Adapted from *The American Journal of Cardiology*, 97 (1), Andreas Rück and Christer Sylvén, "Improvement" in the Placebo Group Could Be Due to Regression to the Mean as Well as to Sociobiologic Factors, pp. 152–153, Copyright (2006), with permission from Elsevier.

constipation, whereas 10% of those who received the placebo had constipation. The crucial point here is that these patients were not selected on the basis of constipation, thus regression to the mean is unlikely to have occurred. These data seem to be consistent with a real placebo effect, whereby constipation increases from 3% to 10% after placebo treatment (see also Davis, 2002).

2.1.4 Signal detection ambiguity can sometimes explain symptom "reduction"

A particular type of error made by either the patient or the physician, a false positive error, may explain the illusory improvement occurring in some circumstances. This is known as "signal detection theory." It is based on the occurrence of errors in detection of ambiguous signals (Clark, 1969; Allan and Siegel, 2002). For example, if the patient or the doctor is trying to detect a change in a symptom, say pain, then he or she can fail to identify it (a false rejection) or they can erroneously identify something that turns out to be something else (a false positive). As indicated by Allan and Siegel (2002), false positives are more likely to occur when the consequences of a false rejection are deemed to be greater than those of a false positive. A patient may erroneously detect symptomatic relief in response to an inert treatment, and certainly the ambiguity of the symptom's intensity, like fluctuations in pain, is important. In other words, small and large fluctuations represent a noisy environment that makes a judgment about a symptom difficult.

Signal detection theory is a model that was developed to explain decision-making in noisy environments, and it simply states that some signals cannot be distinguished from noise on the basis of their magnitude. Clark (1969) investigated the effects of placebo administration on painful radiant thermal stimulation and found that the placebo condition yielded fewer painful responses compared with a control. However, analysis in the context of signal detection theory showed that thermal sensitivity was the same in the placebo and control conditions. The effect of the placebo was to alter the subject's response criteria and not thermal sensitivity. Signal detection theory was also used in a study by Feather et al. (1972), who concluded that placebos did not produce real decreases in pain sensitivity.

Although signal detection theory may explain the effects of placebos in some circumstances, there is now strong neurobiological evidence that symptom reduction is real in some conditions, such as in pain and Parkinson's disease, in which the neural correlates of such reductions have been found (see Chapters 4 and 5). Therefore, signal detection theory must be considered a possible confounding factor in some circumstances, and it needs to be ruled out through the analysis of objective measurements, such as metabolic changes in the brain or changes in neuron activity.

2.1.5 Sometimes patients and doctors give biased reports of the clinical condition

Biases represent an important confounding factor in the evaluation of clinical improvement. This is true for both patients and doctors. For example, there is some evidence that the patient often wants to please the doctor for the time and effort spent helping him, so he may exaggerate his feeling of clinical improvement (Roberts, 1995; Sackett, 1995; Kienle and Kiene, 1997). Other types of bias are represented by the so-called scaling biases, whereby an asymmetrical measurement scale (e.g., many categories for improvement and one or none for deterioration) tempts the patient to give too many positive reports (Kienle and Kiene, 1997). It is also important to consider that some patients may exaggerate their symptoms in order to be included in a clinical trial (Kleinman et al., 2002).

Investigator biases are important as well; he or she may become unblinded during the course of a clinical trial, which may affect his or her expectations about the effectiveness of the therapy under study. Indeed, there is evidence that the doctor's expectations may affect the placebo response of his patients. Gracely et al. (1985) devised an experiment in which doctors knew they had a high or low probability of giving the powerful painkiller fentanyl to their patients. When the physicians knew that fentanyl administration was highly probable, the administration of placebo was more effective than when they knew there was a lower chance of administering fentanyl. Thus, the doctor's knowledge about a therapy may affect the outcome in patients through verbal communication and/or attitudes.

2.1.6 Co-interventions can sometimes be the cause of improvement

Co-interventions and additional treatments are other important confounding factors that are sometimes ignored, thus leading to erroneous interpretation. For example, a concomitant diet may be responsible for a clinical improvement during placebo treatment. There are several examples of neglected co-interventions that may have accounted for the reduction of a symptom. As pointed out by Kienle and Kiene (1997) in one trial on angina pectoris in the Beecher's analysis (Beecher, 1955), the placebo group also received nitrates (Travell et al., 1949). In another trial on the common cold, patients were allowed to take hot baths, gargles, and diets (Diehl, 1953). Similarly, the study by Lichstein et al. (1955) claims substantial placebo effects in the treatment of unstable colon, but all these patients had been put on a special diet. In another study, this time on alcoholism, patients in the placebo group received specialized medical and psychological support (Wells, 1957). Therefore, it is very important to consider all possible co-interventions when assessing the outcome of a therapy.

An interesting example of co-factors that may contribute to therapeutic outcome after placebo administration is the case of placebos for cough given in syrup form. In this regard, Eccles (2006) analyzed the beneficial role of the sweet taste of cough syrups on the cough itself. In fact, cough syrups contain many substances, including sugar, honey, capsicum, and citric acid. These substances may in turn cause reflex salivation and promote mucus secretion, thus lubricating the pharynx and larynx and helping to reduce coughing. In general, sweet gustatory stimuli are also known to have antitussive effects through the facial, glossopharyngeal, and vagus nerves (Eccles, 2006). It is clear that any reduction of cough associated with these substances in syrups is not a real placebo effect, but rather the effect of a co-intervention (the stimulation of the gustatory receptors) and this is often neglected as a possible beneficial factor influencing coughing.

2.1.7 **Classical clinical trials are not good for understanding placebo effects**

All the phenomena analyzed in the previous sections are present in clinical trials. For example, if a symptom subsides in a group that takes placebo, this can be due to spontaneous remission, regression to the mean, some co-intervention, a real placebo effect, and so on, but there is no way to distinguish between all these factors in the absence of adequate control groups. Therefore, clinical trials do not represent a good model for studying and understanding the mechanisms underlying the placebo effect, unless the target of the trial is the investigation of the placebo effect and the use of appropriate controls. Indeed, many results obtained in the classical clinical-trial setting (whereby the only comparison carried out is between an active treatment and a placebo group) differ from those obtained in the laboratory setting. This is not surprising, as in the laboratory setting it is possible to compare a no-treatment group with a placebo group, so that the spontaneous remission of symptoms can be identified. In the laboratory setting, other confounding variables can be controlled as well. For example, the statistical phenomenon of regression to the mean can be ruled out by using "experimental pain," whereby pain intensity can be controlled experimentally and selections can be avoided. Likewise, symptom-detection ambiguity and subject bias can be eliminated through measurement of objective physiological parameters; furthermore, the possible effects of co-interventions can be eliminated by choosing an appropriate experimental model.

In 2001, Hrobjartsson and Goetzsche (2001) conducted a systematic review and meta-analysis of clinical trials in which patients were randomly assigned to either placebo or no treatment. The purpose was to investigate the clinical effect of placebos, discerning whether patients randomized to placebo under blind conditions have better outcomes than those randomized to no treatment. The investigators identified 130 trials in which 40 different clinical outcomes were investigated by selecting binary outcomes (e.g., the proportion of alcohol abusers and nonalcohol abusers) and continuous outcomes (e.g., the amount of alcohol consumed). They considered the effect of three types of placebos—pharmacological (e.g., a pill), physical (e.g., a manipulation), and psychological (e.g., conversation)—and calculated the pooled relative risk for binary outcomes as well as the pooled standardized mean differences for continuous outcomes. The pooled relative risk was defined as the ratio of the number of patients with an unwanted outcome to the total number of patients in the placebo group, divided by the same ratio in the untreated group. The standardized mean difference was defined as the difference between the mean values for unwanted outcomes in the placebo and untreated groups divided by the pooled standard deviation. A negative value indicated a beneficial effect of placebo both for binary and continuous outcomes. The findings by Hrobjartsson and Goetzsche (2001) did not detect a significant effect of placebo, as compared with no treatment, in pooled data from trials with subjective or objective binary or continuous objective outcomes. However, they found a significant difference between placebo and no treatment in trials with subjective outcomes and in trials involving the treatment of pain. There also was some evidence that placebos had greater effect in small trials with continuous outcomes than in large trials, with an inverse relation between trial size and placebo size. Furthermore, in an update of their first review, Hrobjartsson and Goetzsche (2004) argued that when a large effect of a placebo intervention is not present, small effects on continuous outcomes, for example, in pain, could not be clearly distinguished from biases. Therefore, the observed significant effect of placebo on subjective outcomes may have been due to biased reports of the patients rather than to real placebo effects. In a more recent updated meta-analysis, Hrobjartsson and Goetzsche (2010) again found that placebo interventions have no important clinical effects in general. However, in certain settings placebo interventions can influence patient-reported outcomes, especially pain and nausea, though it is difficult to distinguish patient-reported effects of placebo from biased reporting.

The first original meta-analysis by Hrobjartsson and Goetzsche (2001), albeit of great impact when published, was not successful subsequently and now most researchers do not take it very seriously. In fact, it is important to note that they used very broad inclusion criteria and failed to recognize that placebos are not expected to work uniformly across diseases or disorders (Shapiro and Shapiro, 1997; Ader, 2001; Brody and Weismantel, 2001; Di Nubile, 2001; Einarson et al., 2001; Greene et al., 2001; Kaptchuk, 2001; Kirsch and Scoboria, 2001; Kupers, 2001; Lilford and Braunholtz, 2001; Miller, 2001; Papakostas and Daras, 2001; Shrier, 2001; Spiegel et al., 2001; Wickramasekera, 2001). Aggregating without regard to the heterogeneity of disorders means we cannot discern whether a placebo really works. It is as if we wanted to test the effects of morphine across all medical conditions, like pain, schizophrenia, marital discord, asthma, nephritis, and other diseases. Of course a pooled analysis would find no effect of morphine. Another problematic aspect of Hrobjartsson and Goetzsche's study it that it is impossible to consider the critical factors involved in placebo responses, such as patient and physician expectations, the healing context, and the cues and factors that can influence the effectiveness of a therapeutic intervention (Di Blasi et al., 2001; Benedetti, 2002; Moerman and Jonas, 2002; Moerman, 2003; Benedetti et al., 2005; Colloca and Benedetti, 2005).

In 2002, Vase et al. (2002) conducted another meta-analysis that included 23 of the 29 clinical trials from the meta-analysis by Hrobjartsson and Goetzsche (2001) and an additional meta-analysis of 14 studies investigating placebo analgesic mechanisms. Although this study has been criticized by Hrobjartsson and Goetzsche (2006), Vase et al. (2002) found that the magnitudes of the placebo analgesic effects were higher in studies that investigated placebo analgesic mechanisms compared with clinical trials where the placebo was used only as a control condition. These authors suggest that this difference might be due to the different placebo instructions and suggestions given in the clinical trial setting compared to the experimental setting (Vase et al., 2002). In fact, clinical trial investigators typically avoid giving oral suggestions of analgesia in favor of neutral instructions, whereas investigators of the placebo effect typically emphasize the analgesic suggestions.

In general, these two meta-analyses are worthy of consideration because they present the scenario for two different ways of investigating the placebo effect: on the one hand the randomized clinical trial, and on the other the clinical/experimental setting specifically designed to investigate the placebo effect. Clearly in order to understand the magnitude and mechanisms of the placebo effect across different medical conditions and therapeutic interventions, investigations must be carried out under strictly controlled conditions in the laboratory setting, or at least in a clinical trial that is intentionally devised to analyze the placebo group.

Even if the placebo effect is a phenomenon of small magnitude in some circumstances and in some medical conditions, understanding it is necessary within routine medical practice, the clinical trial setting, and the experimental approach to mind–brain–body issues. For example, a recent debate focused on the possible small or large magnitude of placebo effects, omitting some crucial questions about the underlying mechanisms. Starting from the meta-analysis by Hrobjartsson and Goetzsche (2001), Wampold et al. (2005) re-analyzed the same studies and found robust placebo effects both for pharmacotherapies and psychotherapies. In a rebuttal, Hrobjartsson and Goetzsche (2007) presented evidence that claimed that Wampold's re-analysis was wrong.

As emphasized by Hunsley and Westmacott (2007), the meta-analysis results reported by the two sets of authors (Hrobjartsson and Goetzsche, and Wampold's group) are nearly identical, yet their conclusions differ dramatically. Hunsley and Westmacott (2007) also stress that both meta-analyses indicate that placebo effects do exist and cannot be dismissed as unimportant, although their magnitude appears to be small. Interestingly, these authors compared the size of the effect of placebos with those of other treatments by using the NNT index (number needed to treat), which represents the number of patients that one would need to treat in order to have one more successful outcome than would be possible with the control condition. By considering that the NNT value for placebos is approximately 7, Table 2.2 shows that the magnitude of the placebo effect is comparable to that of transfusion to treat stroke in children with sickle-cell anemia or to the value of adding radiotherapy to tamoxifen in the treatment of breast cancer (Hunsley and Westmacott, 2007).

Table 2.2 Examples of effect sizes from individual studies expressed as the number needed to treat (NNT). For comparison, NNT values for placebo are around 7. Data from The Centre for Evidence-Based Medicine

Condition or disorder	Intervention vs. control	Outcome	NNT
Chronic depression	Nefazodone and psychotherapy vs. either treatment alone	Remission	4
Stroke in children with sickle-cell anemia	Transfusion vs. standard care	All strokes	7
Post-menopausal women with breast cancer	Radiotherapy plus tamoxifen vs. tamoxifen alone	Recurrence	8
Patients resuscitated from ventricular arrhythmias	Implantable defibrillator vs. antiarrhythmic drug therapy	All-cause mortality	13
Hip fractures in nursing home patients	External hip protectors vs. control	Hip fracture	24

In more recent times, some authors have tried to reconsider the meta-analytic approach in order to investigate different aspects. For example, Koog et al. (2011) found that randomized three-armed trials (no treatment, active treatment, placebo), which are necessary for estimating the placebo effect, may be subject to publication bias. For the treatment effect, small trials with fewer than 100 patients per arm showed more benefits than large trials with at least 100 patients per arm in acupuncture and acupoint stimulation. For the placebo effect, no differences were found between large and small trials. In addition, the treatment effect was found to be subject to publication bias because study design and any known factors of heterogeneity were not associated with the small study effects. The magnitude of the placebo effect was smaller than that calculated after considering publication bias. Therefore, if the magnitude of the placebo effect is assessed in an intervention, the potential for publication bias should be investigated using data related to the treatment effect.

In another analysis, Howick et al. (2013) performed a direct test for differences between placebo and active treatment effects in three-armed trials (no treatment, active treatment, placebo). In trials with continuous outcomes, the authors found no difference between treatment and placebo effects. In trials with binary outcomes, treatments were significantly more effective than placebos. Treatment and placebo effects were not different in 22 out of 28 predefined subgroup analyses. Of the six subgroups with differences, treatments were more effective than placebos in five. However, when all criteria for reducing bias were ruled out, placebos were more effective than treatments. Thus, placebos and treatments often have similar effect sizes.

As the context around the patient is the crucial factor in placebo responsiveness, and psychological factors are at the core of its magnitude, it is not surprising that placebo effects in clinical trials are highly variable, and often small. By contrast, as discussed throughout this book, when the context and the patient's psychological factors are manipulated under strictly controlled conditions in the laboratory setting, the magnitude of the placebo effect can be modulated like many other physiological parameters. Therefore, despite the usefulness of all these meta-analyses, the clinical trial setting is not a good model for understanding the placebo effect and is likely to lead to erroneous, or at least confusing, interpretations. We should be aware that placebos act through a set of different mechanisms, thus they must be investigated using different approaches for different diseases and therapeutic interventions. For example, if we want to study the placebo effect in the immune and endocrine systems, we cannot elicit it through experimental manipulation of the patient's expectations, as expectation is likely to have small or no effect on immune mediators and hormones. By contrast, if we use a conditioning paradigm, robust placebo effects can be observed in both the immune and endocrine system (see Chapter 7).

2.2 **What they are**

2.2.1 **Is the placebo effect different from the placebo response?**

Today placebo researchers tend to use the term "placebo effect" and "placebo response" interchangeably (Colloca et al., 2008). Accordingly, throughout this book I will use the two terms interchangeably. However, it should be noted that the term "placebo effect" is sometimes considered to be different from "placebo response." This is because, as seen in Chapter 1, the term "placebo effect" was originally used to mean any improvement in the condition of a group of subjects that has received a placebo, thus including everything (spontaneous remission, regression to the mean, biases, co-interventions, real placebo responses, and so forth). By contrast, "placebo response" sometimes refers to the change in an individual caused by placebo manipulation, which represents the real psychophysiological placebo response of a subject to the inert treatment. Unfortunately, it is not easy to identify a placebo response in a single individual, and many control subjects are sometimes necessary to rule out spontaneous remissions, biases, and symptom detection ambiguities. For example, in a situation where someone reports a pain reduction from 7 to 6 on a numerical rating scale of 0 to 10 after the administration of a placebo, there is no way to say whether this small reduction is attributable to a placebo effect or to a spontaneous remission or a bias. For this reason, the placebo effect is better described as a group effect and, indeed, most of the studies on placebo mechanisms consider the mean reduction of a symptom in a group of subjects after placebo administration. There are, however, a few instances in which the natural history of a symptom is straightforward and guarantees safe identification of the placebo response in a single individual. For example, in this sense, postoperative pain is a good model, as this kind of pain either increases or is constant over time during the first hours after surgery. Therefore, it is safe to assume that a reduction of postoperative pain after placebo administration during the first hours after surgery is not due to a spontaneous fluctuation.

I believe that the difference between the words "effect" and "response," which is often present in the literature, is only a matter of definition, and is worthy of consideration only in part. I think that distinguishing between placebo effects and placebo responses is neither advantageous nor useful, because we risk going back to the old concept of placebo effect, which included everything. Therefore, I suggest that we use placebo *effect* and *response* interchangeably to mean a psychobiological phenomenon occurring in an individual or in a group of individuals.

2.2.2 The psychosocial context around the therapy is the crucial factor

For a long time, the word placebo has been equated with "sugar pill," as it was widespread practice to give a carbohydrate tablet as a means of detecting "mystifiers" (identified through the success of the sham therapy) or as a compassionate remedy for the terminally ill. However, the aim of "pleasing" the patient, as the etymology of the word suggests, can clearly be achieved not only with drugs but also with any medical treatment ranging from physical cures to psychotherapy. What matters is not the sugar, of course, but its symbolic significance, which can be attached to practically anything (Brody, 2000). Moerman (2002) went as far as proposing to substitute the term "placebo response" with "meaning response," to underscore the importance of the patient's beliefs about the treatment and stress what is present (something in the environment inducing the expectation of a benefit) rather than what is absent (a chemical or manipulation of

Box 2.1 Moerman's meaning response

Dan Moerman's proposal to replace the term "placebo response" with "meaning response" reminds us that what matters is not the inert treatment per se but rather the meaning of the surrounding context and of the therapeutic ritual. He selected his ten favorite studies that convinced him to use the term "meaning response" (Moerman, 2013), and lists them according to a descending order.

Position n. 10. Both aspirin and placebo work better when they have a highly advertised brand name on them (Branthwaite and Cooper, 1981).

Position n. 9. The physician's knowledge of the context in which placebos are given can change the outcome, which indicates that the physician can transmit his expectations to his patients (Gracely et al., 1985).

Position n. 8. Analgesia following the administration of a placebo can be blocked by antagonizing the opioid receptors with naloxone, and this occurs only when the doctor knows that the patient might get morphine (Levine et al., 1978).

Position n. 7. As in the previous study, analgesia following placebo administration is blocked by naloxone. In addition, it is enhanced by blocking cholecystokinin, an antiopioid peptide (Benedetti, 1996).

Position n. 6. Chinese-Americans and Japanese-Americans have been found to be more likely to die on the 4th day of the month, and this is because "four" is an unlucky number (in Chinese it is similar to the word "death") (Phillips et al., 2001).

Position n. 5. Placebos can be deeply meaningful and can help even if one knows they are inert (Park and Covi, 1965; Kaptchuk et al., 2010).

Position n. 4. In an analysis of 6944 patients with depression, placebos have been found to determine the 80% of the clinical improvement, thus the real drug effect is only 20% (Kirsch et al., 2002).

Position n. 3. The proportion of patients with depression responding to placebos increased from 20% to 35% in the period 1981–2000, and the same increase occurred for antidepressants (from 40% to 55%) (Walsh et al., 2002). Thus, the responses to placebos change, as the meaning of drug effectiveness changes over time.

Position n. 2. Brain responses to placebos across different neuroimaging studies underscore the reality of meaningful treatments (de la Fuente-Fernandez et al. 2001; Leuchter et al., 2002).

Position n. 1. Hidden therapies are less effective than open ones. Therefore, the knowledge about the treatment and its meaning affect the therapeutic outcome (Amanzio et al., 2001; Benedetti et al., 2003a). This is the best example showing that we do not need to administer placebos in order to induce psychological effects; the meaning response is always there, in any therapy.

proven specific efficacy). Therefore, the concept of placebo has shifted from the "inert" content of the placebo agent (e.g., sugar pills) to the concept of a simulation of an active therapy within a psychosocial context. In this regard, Moerman's meaning response makes us understand that what matters is the meaning of the therapeutic ritual and not the inert substance per se (Box 2.1).

On the basis of these considerations, when a medical treatment (for instance, a drug) is given to a patient, it is not administered in a vacuum, but in a complex set of psychological states that varies from patient to patient and from situation to situation. For example, when morphine is given to relieve pain, it is administered along with a complex set of psychosocial stimuli which tell the patient that a benefit or worsening may occur shortly (Fig. 2.3). These psychosocial stimuli represent the context around the therapy and the patient and such a context may be as important as the specific pharmacodynamic effect of a drug. Di Blasi et al. (2001) listed a series of contextual factors that might affect the therapeutic outcome. These range from the treatment characteristics (color and shape of a pill) to the patient's and provider's characteristics (treatment and illness beliefs, status, and sex) and from the patient–provider relationship (suggestion, reassurance, and compassion) to the healthcare setting (home or hospital) and room layout. Thus, the context is made up of anything that surrounds the patient under treatment, what can be defined as "the ritual of the therapeutic act," including doctors, nurses, hospitals, syringes, pills, machines, and such like, but certainly doctors and nurses are a very important component of the context, as they can transmit a lot of information to the patient through their words, attitudes and behaviors (Benedetti, 2002). By using a single word, Balint (1955) referred to this context as the whole atmosphere around the treatment. In order to highlight the important role of the context in the placebo effect, Miller and Kaptchuk (2008) have proposed using the term "contextual healing."

Thomas (1987) found that positive and negative consultations in general practice have an important impact on patients who present with minor illness (see section 10.5). Likewise, Di Blasi et al. (2001) examined 25 randomized clinical trials in

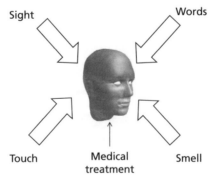

Fig. 2.3 When a medical treatment is being administered, it is surrounded by a complex psychosocial context—the sight of medical personnel and the hospital environment, the touch of machines, the words used by doctors and nurses, and the smell of drugs. All these sensory stimuli tell the patient that a therapy is being carried out. A positive context may improve the therapeutic outcome, whereas a negative context may worsen it.

which the context about the treatment and the patient's expectations about the therapeutic outcome were manipulated. A consistent finding was that those doctors who adopt a friendly and reassuring manner are more effective than those who are formal and do not offer reassurance.

Interestingly, marketing may affect the magnitude of the placebo effect. In a study in 835 patients suffering from headache, the participants were randomized to branded aspirin, unbranded aspirin, branded placebos, and unbranded placebos (Branthwaite and Cooper, 1981). Pills were dispensed in either a plain bottle or a bottle with a prominent brand name on the label. Results showed that branded aspirin was the most effective, followed by the unbranded aspirin, then by branded placebo, and finally by unbranded placebo. Similarly, Faasse et al. (2013) found that medication formulation change from branded to generic is associated with reduced subjective and objective measures of medication effectiveness and increased side effects.

More recently, Waber et al. (2008) investigated the effects of price on analgesic response to placebo pills. After randomization, half the participants were told that the drug (actually a placebo) had a regular price of US$2.50 per pill and half were told that the price had been discounted to US$0.10 per pill. Overall, the participants in the regular price group experienced a larger reduction in pain compared to the low-price (discounted) group. These results are consistent with described phenomena of commercial variables affecting patients' expectations, and expectations influencing therapeutic efficacy. This may explain the popularity of high-cost medical therapies over inexpensive, widely available alternatives such as over-the-counter drugs (Waber et al., 2008).

The placebo effect is therefore a context effect (Di Blasi et al., 2001; Benedetti, 2002). Not only is the context around a treatment associated with positive outcomes, but to negative outcomes as well. For example, distrust in a therapy and/or in medical personnel can make a patient expect a negative outcome, which is called nocebo effect (see later sections). It is important, therefore, to realize that the study of the placebo effect is the study of the psychosocial context around the treatment—whether it is positive or negative—and how these social stimuli and therapeutic rituals may affect the patient's brain (see the most common therapeutic rituals in Box 2.2). This, in turn, may have either beneficial or negative effects on the course of a disease and/or the response to a therapy.

2.2.3 Placebo and nocebo effects occur when inert treatments are given

By definition, a placebo effect is the effect that follows the administration of a placebo, that is, of an inert treatment. Therefore, any psychobiological effect on the brain and/or the body that follows the administration of a placebo can be called, in its own rights, placebo effect or placebo response (Table 2.3). It is important to stress that the inert treatment is given along with contextual stimuli, for example, verbal suggestions of clinical improvement which make the patient believe that the treatment is real and effective. As described earlier, it is crucial to point out that the inert treatment (e.g., a sugar pill or a saline solution) will never acquire therapeutic properties, so that a pharmacologically inert substance will always remain inert. What matters is the context and

Box 2.2 Therapeutic rituals in medical practice

Both conventional and alternative medicine are full of therapeutic rituals. Often there is no difference between these two medical approaches, because in both cases pills are administered, substances injected, and physical procedures performed. Rituals convey the meaningful information that a therapy is being carried out, thus patients expect a therapeutic benefit with the subsequent clinical amelioration of their symptoms. The most common therapeutic rituals are: taking a pill (Fig. 2.4), receiving an injection (Fig. 2.5), undergoing surgery (Fig. 2.6), being touched by a medical device (Fig. 2.7). In nonconventional medicine, many complex rituals are often performed, such as piercing the skin in specific points with acupuncture needles (Fig. 2.8), placing talismans and magnets over the body, praying, and worship. Shamanic procedures, both in Western and non-Western societies, involve even more complicated rituals, such as singing, playing, drumming, and dancing.

It is crucial to understand that, from the perspective of the sufferer, it makes no difference where the ritual comes from. What matters is his/her trust and belief in the ritual itself. Rituals are at the very heart of placebo effects, for they are made of sensory and social stimuli that tell the sick person that a treatment is in progress and that an improvement should be taking place shortly. Throughout this book, we will see that all these social stimuli can activate the same biochemical and receptorial pathways that are activated by drugs.

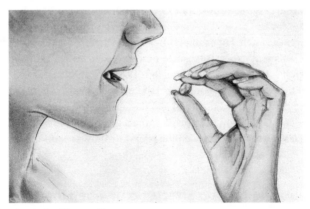

Fig. 2.4 The ritual of taking a pill.

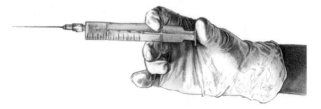

Fig. 2.5 The ritual of an injection.

Box 2.2 Therapeutic rituals in medical practice (continued)

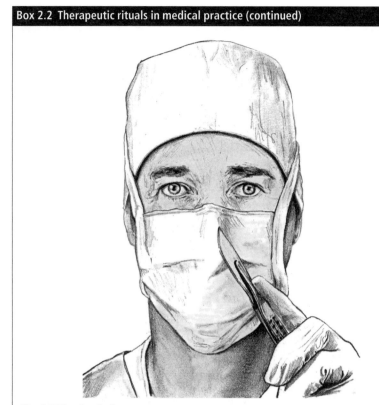

Fig. 2.6 The ritual of surgery.

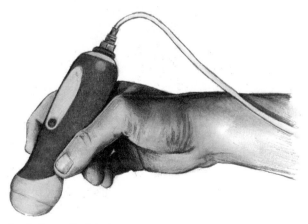

Fig. 2.7 The ritual of a medical device.

Box 2.2 Therapeutic rituals in medical practice (continued)

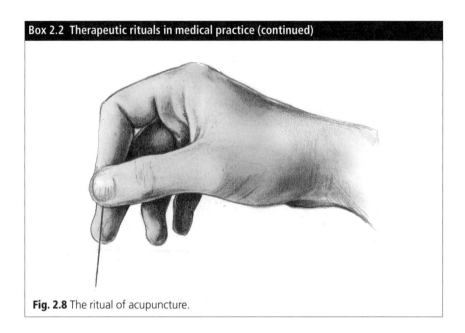

Fig. 2.8 The ritual of acupuncture.

the verbal suggestions of clinical benefit. Therefore, a placebo would be better defined as an inert treatment plus the context that tells the patient a therapeutic act is being performed.

The nocebo effect is a placebo effect because an inert substance is administered. However, in order to induce a nocebo effect, the inert substance is given along with a negative context, for example, verbal suggestions of clinical worsening, so as to induce negative expectations about the outcome. The term *nocebo* ("I shall harm") was introduced in contrast to the term placebo ("I shall please") by some authors to distinguish the pleasing from the noxious effects of placebos (Kennedy, 1961; Pogge, 1963; Kissel and Barrucand, 1964; Hahn, 1985, 1997). If the positive psychosocial context, which is typical of the placebo effect, is reversed in the opposite direction, the nocebo effect can be studied.

Table 2.3 Main differences between placebo and placebo-related effects

Placebo effects	Placebo-related effects
Inert treatments are given	No inert treatments are given
Expectation induced by administration of inert treatments	Suggestions of improvement or worsening without administration of inert treatments
Conditioning, whereby the conditioned stimulus is neutral (inert)	Difference between expected (open) and unexpected (hidden) treatments
Nocebo effect, whereby the administration of inert treatments induces negative expectations	Expectation of belonging to either the placebo or active treatment group in a clinical trial

From an ethical point of view, the investigation of the nocebo effect is difficult to carry out. In fact, whereas the induction of placebo responses is certainly ethical in many circumstances (Benedetti and Colloca, 2004), the induction of nocebo responses represents a stressful and anxiogenic procedure, because verbally induced negative expectations of symptom worsening may lead to a real worsening. Certainly, a nocebo procedure is unethical in patients, and this is one of the main reasons why much less is known about nocebo phenomena.

2.2.4 Placebo- and nocebo-related effects do not involve the administration of inert treatments

By definition, if no placebo is administered, the effect that follows its administration cannot be called a placebo or nocebo effect. However, it has become clear in recent times that the term placebo effect is too restrictive and does not help explain the underlying mechanisms (Benedetti, 2008). Indeed, there are several placebo-like effects, whereby no placebo is given, which are due to the influence of the context surrounding the treatment on the patient's brain (Table 2.3). For example, although a placebo is usually given along with verbal suggestions of clinical improvement, verbal suggestions of either improvement or worsening can be given alone, without administering any inert treatment, so as to induce expectancies about the outcome.

Another example of placebo-related effect is represented by the decreased effectiveness of hidden treatments. It is possible to eliminate the placebo (psychosocial) component and analyze the specific effect of the treatment, free of any psychological contamination, by making the patient completely unaware that a medical therapy is being carried out (Colloca et al., 2004; Benedetti et al., 2011). To do this, drugs are administered through hidden infusions by machines. A hidden infusion of a drug is delivered by a computer-controlled infusion pump, preprogrammed to deliver the drug at the desired time. The crucial point here is that the patients do not know that any drug is being injected, so that they do not expect anything. By contrast, an open administration represents routine medical practice, whereby drugs are given overtly and the patients expect a clinical benefit. Therefore, an open injection of a drug represents an expected treatment, whereas a hidden injection represents an unexpected therapy. The difference between the outcomes following administration of the expected and unexpected therapy is the placebo (psychological) component, even though no placebo has been given (Colloca et al., 2004; Benedetti et al., 2011).

Regardless of placebo administration, expectations can make a big difference in a clinical trial. In fact, what the subjects expect in a clinical trial may influence the outcome, irrespective of whether they belong to the placebo group or to the active treatment group (Benedetti, 2005, 2007). For example, in one clinical trial, real acupuncture was compared with placebo acupuncture and patients were asked which group they believed they belonged to (either placebo or real treatment). Patients who believed they belonged to the real acupuncture group experienced greater clinical improvement than those who believed they belonged to the placebo acupuncture group (Bausell et al., 2005) (see also sections 4.1.3 and 5.1.2).

Placebo- and nocebo-related effects, therefore, do not involve the administration of any inert treatment (placebo). However, it appears clear that in many circumstances similar mechanisms are at work. For example, is there any difference between placebo administration along with suggestions of analgesia and suggestions of analgesia alone? Maybe the administration of a placebo, which is nothing but the simulation of the therapeutic act, enhances the suggestions of improvement because it makes the verbal suggestions more credible. Although this point is still unknown, it appears clear that it is neither useful nor advantageous to restrict the study of the placebo effect to the procedure of giving a placebo.

2.2.5 Are subjective outcomes different from objective outcomes?

One of the most debated issues in the history of placebo research is about subjective versus objective measurements. The specific reason for this debate is that the subjective reports by patients about their clinical condition are often considered to be strongly influenced by biases (see section 2.1.5). Indeed, Hrobjartsson and Goetzsche (2001) found a difference between subjective and objective measurements. They did not detect a significant effect of placebo (as compared with no treatment) in trials with subjective or objective binary or continuous objective outcomes, but they did find a significant difference between placebo and no treatment in trials with subjective outcomes and in trials involving the treatment of pain. There also was some evidence that placebos had a greater effect in small trials with continuous outcomes than in large trials, which may be due to biased reports of patients rather than to real placebo effects.

Although this issue is clearly an important one, today there is no reason to believe that subjective placebo responses can be dismissed as report biases. In fact, with a typical subjective symptom like pain, there are now a number of brain imaging studies that indicate the subjective experience of pain reduction following placebo administration is accompanied by objective changes in several brain regions where pain transmission is inhibited (see Chapter 4). Likewise, substantial placebo responses can be observed in motor disorders such as Parkinson's disease, in which motor performance can be measured objectively (see Chapter 5), and in the immune and endocrine systems, in which objective measurements of immune mediators and hormone plasma concentrations can be obtained (Chapter 7).

Therefore, the question of whether placebos induce subjective or objective changes has been reframed with respect to identifying the neural substrates of the subjective changes. In other words, subjective reports by patients are as important as the objective changes, provided that other phenomena, like the patient's biases, can be ruled out. For example, a subjective report of well-being after placebo administration is worthy of scientific inquiry in the same way as an objective change in motor performance. One good example is seen in a study in Parkinson's disease, in which subjective reports of well-being were recorded following administration of a placebo, such as "I feel good, I want to stand up" or "I feel like the usual therapy" or "I feel much better" (Benedetti et al., 2004). Without the appropriate controls and objective measurements, these reports could not be distinguished from biases, such as the patient's desire to please the experimenter. An in-depth analysis of these subjective effects revealed that the subjective reports of well-being were accompanied by the objective reduction of muscle rigidity, as assessed by a blinded neurologist, as well as by a reduction of the firing rate and bursting activity of subthalamic nucleus neurons, as assessed by intraoperative single-unit recording (Benedetti et al., 2004).

Thus, a clear-cut distinction between subjective and objective measurements is neither advantageous nor useful, provided that the correct methodology is applied to rule out possible biases and other phenomena. Whenever a subjective report of well-being is reported by patients after placebo administration, before dismissing it as a bias or a subjective experience that is not worthy of consideration we should devise the appropriate experimental approach in order to uncover the underlying mechanisms.

2.3 How they work

2.3.1 There is not a single placebo effect but many

There is not a single mechanism of the placebo effect and not a single placebo effect—but many. So we have to look for different mechanisms in different medical conditions and in different therapeutic interventions. Expectation and anticipation of clinical benefit play a crucial role when conscious physiological functions are involved, whereas classical conditioning is the main element in unconscious physiological functions (Benedetti et al., 2003b) (Fig. 2.9). For example, expectations have no effect on hormone secretion, whereas a conditioning procedure can induce conditioned placebo hormonal responses. Therefore, different systems and apparatuses as well as different diseases and treatments are affected by placebos in different ways. Indeed, this book aims to describe the different placebo and placebo-like effects across different medical conditions in order to make it clear that the placebo effect is a general phenomenon that involves different mechanisms.

The existence and occurrence of many placebo effects across diseases has also an important methodological meaning. It is necessary to adopt the appropriate methodology and procedure in order to study different placebo effects. For example, if a procedure that induces strong expectations is used to elicit hormonal placebo responses, no effect will be observed, as hormone secretion is not affected by expectations in most of the cases (see section 7.3). Of course, until all the mechanisms involved in different conditions are identified, it is not possible to rule out the possibility of some common mechanisms across medical conditions. For example, reward mechanisms as well as classical conditioning may represent a common substrate in different diseases and different systems.

Therefore, one of the main problems in current placebo research is how these different mechanisms should be considered and classified. A first approach to the classification of different placebo responses might be based on the mechanism that is involved. On the other hand, today we do not know exactly when and in which conditions these mechanisms take place: anxiety reduction might be important only in some medical conditions but not in others, or otherwise learning might be a common mechanism across all medical conditions. Reasoning in this way, a second approach to the classification of different placebo responses, is a disease-based classification whereby the biological underpinnings are investigated in different conditions such as pain and Parkinson's disease. Therefore, it is not clear whether we should differentiate the placebo responses on the basis of the mechanism or rather on the basis of the disease. This will be a future challenge in placebo research, that is, to understand where (in which disease), when (in which circumstance), and how (with which mechanism) placebos work. Thus, due to our limited understanding of the relationship between mechanisms and diseases, I will present both approaches. In the next few sections of this Part 1 of the book, the general mechanisms that have been identified are described, whereas in Parts 2 and 3 a systematic description across different diseases will be performed.

2.3.2 Expectation of a future outcome is one of the principal mechanisms

Most of the research on placebos has focused on expectations as the main factor involved in placebo responsiveness (Fig. 2.9). Indeed, the literature is full of studies that analyze expectations (Tracey, 2010; Colloca and Miller, 2011; Atlas and Wager, 2012), and the terms "effects of placebos" and "effects of expectations" are frequently used interchangeably, as described many times throughout this book.

In general, expectations of a future outcome and of a future response—the so-called response expectancies—are held by each individual about his or her own emotional and physiological responses such as pain, anxiety and sexual arousal (Kirsch, 1985, 1990, 1999). Expectations may lead to a cognitive readjustment of the appropriate behavior. Thus, it is not surprising that positive expectations lead to adoption of a particular behavior, for instance, resuming a normal daily schedule, whereas negative expectations lead to its inhibition (Bandura, 1977, 1997; Bootzin, 1985). Otherwise, the effects of expectations may be mediated by changes in other cognitions, such as a decrease in self-defeating thoughts when expecting analgesia (Stewart-Williams and Podd, 2004). Expectations are unlikely to operate alone, and several other factors have been identified and described, such as memory and motivation (Price et al., 1985, 2001, 2008; 2000; Geers et al., 2005a) and meaning of the illness experience (Pennebaker, 1997; Brody, 2000). According to Brody (2000) the meaning precedes other causal mechanisms, like expectation. In an attempt to explain the causal mechanisms of the placebo effect, Bootzin and Caspi (2002) and Caspi and Bootzin (2002) integrate multiple explanatory mechanisms in a model that involves factors which are both internal and external to the individual, including expectation.

Expectation is certainly a difficult issue, as it can involve different factors and mechanisms. For example, Frank (1961, 1971, 1981) analyzed the healing process within the context of patient's expectations, though he proposed that *hope* is the primary mechanism of change in the folk tradition of healing and in psychotherapy. Indeed, hope can be defined as the desire and expectation that the future will be better than the present. Expectations may also play a role in the so-called Hawthorne effect. This describes the clinical improvement in a group of patients in a clinical trial that is attributable to the fact they are being observed (Last, 1983). In other words, a patient who knows he is being studied may expect a better therapeutic benefit because of the

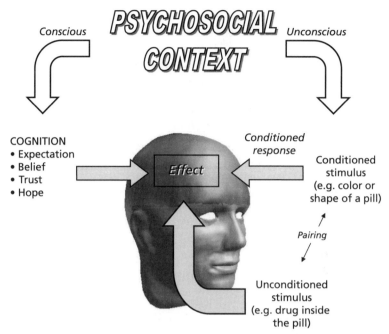

Fig. 2.9 The psychosocial context around the treatment may act on the patient's brain through unconscious and conscious mechanisms. Conscious mechanisms involve complex cognitive factors, such as expectation and anticipation of benefit, belief in the treatment, and trust and hope. Unconscious mechanisms involve classical conditioning whereby, after repeated pairings between a conditioned contextual stimulus (e.g., the color and the shape of a pill) with an unconditioned stimulus (the pharmacological agent inside the pill), the conditioned stimulus alone can produce an effect (a conditioned response).

many examinations he undergoes, the special attention he receives from the medical personnel, and the trust in the new therapy under investigation. It appears therefore clear that expectation is a general term that can be considered from many different perspectives.

From a neuroscientific point of view, expecting a future event may involve several brain mechanisms aimed at preparing the body to anticipate that event. For example, the expectation of a future positive outcome may reduce anxiety and/or activate the neuronal networks of reward mechanisms, whereas the expectation of a negative outcome may result in anticipation of a possible threat, thus increasing anxiety. Indeed, anxiety has been found to be reduced after placebo administration in some studies. In other words, if one expects a distressing symptom to subside shortly, anxiety tends to decrease. For example, McGlashan et al. (1969) and Evans (1977) studied experimental pain in both "trait" and "state" anxiety subjects. Trait anxiety represents a personality trait which can be found throughout life; state anxiety may be present in specific stressful situations, representing an adaptive and transitory response to stress. These researchers gave the subjects a placebo which they believed to be a painkiller. There was no correlation between trait anxiety and pain tolerance after placebo administration, but there was a strict correlation between situational anxiety and pain tolerance during the placebo session. In fact, subjects who showed decreased anxiety had better pain tolerance than those who experienced increased anxiety. Similar results were also obtained by Vase et al. (2005), who found decreased anxiety in patients with irritable bowel syndrome who received a placebo treatment. Moreover, brain imaging studies have found reduced activation of anxiety-related areas during a placebo response (Petrovic et al., 2005) (see also section 6.2.2).

Expectations may also induce changes through reward mechanisms, which ensure future reward acquisition. These mechanisms are mediated by specific neuronal circuits that link cognitive, emotional, and motor responses; they are traditionally studied in the context of the pursuit of natural (e.g., food), monetary, and drug rewards (Mogenson and Yang, 1991; Kalivas et al., 1999). In animals, dopaminergic cells in the brainstem ventral tegmental area that project to the nucleus accumbens of the ventral basal ganglia respond to both the magnitude of anticipated rewards and deviations from the predicted outcomes, thus representing an adaptive system modulating behavioral responses (Setlow et al., 2003; Tobler et al., 2005; Schultz, 2006). A simplified schema of the reward circuitry is shown in Fig. 2.10. The nucleus accumbens plays a central role in the dopamine-mediated reward mechanism, together with the ventral tegmental area, the amygdala, the periaqueductal gray, and other areas in the thalamic, hypothalamic, and subthalamic (pallidum) regions.

In 2001, de la Fuente-Fernandez et al. (2001, 2002) used positron emission tomography to show dopamine activation in the nucleus accumbens following administration of a placebo in patients with Parkinson's disease. Interestingly, no relationship was found between dopamine activity in the nucleus accumbens and the actual placebo effects on motor function; this suggests that dopamine activation was better related to

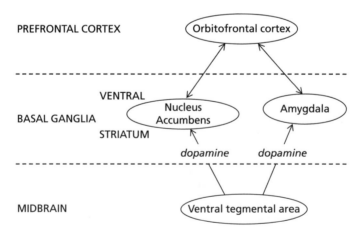

Fig. 2.10 A simplified schema of the reward system. It has been found to be activated by placebos in some circumstances, as assessed by an increase in dopamine activity in the nucleus accumbens. In the case of placebo administration, the reward is represented by the clinical improvement.

the expectation of reward (see section 5.1). Likewise, Mayberg et al. (2002) observed activation of the nucleus accumbens in depressed patients after 1 week of placebo treatment, and Petrovic et al. (2005) described a correlation between ratings of negative-affect improvement during preconditioning with a benzodiazepine and ventral basal ganglia synaptic activity after receiving a placebo (see also sections 6.1 and 6.2). In addition, Scott et al. (2007) found a correlation between responsiveness to placebo and responsiveness to monetary reward in a model of experimental pain in healthy subjects; they also found that placebo responsiveness was related to the activation of dopamine in the nucleus accumbens (see section 4.1.8). All these studies seem to confirm involvement of dopamine activity in the nucleus accumbens, and the general reward circuitry, in the expectations induced by administration of a placebo (de la Fuente-Fernandez, 2009). Detailed accounts of this are covered in other chapters.

Expectations may also enhance the identification of somatic information. Indeed, Geers et al. (2011) studied three expectation groups. In the first group, participants ingested a placebo and were told it was caffeine (deceptive expectation). In a second group, participants ingested a placebo and were told it may be either caffeine or placebo (double-blind expectation). Participants in the third group were given no expectation. All participants then tallied the placebo-relevant and placebo-irrelevant sensations they experienced during a 7-minute period. The deceptive expectation group identified more placebo-relevant sensations than placebo-irrelevant sensations, whereas the no-expectation group identified more placebo-irrelevant sensations than placebo-relevant sensations. The double-blind expectation group identified an equal amount of placebo-relevant and irrelevant sensations. The amount of both placebo-relevant and placebo-irrelevant sensations detected mediated the relationship between the expectation manipulation and subsequent symptom reports. Therefore, in this study, expectations caused placebo responding, in part, by altering how one identifies bodily sensations.

2.3.3 The placebo effect is a learning phenomenon

Subjects who suffer from a painful condition, such as a headache, and who regularly consume aspirin, can associate the shape, color, and taste of that pill to a decrease in their pain. After repeated associations, a sugar pill that looks like aspirin can also decrease their pain (Fig. 2.9). In place of the shape, color, and taste of pills, several other stimuli can be associated with clinical improvement, such as syringes, stethoscopes, white coats, hospitals, doctors, nurses, and so on. The mechanism that underlies this effect is "conditioning" whereby a conditioned (neutral) stimulus (like the color or shape of a pill) can be effective in inducing the reduction of a symptom if it is repeatedly associated with an unconditioned stimulus (like the drug inside the pill). This type of associative learning may represent the basis of many placebo effects—the placebo is the conditioned (neutral) stimulus itself. Indeed, in the 1960s, Herrnstein (1962) found that injection of scopolamine induced motor changes in rats, and these motor changes also occurred after injection of a saline solution (placebo) which was performed after the scopolamine injection.

A sequence effect of this sort also occurs in humans. For example, it has long been known that placebos given after drugs are more effective than when they are given for

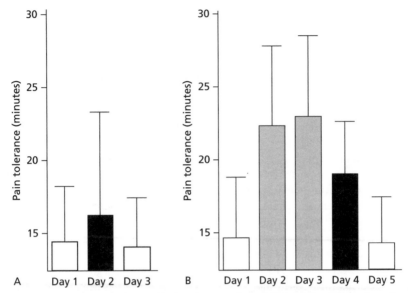

Fig. 2.11 Tolerance to experimental ischemic arm pain. In (A) a placebo (suggestion of analgesia) is given for the first time on day 2 (days 1 and 3 represent control conditions) as shown by the black column. In (B) the placebo is given on day 4 after administration of the painkiller ketorolac on days 2 and 3 (shaded columns). Days 1 and 5 represent control conditions. It can be seen that the placebo given after pharmacological preconditioning induces greater placebo analgesia than placebo given without preconditioning. Reproduced from Amanzio M and Benedetti F, Neuropharmacological dissection of placebo analgesia: expectation-activated opioid systems versus conditioning-activated specific subsystems, *Journal of Neuroscience*, 19, pp. 484–97 Copyright 1999, The Society for Neuroscience.

the first time (Sunshine et al., 1964; Batterman, 1966; Batterman and Lower, 1968; Laska and Sunshine, 1973). Figure 2.11 shows that if a placebo is given for the first time, the placebo response is present but small. If the placebo is administered after two prior administrations of an effective painkiller, the placebo analgesic response is much larger (Amanzio and Benedetti, 1999), thus indicating that the placebo effect is a learning phenomenon. This holds true for nonpharmacological treatments as well (André-Obadia et al., 2011).

These clinical and pharmacological observations are in keeping with studies conducted in the laboratory setting by Voudouris et al. (1989, 1990). They showed that the placebo effect can indeed be conditioned. They applied a neutral nonanesthetic cream (placebo) to one group of subjects who were assured that it was a local anesthetic; not surprisingly, some of these subjects showed a placebo response after painful electrical stimulation. In a second group, the application of the same placebo cream was associated with surreptitious reduction of the intensity of stimulation, so as to make them believe that it was a powerful painkiller. These subjects, who had experienced a "true analgesic effect," became strong placebo responders. Voudouris et al. (1989, 1990) concluded that conditioning is the main mechanism involved in the placebo effect.

These experiments were replicated by other authors, however a cognitive component was found to contribute to the conditioning-induced placebo responses. For example, De Jong et al. (1996) found a correlation between the expected and the actual level of analgesia in a similar experimental situation, thus suggesting that expectation is involved. Montgomery and Kirsch (1997) used a design in which subjects were given cutaneous pain via iontophoretic stimuli (see also Chapter 4). Subjects were surreptitiously given stimuli with reduced intensities in the presence of a placebo cream (the conditioning procedure) and were divided into two groups. The first did not know about the manipulation of the stimulus; the second group was informed about the experimental design and learned that the cream was inert. There was no placebo analgesic effect in this second group. This suggests that conscious expectation is necessary for placebo analgesia. This is a very important point because it suggests that expectation plays a major role, even in the presence of a conditioning procedure. In other words, expectation and conditioning are not mutually exclusive—they may represent two sides of the same coin (Stewart-Williams and Podd, 2004).

Early in the 1930s, Tolman (1932) dissented from the view that conditioning is an automatic nonconscious event, due to the temporal contiguity between the conditioned and the unconditioned stimulus. Indeed, in the 1960s, conditioning was reinterpreted in cognitive terms on the basis that conditioned learning does not depend simply on pairing of the conditioned and unconditioned stimuli (see Box 2.3), but on the information that is contained in the conditioned stimulus (Rescorla, 1988). In other words, conditioning would lead to the expectation that a given event will follow another event,

Box 2.3 The "blocking" experiment and the cognitive reinterpretation of conditioning

In 1968, Leon Kamin performed the following experiment (Kamin, 1968). Two groups of rats receive the same eight pairings of light (conditioned stimulus: CS) with an aversive electric shock (unconditioned stimulus: US). A second CS, a white noise, is presented simultaneously with the light. However, for one group, the noise is paired with shock in an earlier phase of the experiment; for the other, the noise has no pre-training (Table 2.4). It is important to note that both groups receive the exact same experience with the light and they differ only with the noise pre-training. The rats with no prior experience with the noise show near maximal conditioned response (fear) to the light, but those that had received noise–shock pairings earlier exhibit almost no conditioned fear response. Therefore, pre-training to the noise blocks conditioning to the light. The critical point here is that both groups experience identical temporal contiguity between the light and shock, yet conditioned responses to the light in the two groups are different. Thus, temporal contiguity between light and shock is not a sufficient requirement to elicit conditioned responses.

Box 2.3 The "blocking" experiment and the cognitive reinterpretation of conditioning (continued)

Table 2.4 Design of the blocking experiment

	Phase 1: pre-training	Phase 2: blocking	Phase 3: testing
Control group	No training	8 pairings of noise/light with shock	90% of maximum response to light
Blocking group	16 pairings of noise with shock	8 pairings of noise/light with shock	10% of maximum response to light

One possible explanation for this difference is that surprise plays a critical role in conditioning. Surprise can be defined as the difference between what one gets and what one expects to get. This finding provided the impetus for the development of a number of new cognitive conceptualizations of the conditioning process. This cognitive reinterpretation of conditioning can be conceptualized in the following way: what matters in the conditioning process is not so much the temporal contiguity between the CS and the US, but rather the information that the CS provides about the US. In other words, conditioning would lead to the expectation that a given event will follow another event.

and this occurs on the basis of the information that the conditioned stimulus provides about the unconditioned stimulus (Reiss, 1980; Rescorla, 1988; Kirsch et al., 2004).

Despite the reinterpretation of conditioning in cognitive terms, conditioning in humans is not always cognitively mediated, particularly when considering conditioned placebo responses (Stewart-Williams and Podd, 2004). For example, there is experimental evidence in humans that unconscious conditioned placebo responses are present in the immune and endocrine system (Chapter 7) and in the cardiovascular and respiratory system (Chapter 8). It has also been suggested that unconscious conditioning is important in placebo responses that involve unconscious physiological functions, whereas it is cognitively mediated when conscious processes come into play (Benedetti et al., 2003b). According to this model, expectation has no effect on unconscious processes (Fig. 2.12). It is also worth noting that even in placebo analgesia some noncognitive unconscious components may be present. For example, Amanzio and Benedetti (1999) showed that a placebo analgesic response is still present, albeit reduced, in the absence of expectation after prior conditioning, thus suggesting that a small portion of the placebo effect may occur unconsciously.

Indeed, Jensen et al. (2012) confirmed an important nonconscious component of placebo analgesia. They performed two experiments in which the responses to thermal pain stimuli were assessed. In the first experiment they assessed whether a conditioning paradigm, using clearly visible cues for high and low pain, could induce placebo and nocebo responses. In the second experiment they assessed in a separate group of subjects whether conditioned placebo and nocebo responses could be triggered in

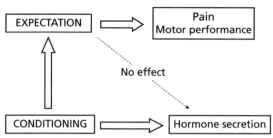

Fig. 2.12 Different action of expectation and conditioning on physiological functions. During a placebo procedure, conscious physiological processes like pain and motor performance are affected by verbally induced expectations, even though a conditioning procedure is performed. By contrast, unconscious physiological processes like hormone secretion are totally unaffected by expectations, but are influenced by placebos through unconscious conditioning mechanisms. Reproduced from Benedetti F, Pollo A, Lopiano L, Lanotte M, Vighetti S, and Rainero I, Conscious expectation and unconscious conditioning in analgesic, motor and hormonal placebo/nocebo responses, *Journal of Neuroscience*, 23 (10), pp. 4315–23, figure 7 Copyright 2003, The Society for Neuroscience.

response to nonconscious (masked) exposures to the same cues. Significant placebo and nocebo responses were found in both the first (using clearly visible stimuli) and second experiment (using nonconscious stimuli), indicating that the mechanisms responsible for placebo and nocebo effects can operate without conscious awareness of the triggering cues.

As pointed out many times (Ader, 1997; Siegel, 2002; Enck et al., 2008), many placebo effects can be explained in the context of conditioning theories. In fact, a placebo is by definition a neutral stimulus with no therapeutic effects, in the same way that a conditioned stimulus is by definition neutral. Likewise, a placebo response is by definition elicited by a neutral stimulus, in the same way that a conditioned response is induced by a neutral stimulus. The specific experimental settings and effects are described elsewhere in this book.

A central point in the conditioning mechanisms that underlie the placebo effect is represented by the nature of the unconditioned response (Siegel, 2002; see also section 7.3.1). There are, in fact, some examples of conditioned responses that do not go in the same direction as the unconditioned response. For example, the unconditioned response to insulin is hypoglycemia, while the conditioned response has also been hyperglycemia in some conditions (Siegel, 1972, 1975). Whenever the conditioned response is opposite to the unconditioned response, the unconditioned response must be defined correctly. In fact, administration of insulin produces hypoglycemia which is not, however, the unconditioned response, but rather the unconditioned stimulus that is detected by receptors in the central nervous system. The real unconditioned response is the compensatory hyperglycemia that the central nervous system adopts once the hypoglycemia has been detected. Thus, by defining the unconditioned response correctly, the apparent contrasting outcomes can be resolved.

An important point emphasized by Ader (1997) is that the typical studies of conditioning use an experimental approach whereby the unconditioned response is a response that goes outside the boundaries of normal homeostasis. For example, painful stimulation is usually adopted as an unconditioned stimulus in animals and healthy human volunteers, and pain is a typical situation outside normal homeostasis. A patient is usually in the opposite situation. In fact, the starting point of a patient in pain is outside homeostasis, and a placebo tends to restore the normal homeostatic condition, that is, no pain. This might be an important difference between the experimental setting and the real clinical situation.

Conditioning is not the only learning mechanism that might be involved in placebo phenomena. Social learning is another form of learning, where people learn from one another by observational learning and imitation. The placebo effect may involve social learning as well, as expectations of future positive or negative outcomes may have a major effect in social learning (Bootzin and Caspi, 2002).

Indeed, Colloca and Benedetti (2009) compared placebo analgesia induced through social observation (Group 1) with first-hand experience via a typical conditioning procedure (Group 2) and verbal suggestion alone (Group 3). In Group 1, subjects underwent painful stimuli and placebo treatment after they had observed a demonstrator showing analgesic effect when the painful stimuli were paired to a green light. In Group 2, subjects were conditioned according to the typical association between a green light and the surreptitious reduction of stimulus intensity, so as to make them believe that the treatment worked. In Group 3, subjects received painful stimuli and were verbally instructed to expect a benefit from a green light. It was found that observing the beneficial effects in the demonstrator induced substantial placebo analgesic responses, which were positively correlated with empathy scores. Moreover, observational social learning produced placebo responses that were similar to those induced by directly experiencing the benefit through the conditioning procedure, whereas verbal suggestions alone produced significantly smaller effects. Thus placebo analgesia is finely tuned by social observation, indicating that different forms of learning take part in the placebo phenomenon.

In two more recent studies, which were performed independently by two groups (Swider and Babel, 2013; Vögtle et al., 2013), observational social learning was also found to play a fundamental role in nocebo hyperalgesia, which can be interpreted as a true social contagion of negative emotions (Benedetti, 2013) (see section 4.2.2 for more details).

2.3.4 Some personality traits may be associated with placebo responsiveness

Although there are some inconsistencies in findings about the relationship between personality and placebo responsiveness (Geers et al., 2005b), some studies indicate that certain personality traits can predict placebo responsiveness. For example, De Pascalis et al. (2002) found that individual differences in suggestibility contribute significantly to the magnitude of placebo analgesia. The highest placebo effect was found in highly suggestible subjects who received suggestions that were presumed to elicit high expectations for drug efficacy. A specific relation between suggestibility, hypnotic susceptibility, and placebo analgesia has been described in other studies, which favor a possible shared mechanism in hypnosis and placebo response (Derbyshire and Oakley 2013; Huber et al., 2013).

Geers et al., (2005b) found that personality and situational variables interact to determine placebo responding. In this study, optimists and pessimists were randomly assigned to one of three groups. The first group was told they were to ingest a pill that would make them feel unpleasant (deceptive expectation); the second group was told they were to ingest either a real or an inactive pill (conditional expectation); the third was told they were to ingest an inactive pill (control). The pessimists were more likely than the optimists to follow a negative placebo (nocebo) expectation when given a deceptive expectation, but not when given a conditional expectation. This suggests that the personality variable "optimism–pessimism" relates to placebo responding when people are given a deceptive, but not a conditional, expectation. Thus, personality and situational variables seem to interact to determine placebo responding.

In a subsequent study, Geers et al. (2007) tested people who varied in their level of optimism. In the first condition, they were given the expectation that a placebo sleep treatment would improve their sleep quality. In the second condition, they underwent the same sleep treatment but were not given the positive placebo expectation. In the third condition, they received neither the positive placebo expectation nor underwent the placebo sleep treatment. Optimism was positively associated with better sleep quality in the first condition, suggesting that optimism relates to placebo responding. These data have been confirmed in another study by the same group (Geers et al., 2010), as well as by Morton et al. (2009), who found that both high dispositional optimism and low state anxiety are significant predictors of the placebo response.

Schweinhardt et al. (2009) examined the relationships between brain gray matter, placebo analgesic response, and personality traits associated with dopaminergic neurotransmission, which are usually related to more positive attitudes and higher sensitivity to incentives and rewards, that is, more desire to go after goals or rewards, such as food, sex, money, education, or professional achievements. These investigators reported that dopamine-related traits predict a substantial portion of the pain relief an individual gains from a sham treatment. Voxel-based morphometry of magnetic resonance images showed that the magnitude of placebo analgesia was related to gray matter density in several brain regions, including the ventral striatum, insula, and prefrontal cortex. Likewise, gray matter density in ventral striatum and prefrontal cortex was related to dopamine-related personality traits.

In a different study, Pecina et al. (2013) assessed psychological traits in healthy controls as to their capacity to predict placebo analgesic effects, placebo-induced activation of μ-opioid neurotransmission, and changes in cortisol plasma levels during an experimental pain challenge with and without placebo administration. The results showed that an aggregate of scores from Ego-Resiliency, Altruism, Straightforwardness (positive predictors), and Angry Hostility (negative predictor) scales accounted for 25% of the variance in placebo analgesic responses. The subjects scoring above the median in a composite of those trait measures also presented greater placebo-induced activation of μ-opioid neurotransmission in the subgenual and dorsal anterior cingulate cortex, orbitofrontal cortex, insula, nucleus accumbens, amygdala, and periaqueductal gray. Significant reductions in cortisol levels were observed during placebo administration and were positively correlated with decreases in pain ratings, μ-opioid system activation in the dorsal anterior cingulate cortex and periaqueductal gray, and as a trend, negatively with Angry Hostility scores. Therefore, personality traits explain a substantial proportion of the variance in placebo analgesic responses, and are associated with activations in endogenous opioid neurotransmission and, as a trend, with cortisol plasma levels.

2.3.5 Genetics may affect placebo responding

Substantial placebo responses have been found for some genetic variants but not for others, for example, in some psychiatric disorders (Rausch et al., 2002; Furmark et al., 2008). In one study (Furmark et al., 2008), patients with social anxiety disorder were genotyped with respect to the serotonin transporter-linked polymorphic region (5-HTTLPR) and the G-703T polymorphism in the tryptophan hydroxylase-2 (TPH2) gene promoter. It was found that only those patients who were homozygous for the long allele of the 5-HTTLPR or the G variant of the TPH2 G-703T polymorphism showed robust placebo responses and reduced activity in the amygdala, as assessed by functional magnetic resonance imaging. Conversely, carriers of short or T alleles did not show placebo responses.

In patients with major depressive disorder (Leuchter et al., 2009), polymorphisms in genes encoding the catabolic enzymes catechol-O-methyltransferase (COMT) and monoamine oxidase A were examined. Small placebo responses were found in those patients with monoamine oxidase A G/T polymorphisms (rs6323) coding for the highest activity form of the enzyme (G or G/G). Similarly, lower placebo responses were found in those patients with ValMet catechol-O-methyltransferase polymorphisms coding for a lower-activity form of the enzyme (2 Met alleles). In addition, the COMT functional val158met polymorphism was found to be associated to the placebo effect in irritable bowel syndrome. The strongest placebo response occurred in met/met homozygotes (Hall et al., 2012). Therefore, the role of genetic factors in placebo responding appears to be an important factor across a number of diseases, ranging from neuropsychiatric to gastrointestinal/psychosomatic disorders, and will be further discussed in the relative chapters. The study of single-nucleotide polymorphisms has been crucial in this regard (Box 2.4).

2.3.6 Other possible explanations have been proposed

Many new hypotheses, mechanisms, and models have been proposed over the past years, and these may account for different placebo responses across a variety of conditions. Whereas some of these proposals use a philosophical and anthropological perspective, others rely on a more neuroscientific approach. Albeit interesting, these hypotheses and theories need confirmation. Here, only a few of them are presented.

Medical anthropologists have proposed a constructionist view of the placebo experience which has at its core the concept of embodiment. According to this idea, the human mind is strongly influenced and shaped by aspects of the body, such as the

Box 2.4 Single-nucleotide polymorphisms

A single-nucleotide polymorphism (SNP) is a variation in the DNA sequence occurring when a single nucleotide—adenine (A), thymine (T), cytosine (C), or guanine (G)—differs between members of a biological species or paired chromosomes in a human. For example, two individuals may have the following two sequences in a fragment of DNA:

CATC<u>G</u>AA   CATC<u>T</u>AA

These are different only for a single nucleotide (underlined). The study of SNPs is useful to understand the relationship between different genetic variants and different physiological functions and behaviors. In fact, the difference even of a single nucleotide can produce the substitution of one amino acid with another in the sequence of a protein, with the subsequent change of the protein function. For example, the μ-opioid receptor may show the following polymorphisms:

A118G   C17T

which correspond to a substitution of adenine (A) with guanine (G) in position 118 and of cytosine (C) with thymine (T) in position 17, respectively, of the DNA sequence. These changes in the DNA sequence lead to the following changes in the amino acid sequence in the mu opioid receptor:

A118G → Asn40Asp (N40D)   C17T → Ala6Val (A6V)

which correspond to a substitution of asparagine (Asn) with aspartic acid (Asp) in position 40 and of alanine (Ala) with valine (Val) in position 6, respectively, of the μ-opioid receptor.

The effects of these substitutions may be important in a number of conditions, from the action of the μ-opioid receptor across different physiological functions to the binding affinity of different opioid agonists such as morphine. For example, the polymorphism A118G shows higher binding affinity for endogenous ligands such as β-endorphin, and this genetic variation may account for different analgesic responses across different individuals (Bond et al., 1998). The study of SNPs has been useful to investigate the role of genetic factors in the placebo response in different medical conditions, like social anxiety, depression, and irritable bowel syndrome.

sensory systems and interactions between the environment and the society. Thus, our experiences can not only be consciously stored as memories, but also imprinted straight onto our body, without involvement of any cognitive process. An example of how sociocultural experiences and processes can impact on the individual's physiology is offered by studies of trauma or stress, as in post-traumatic stress disorder (PTSD), where symptoms like frightening thoughts or sleep disorders are the result of an implicit perception, the literal "incorporation" of a terrifying event from the external world, which has bypassed conscious awareness. According to this theory, the placebo effect is a positive effect of embodiment and the nocebo effect a negative one. Lived positive experiences can be channeled into objects or places, which then acquire the potential to trigger healing responses. Importantly, this process needs not involve conscious expectation or conscious attribution of symbolic meaning to the object or place (Thompson et al., 2009). When a symbolic meaning is indeed attributed to an object or place, we enter the domain of the performative efficacy theory. Therapeutic performances may have per se a convincing, persuading effect. A change in the body or mind can be achieved just by the *ritual* of the therapeutic act. The performance inducing a placebo effect may be social, as in sham surgery in clinical trials producing positive outcomes in the placebo arm, or in the case of a mother's kiss on a child wound; or it may be internal, as for athletes mentally rehearsing before a competition. In this framework, a placebo effect could result from the internal act of imagining a specific change of state of the body. Central to the performative efficacy of the ritual is the patient–provider relationship, with factors such as empathy, prestige of the healer, gesture, and recitation all contributing to the treatment success (Thompson et al., 2009).

A different perspective is considered by Kradin (2011), who argues that the placebo response is a developmental achievement, rooted in implicit procedural memories that are linked to background affects of well-being evoked by the relation with a caregiver. He goes further, suggesting that the placebo response represents a brain response aimed at countering the dysphoric effects attributable to chronic stress, and that it is dependent on developmental attachment dynamics.

With a more neuroscientific approach, Koban et al. (2012) recorded event-related potentials to response errors in a go/no-go task during placebo versus a matched control condition. Error commission was associated with two well-described components, the error-related negativity and the error positivity. These investigators found that the error positivity, but not the error-related negativity, was amplified during placebo analgesia compared to the control condition, with neural sources in the lateral and medial prefrontal cortex. This increase in error positivity was driven by participants showing a placebo-induced change in pain tolerance, but was absent in nonresponders. These results suggest a possible new functional mechanisms underlying placebo analgesia, that is a placebo-induced transient change in prefrontal error monitoring and control functions.

In a more recent study, placebo analgesia has been found to be enhanced by oxytocin, a hormone known to be involved in empathy, trust, and social learning. Subjects who received intranasal administration of oxytocin showed larger placebo analgesic responses compared to controls, suggesting an important role of prosocial behavior in the placebo effect and the possibility to exploit this effect in clinical practice (Kessner et al., 2013).

2.3.7 **Placebo effects are also present in animals**

If an injection of saline solution is performed in a rat that had previously received an injection of scopolamine, the saline solution can mimic the motor changes produced by scopolamine (Herrnstein, 1962). As discussed in other sections (e.g., section 2.3.3) and chapters (e.g., Chapter 4), the underlying mechanism is likely to be classical, or Pavlovian, conditioning, although the original interpretation of conditioning has been reframed in cognitive terms (section 2.3.3 and Box 2.3).

Indeed, one of the most common questions arising among neuroscientists and clinician scientists is whether placebo responses are also present in animals. Some investigations of the effects of placebos in animals have been started, such as pharmacological conditioning and blockade with specific antagonists of opioid receptors (Bryant et al., 2009; Guo et al., 2010; Zhang et al., 2013). Not surprisingly, as most of our knowledge about the biological mechanisms of the placebo response comes from the study of placebo analgesia, these studies in animals have been carried out in the field of pain and analgesia, and a more detailed account will be given in Chapter 4.

What is emerging today is that animal models might represent an interesting approach to understand some mechanisms of different placebo effects, including the identification of some biochemical pathways that are more difficult to study in humans. For example, Nolan et al. (2012) used an elegant model of operant conditioning with an affective behavioral endpoint. The authors used a conflict–reward assay, in which rodents express their willingness to withstand thermal pain to obtain a sweet reward. This paradigm tests mild noninjurious pain and, unlike other models, such as the hot plate, it is likely to incorporate cognitive and affective components of pain, which often represent the most common and debilitating aspects of chronic pain sufferers. In this model, a reward bottle with sweetened milk was positioned such that access to the milk reward was possible, but access was contingent on facial contact with a thermode. The rats were conditioned by pairing thermal pain with a subcutaneous injection of morphine. After two conditioning trials, morphine was replaced with saline solution, and then the analgesic response was tested by assessing the ratio of successful licks to lick attempts. Placebo analgesic responses resembled in all respects those in humans. First, as in humans, there was strong interindividual variability in the response, which allows subdivision into responders and nonresponders. Second, there was a positive relationship between the unconditioned analgesic effect by morphine and the conditioned effect by the placebo, which may reflect individual differences in morphine efficacy or in learning capabilities, as also found in humans (Amanzio and Benedetti, 1999). Third, the conditioned placebo response was suppressed by the opioid antagonist naloxone, thus showing that this response is mediated by endogenous opioids, as described in detail in Chapter 4. Fourth, in the study by Nolan et al. (2012), no real conditioned stimuli, such as lights or sounds, were presented, as is usually done in conditioning paradigms in animals. In other words, the mere act of performing an injection is enough to induce conditioned placebo responses. This is an important point, as it resembles a real clinical situation in humans, whereby the whole context around the patient and the therapeutic act itself represent the conditioned stimuli (Benedetti, 2012).

Although a cognitive component may be present also in animals, expectations are likely to play a minor role in animals compared to humans. It follows that an animal model of placebo analgesia is likely not to be appropriate to investigate the involvement of higher brain functions in placebo responsiveness. Nonetheless, the investigation of placebo responses in animals represents a window into the brain mechanisms of pain modulation as well as into some of the unsolved questions that arise in clinical trials, such as pharmacological conditioning in crossover designs.

2.3.8 What is the difference between placebo responders and nonresponders?

In light of the mechanisms reviewed in previous sections, it appears that placebo responsiveness may depend on many factors, and on the mechanisms involved in a given type of placebo effect (e.g., learning and reward). It should be emphasized once again, therefore, that there is not a single placebo effect but many, so there also are many reasons why some people respond to placebos while others do not. Learning is certainly an important factor, as people who have had prior positive therapeutic experiences show larger placebo responses than those who have not (Fig. 2.11). In a study by Colloca and Benedetti (2006), small, medium, and large placebo responses were observed, depending on several factors like their previous positive or negative experiences of analgesic treatment and the time lag between treatment and the placebo responses, further indicating that placebo analgesia is finely tuned by prior experience (see Fig. 4.2C).

Another important determinant of placebo responsiveness may be individual differences in the efficiency of the neural mechanisms of reward. In fact, a correlation between expectation of reward and dopamine activation in the nucleus accumbens has been found in people with Parkinson's disease (de la Fuente-Fernandez et al., 2001, 2002). In another imaging study that used both positron emission tomography and functional magnetic resonance, Scott et al. (2007) tested the correlation between responsiveness to placebo and responsiveness to monetary reward. They found that responsiveness to placebo was related to activation of dopamine in the nucleus accumbens. In addition, these subjects were then tested for monetary responses in the nucleus accumbens. A correlation between placebo and monetary responses was found, thus suggesting that the efficiency of the nucleus accumbens reward system may play a role in placebo responsiveness (see section 4.1.8).

Another approach to understanding the differences between placebo responders and nonresponders is to analyze the biological changes occurring in the brain and/or body following placebo administration. However, these phenomenological findings fail to unravel exactly what determines such differences in responsiveness. For example, Lipman et al. (1990) found an increase in plasma endorphins in patients with low back pain who responded to a placebo treatment, but patients who did not respond showed no changes in plasma endorphins. Similarly, Petrovic et al. (2002) found that the anterior cingulate cortex was activated in placebo responders but not in nonresponders. Benedetti et al. (2004) observed changes in the firing pattern of neurons in the subthalamic nucleus in placebo responders, but not in nonresponders (see also Chapters 4 and 5). As discussed earlier, although these differences in biochemical and brain responses show that some biological responses to placebos are different in responders and nonresponders, they give little information about the determinants of these differences.

As discussed in section 2.3.5, different genetic variants may account for the differences between placebo responders and nonresponders, for example, in social anxiety (Furmark et al., 2008), depression (Leuchter et al., 2009), and irritable bowel syndrome (Hall et al., 2012). In light of the numerous neurotransmitters that are involved in placebo and nocebo responsiveness, this is not surprising. The main challenge of future research will be to broaden our knowledge on the genetic determinants of different placebo effects, in order to better understand good and poor responsiveness to placebos across different individuals.

2.4 **Why they occur**

2.4.1 **Expectation-mediated placebo effects may be related to other self-regulatory processes**

By considering other self-regulatory processes, the brain regions engaged by placebos that involve manipulation of expectations may be part of a general circuit underlying the voluntary regulation of affective–emotional responses. A summary of data obtained from 15 studies on the placebo effect, regulation of emotions, and activation by opioid drugs is shown in Fig. 2.13. The superposition of peak coordinates of increased activation in each of these conditions reveals that several frontal areas are consistently engaged during different tasks in which negative affect must be suppressed. On the lateral surface, these regions include the dorsolateral and ventrolateral prefrontal cortex, and the rostral prefrontal cortex. On the medial surface, the midstral dorsal anterior cingulate and the neighboring superior medial prefrontal cortex are involved. On the orbital surface, the peaks of increased activation are located around the medial orbital sulcus bilaterally. All these regions, with the notable exception of the orbitofrontal cortex and right ventrolateral prefrontal cortex, have been found to be activated following administration of an opioid analgesic (Firestone et al., 1996; Adler et al., 1997; Wagner et al., 2001; Petrovic et al., 2002). Both the dorsal and ventral prefrontal cortex have also been shown to be consistently activated in the voluntary positive reinterpretation of the meaning of aversive visual stimuli (Ochsner et al., 2002, 2004; Levesque et al., 2003; Phan et al., 2005) and correlated with reduced activation of the amygdala (Lieberman et al., 2005) and anxiety (Bishop et al., 2004).

In a study of placebo modulation of affective responses to pictures, Petrovic et al. (2005) found placebo-induced activity in both the dorsolateral and ventrolateral prefrontal cortex and the midstral cingulate. Both increased activation in these regions and placebo-induced decreases in the amygdala were correlated with larger placebo effects in reported emotion. Interestingly, Rainville et al. (1997) found that the same region of the cingulate cortex was modulated by hypnotic analgesia. It is important to point out that these different varieties of self-regulation have not been tested in the same study. Nonetheless, the co-localization shown in Fig. 2.13 suggests there may be a general system for self-regulation that applies to both emotions and pain, as well as both voluntary strategies and the externally generated appraisals that produce placebo effects.

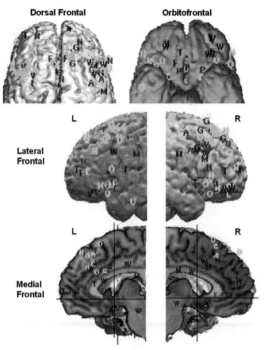

Fig. 2.13 Regions of the frontal lobes showing increased activity in recent studies of self-regulation. Increases are shown for delivery of opiate analgesics compared with resting nondrug control states (blue letters), downregulation of aversive emotional experience (green letters) through emotional reappraisal, and placebo effects on pain or emotional processing (red letters). Some peaks reflect regions for which increases in activity are correlated with reductions in negative emotional experience or pain. One exception is the study by Bishop et al. (2004) in which frontal activation was correlated with a reduced state of anxiety. Peak locations from the same study within 12 mm were averaged together for clarity of presentation. Reproduced from Fabrizio Benedetti, Helen S. Mayberg, Tor D. Wager, Christian S. Stohler, and Jon-Kar Zubieta, Neurobiological mechanisms of the placebo effect, *Journal of Neuroscience*, 25 (45), pp. 10390–402 Copyright 2005, The Society for Neuroscience. (See Plate 1.)

Studies on opioid increases:

F—Firestone et al. 1996
A—Adler et al. 1997
N—Wagner et al. 2001
P—Petrovic and Ingvar 2002

Studies on placebo:

W—Wager et al. 2004b (anticipation)
G—Wager et al. 2004b (pain)
I—Lieberman et al. 2004
V—Petrovic et al. 2002
T—Petrovic et al. 2005
M—Mayberg et al. 2002

Studies on emotion regulation:

L—Levesque et al. 2003
C—Ochsner et al. 2002
O—Ochsner et al. 2004
H—Phan et al. 2005
B—Bishop et al. 2004

Taking all these factors into account, one possibility is that placebo and placebo-related effects, in which expectations are involved, are driven by executive control. For example, the dorsal and ventral prefrontal cortex is activated by a large class of cognitively demanding conditions. Distraction from pain also produces activation in these regions (Petrovic and Ingvar, 2002) and working memory and executive attention have also revealed similar activation patterns (Wager and Smith, 2003; Wager et al., 2004a). Another possibility is that this neural network subserves the process of meaning generation and appraisal of current and predicted events (Lazarus, 1991). Effective placebo treatment may engender and active re-evaluation of the significance of pain, which engages both the orbitofrontal cortex and the lateral prefrontal systems in generation and maintenance of short-term context that biases ongoing nociceptive and affective processing (Miller and Cohen, 2001).

The executive functions of the prefrontal areas may generate these self-regulatory processes, including expectation-related placebo effects; this is supported by the disruption of placebo-like responses in people with Alzheimer's disease, who show impairment of their prefrontal executive control (as assessed by the Frontal Assessment Battery) and functional disconnection of their prefrontal lobes (as assessed by electroencephalographic connectivity analysis) (Benedetti et al., 2006) (see section 4.1.10 and 6.3.2). Therefore, placebo and placebo-like effects that involve expectation mechanisms may be phenomena that emerge from the ability of the prefrontal self-regulatory network to suppress negative emotions.

2.4.2 Are placebo and placebo-related effects a product of evolution?

There are many endogenous defense mechanisms in the body, ranging from cellular immune responses and antibody production to wound healing and nerve regeneration. One of the crucial issues for understanding why placebo and placebo-related effects exist at all is whether they represent a sort of endogenous healthcare system that has emerged in humans during evolution. As explained earlier, there is not a single placebo effect, but many. For example, when the placebo is a neutral stimulus that is repeatedly associated with an unconditioned stimulus, the conditioned placebo response must be viewed in the context of conditioning mechanisms. In this case, associations between stimuli (conditioned and unconditioned) occur in the clinical setting, but the meaning is the same as in other contexts—that is, learning to anticipate an event.

When placebo and placebo-related effects are related to expectations, the role of cognition in social interaction plays a key role. It has been suggested, for example, that the facial expression of pain evolved for eliciting medical attention from others (Williams, 2002). In this respect, as suggested by Evans (2002), it is important to know when medical care first emerged, when special care to a sick individual was provided for the first time. Evans (2002) suggests that "medicine" must have originated some time between 5,000,000 and 10,000 years ago (a huge span of time). In fact, the remains of skulls that have undergone complex surgery have been found, dating back more than 7000 years, which suggests sophisticated forms of medical care had evolved at that time. Maybe the first provision of special care to the sick dates back to the very early hominids, the

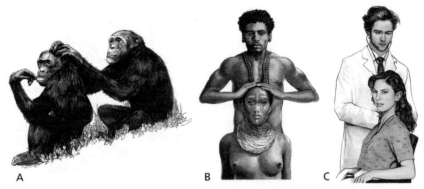

Fig. 2.14 During the course of evolution, social interactions may have evolved from grooming in nonhuman primates or early hominids (A), to shamanism in primitive societies (B), to modern doctors (C). The act of taking care of somebody in the social group may have been very important in the emergence of placebo and placebo-related effects. As soon as the act of giving special care to a sick individual emerged (what we call medical care today), those who trusted a member of their social group (whether a chimpanzee, shaman, or doctor) were likely to have greater advantages than those who did not.

Australopithecus or *Homo habilis*. Indeed, nonhuman primates demonstrate forms of social interactions that resemble medical care, such as grooming and picking ticks off each other's backs (Fig. 2.14).

Reasoning in this way, health management may have evolved in a social context among different groups of hominids. The acts of caring and curing must have become a powerful social stimulus that induced beliefs, trust, hope, and expectations of recovery. If one member of a social group trusts just one other member of that group, he or she may have an improved quality of life and may survive longer. In primitive societies, this trusted group member was the "shaman," but in our modern human society this is a "doctor" (Fig. 2.14). Therefore, individuals who trust a member of their social group, whether a chimpanzee, shaman, or doctor, are better placed than those who do not. Expectation-related placebo effects may be part of the evolution of these complex social interactions (Humphrey, 2002). To become activated, these placebo responses require social contact with the person who is trusted. While the placebo effects require the act of curing (the placebo), the placebo-like effects occur without any act of curing, but simply with the human interaction, both verbal and nonverbal forms.

Interestingly, Wall (1999) claimed that pain is a "need" state, which can be terminated by specific consummatory acts like hunger and thirst. According to Wall (1999) the consummatory acts that terminate pain can be, for instance, either withdrawing one's hand from a noxious stimulus or care and attention from others (the act of caring and the placebo). It is this purely social event that represents the evolutionary novelty in humans (Evans, 2002). A person whose brain is capable of shutting down pain when the presence of medical help is detected may have an advantage over someone whose brain lacks this capacity (Evans, 2003). In Chapter 4, we will see that specific endogenous mechanisms are activated by this social act, resulting in suppressed pain transmission.

The conceptualization of the placebo effect as a product of evolution can be better understood if considered within the context of the doctor–patient relationship. In the next chapter (Chapter 3), the interaction between the healer and the sick is considered as a special and unique social encounter that has emerged during evolution. On the one hand, the patient seeks relief from his own discomfort, such as pain. On the other, the healer activates a compassionate behavior that is aimed at relieving suffering. In this sense, the placebo effect can be seen as the final act of a complex and intricate social interaction which represents today an excellent model to investigate several issues belonging to the domain of social neuroscience.

2.5 **Points for further discussion**

1 We need to know where, when, and how placebo effects work. In particular, it is crucial to understand whether some mechanisms, such as reward and learning, are common in different conditions.

2 We know that conditioning is important in unconscious physiological functions like immune responses and hormone secretion. However, according to modern theories of learning, cognitive factors are essential for classical conditioning. It would be interesting to address this issue, particularly within the context of the broader literature on conditioning. Beyond the placebo effect, a key question is: Does unconscious conditioning exist in humans?

3 Although it is clear that prior experience plays a role in many placebo effects, we need to know how this occurs. For example, what kind of learning is involved in different conditions? Unconscious Pavlovian conditioning, or reinforced expectations, or social learning through observation?

4 Is it possible to increase the magnitude and duration of placebo responses through learning, so as to maximize them in the clinical setting and minimize them in clinical trials?

5 Placebo-related effects may need to be extended further to include a variety of psychosocial factors. Harrington (2002) tried to compare placebo effects with a broad range of phenomena, for example, the influence of hospital rooms on recovery, or the influence of cultural and religious beliefs on mortality.

6 Today we know that placebo responders and nonresponders may differ in terms of either previous experience (learning), or efficiency of reward mechanisms, or genetic variations. It is necessary to further investigate these factors, for example, the different genetic polymorphisms across different individuals.

7 A further challenge is to determine whether socially activated placebo mechanisms emerged during evolution as a defense system of the body (in the same way as the immune system and wound healing evolved). Are placebo and placebo-like effects related to trust, beliefs, and hope that emerged in social groups?

References

Ader R (1997). The role of conditioning in pharmacotherapy. In A Harrington, ed. *The placebo effect: an interdisciplinary exploration*, pp. 138–65. Harvard University Press, Cambridge, MA.

Ader R (2001). Much ado about nothing. *Advances in Mind-Body Medicine*, 17, 293–5.

Adler LJ, Gyulai FE, Diehl DJ, Mintun MA, Winter PM and Firestone LL (1997). Regional brain activity changes associated with fentanyl analgesia elucidated by positron emission tomography. *Anesthesiology and Analgesia*, 84, 120–6.

Allan LG and Siegel S (2002). A signal detection theory analysis of the placebo effect. *Evaluation & the Health Professions*, 25, 410–20.

Amanzio M and Benedetti F (1999). Neuropharmacological dissection of placebo analgesia: expectation-activated opioid systems versus conditioning-activated specific subsystems. *Journal of Neuroscience*, 19, 484–94.

Amanzio M, Pollo A, Maggi G and Benedetti F (2001). Response variability to analgesics: a role for non-specific activation of endogenous opioids. *Pain*, 90, 205–15.

André-Obadia N, Magnin M and Garcia-Larrea L (2011). On the importance of placebo timing in rTMS studies for pain relief. *Pain*, 152, 1233–7.

Atlas LY and Wager TD (2012). How expectations shape pain. *Neuroscience Letters*, 520, 140–8.

Balint M (1955). The doctor, his patient, and the illness. *Lancet*, 1, 683–8.

Bandura A (1977). Self-efficacy: toward a unifying theory of behavior change. *Psychological Review*, 84, 191–215.

Bandura A (1997). *Self-efficacy: the exercise of control*. Cambridge University Press, New York.

Batterman RC (1966). Persistence of responsiveness with placebo therapy following an effective drug trial. *Journal of New Drugs*, 6, 137–41.

Batterman RC and Lower WR (1968). Placebo responsiveness—influence of previous therapy. *Current Therapeutic Research*, 10, 136–43.

Bausell RB, Lao L, Bergman S, Lee WL and Berman BM (2005). Is acupuncture analgesia an expectancy effect? Preliminary evidence based on participants' perceived assignments in two placebo-controlled trials. *Evaluation & Health Professions*, 28, 9–26

Beecher HK (1955). The powerful placebo. *Journal of the American Medical Association*, 159, 1602–6.

Benedetti F (1996). The opposite effects of the opiate antagonist naloxone and the cholecystokinin antagonist proglumide on placebo analgesia. *Pain*, 64, 535–43.

Benedetti F (2002). How the doctor' s words affect the patient' s brain. *Evaluation & Health Professions*, 25, 369–86.

Benedetti F (2005). The importance of considering the effects of perceived group assignment in placebo-controlled trials. *Evaluation & Health Professions*, 28, 5–6.

Benedetti F (2007). What do you expect from this treatment? Changing our mind about clinical trials. *Pain*, 128, 193–4.

Benedetti F (2008). Mechanisms of placebo and placebo-related effects across diseases and treatments. *Annual Review of Pharmacology and Toxicology*, 48, 33–60.

Benedetti F (2012). Placebo responses in animals. *Pain*, 153, 1983–4.

Benedetti F (2013). Responding to nocebos through observation: social contagion of negative emotions. *Pain*, 154, 1165.

Benedetti F, Arduino C, Costa S et al. (2006). Loss of expectation-related mechanisms in Alzheimer's disease makes analgesic therapies less effective. *Pain*, 121, 133–44.

Benedetti F, Carlino E and Pollo A (2011). Hidden administration of drugs. *Clinical Pharmacology and Therapeutics*, **90**, 651–61.

Benedetti F and Colloca L (2004). Placebo-induced analgesia: methodology, neurobiology, clinical use, and ethics. *Reviews in Analgesia*, **7**, 129–43.

Benedetti F, Colloca L, Torre E *et al.* (2004). Placebo-responsive Parkinson patients show decreased activity in single neurons of subthalamic nucleus. *Nature Neuroscience*, **7**, 587–8.

Benedetti F, Maggi G, Lopiano L *et al.* (2003a). Open versus hidden medical treatments: the patient's knowledge about a therapy affects the therapy outcome. *Prevention & Treatment*, **6**(1).

Benedetti F, Mayberg HS, Wager TD, Stohler CS, and Zubieta J-K (2005). Neurobiological mechanisms of the placebo effect. *Journal of Neuroscience*, **25**(45), 10390–402.

Benedetti F, Pollo A, Lopiano L, Lanotte M, Vighetti S and Rainero I (2003b). Conscious expectation and unconscious conditioning in analgesic, motor and hormonal placebo/nocebo responses. *Journal of Neuroscience*, **23**, 4315–23.

Bishop S, Duncan J, Brett M and Lawrence AD (2004). Prefrontal cortical function and anxiety: controlling attention to threat-related stimuli. *Nature Neuroscience*, **7**, 184–8.

Bond C, LaForge KS, Tian M *et al.* (1998). Single-nucleotide polymorphism in the human mu opioid receptor gene alters mu-endorphin binding and activity: possible implications for opiate addiction. *Proceedings of the National Academy of Science of the United States of America*, **95**, 9608–13.

Bootzin RR (1985). The role of expectancy in behavior change. In L White, B Tursky and GE Schwartz, eds. *Placebo: theory, research, and mechanisms*, pp. 196–210. Guilford Press, New York.

Bootzin RR and Caspi O (2002). Explanatory mechanisms for placebo effects: cognition, personality and social learning. In HA Guess, A Kleinman, JW Kusek and LW Engel, eds. *The science of the placebo: toward an interdisciplinary research agenda*, pp. 108–32. British Medical Journal Books, London.

Branthwaite A and Cooper P (1981). Analgesic effects of branding in treatment of headaches. *British Medical Journal*, **282**, 1576–8.

Brody H (2000). *The placebo response.* Harper-Collins, New York.

Brody H and Weismantel D (2001). A challenge to core beliefs. *Advances in Mind-Body Medicine*, **17**, 296–8.

Bryant CD, Roberts KW, Culbertson CS, Le A, Evans CJ and Fanselow MS (2009). Pavlovian conditioning of multiple opioid-like responses in mice. *Drug and Alcohol Dependence*, **103**, 74–83.

Caspi O and Bootzin RR (2002). Evaluating how placebos produce change. *Evaluation & the Health Professions*, **25**, 436–64.

Clark WC (1969). Sensory-decision theory analysis of the placebo effect on the criterion for pain and thermal sensitivity. *Journal of Abnormal Psychology*, **74**, 363–71.

Colloca L and Benedetti F (2005). Placebos and painkillers: is mind as real as matter? *Nature Reviews Neuroscience*, **6**, 545–52.

Colloca L and Benedetti F (2006). How prior experience shapes placebo analgesia. *Pain*, **124**, 126–33.

Colloca L and Benedetti F (2009). Placebo analgesia induced by social observational learning. *Pain*, **144**, 28–34.

Colloca L, Finniss DG and Benedetti F (2008). Placebo and nocebo. In A Rice, R Howard, D Justins, C Miaskowski, and T Newton-John, eds. *Textbook of Clinical Pain Management*, pp. 499–513. Hodder Arnold, London.

Colloca L, Lopiano L, Lanotte M and Benedetti F (2004). Overt versus covert treatment for pain, anxiety, and Parkinson's disease. *Lancet Neurology*, **3**, 679–84.

Colloca L and Miller FG (2011). Role of expectations in health. *Current Opinion in Psychiatry*, **24**, 149–55.

Davis CE (2002). Regression to the mean or placebo effect? In HA Guess, A Kleinman, JW Kusek and LW Engel, eds. *The science of the placebo: toward an interdisciplinary research agenda*, pp. 158–66. British Medical Journal Books, London.

De Jong PJ, van Baast R, Arntz A and Merkelbach H (1996). The placebo effect in pain reduction: the influence of conditioning experiences and response expectancies. *International Journal of Behavioral Medicine*, **3**, 14–29.

de la Fuente-Fernández R (2009). The placebo-reward hypothesis: dopamine and the placebo effect. *Parkinsonism and Related Disorders*, **15**(Suppl 3), S72–4.

de la Fuente-Fernandez R, Phillips AG, Zamburlini *et al.* (2002). Dopamine release in human ventral striatum and expectation of reward. *Behavioral Brain Research*, **136**, 359–63.

de la Fuente-Fernandez R, Ruth TJ, Sossi V, Schulzer M, Calne DB and Stoessl AJ (2001). Expectation and dopamine release: mechanism of the placebo effect in Parkinson's disease. *Science*, **293**, 1164–6.

De Pascalis V, Chiaradia C and Carotenuto E (2002). The contribution of suggestibility and expectation to placebo analgesia phenomenon in an experimental setting. *Pain*, **96**, 393–402.

Derbyshire SW and Oakley DA (2013). A role for suggestion in differences in brain responses after placebo conditioning in high and low hypnotizable subjects. *Pain*, **154**, 1487–8.

Di Blasi Z, Harkness E, Ernst E, Georgiou A and Kleijnen J (2001). Influence of context effect on health outcomes: a systematic review. *Lancet*, **357**, 757–62.

Diehl HS (1953). Medicinal treatment of the common cold. *Journal of the American Medical Association*, **101**, 2042–9.

DiNubile MJ (2001). Is the placebo powerless? *New England Journal of Medicine*, **345**, 1278.

Eccles R (2006). Mechanisms of the placebo effect of sweet cough syrups. *Respiratory Physiology & Neurobiology*, **152**, 340–8.

Einarson TE, Helmes M and Stolk P (2001). Is the placebo powerless? *New England Journal of Medicine*, **345**, 1277.

Enck P, Benedetti F and Schedlowski M (2008). New insights into the placebo and nocebo responses. *Neuron*, **59**, 195–206.

Evans FJ (1977). The placebo control of pain: a paradigm for investigating non-specific effects in psychotherapy. In JP Brady, J Mendels, WR Reiger and MT Orne, eds. *Psychiatry: areas of promise and advancement*, pp. 249–71. Plenum Press, New York.

Evans D (2002). Pain, evolution, and the placebo response. *Behavioral and Brain Sciences*, **25**, 459–60.

Evans D (2003). *Placebo: the belief effect*. Harper Collins, London.

Faasse K, Cundy T, Gamble G and Petrie KJ (2013). The effect of an apparent change to a branded or generic medication on drug effectiveness and side effects. *Psychosomatic Medicine*, **75**, 90–6.

Feather BW, Chapman CR and Fisher SB (1972). The effect of a placebo on the perception of painful radiant heat stimuli. *Psychosomatic Medicine*, **34**, 290–4.

Fields HL and Levine JD (1984). Placebo analgesia—a role for endorphins? *Trends in Neuroscience*, **7**, 271–3.

Firestone L, Gyulai F, Mintun M, Adler L, Urso K and Winter P (1996). Human brain activity response to fentanyl imaged by positron emission tomography. *Anesthesia and Analgesia*, **82**, 1247–51.

Frank JD (1961). *Persuasion and healing: a comparative study of psychotherapy*. Schocken Books, New York (rev. ed.: Johns Hopkins University Press, Baltimore, MD, 1973).

Frank JD (1971). Therapeutic factors in psychotherapy. *American Journal of Psychotherapy*, **25**, 350–61.

Frank JD (1981). Therapeutic components shared by all psychotherapies. In JH Hawey and MM Parks, eds. *Psychotherapy research and behavior change*, pp. 9–37. American Psychological Association, Washington, DC.

Furmark T, Appel L, Henningsson S *et al.* (2008) A link between serotonin-related gene polymorphisms, amygdala activity, and placebo-induced relief from social anxiety *Journal of Neuroscience*, **28**, 13066–74.

Geers AL, Helfer SG, Kosbab K, Weiland PE and Landry SJ (2005b). Reconsidering the role of personality in placebo effects: dispositional optimism, situational expectations, and the placebo response. *Journal of Psychosomatic Research*, **58**, 121–7.

Geers AL, Kosbab K, Helfer SG, Weiland PE and Wellman JA (2007). Further evidence for individual differences in placebo responding: an interactionist perspective. *Journal of Psychosomatic Research*, **62**, 563–70.

Geers AL, Weiland PE, Kosbab K, Landry SJ and Helfer SG (2005a). Goal activation, expectations, and the placebo effect. *Journal of Personality and Social Psychology*, **89**, 143–59.

Geers AL, Wellman JA, Fowler SL, Helfer SG and France CR (2010). Dispositional optimism predicts placebo analgesia. *Journal of Pain*, **11**, 1165–71.

Geers AL, Wellman JA, Fowler SL, Rasinski HM and Helfer SG (2011). Placebo expectations and the detection of somatic information. *Journal of Behavioral Medicine*, **34**, 208–17.

Gracely RH, Dubner R, Deeter WD and Wolskee PJ (1985). Clinicians' expectations influence placebo analgesia. *Lancet*, **1**, 43.

Greene PJ, Wayne PM, Kerr CE *et al.* (2001). The powerful placebo: doubting the doubters. *Advances in Mind-Body Medicine*, **17**, 298–307.

Guo JY, Wang JY and Luo F (2010). Dissection of placebo analgesia in mice: the conditions for activation of opioid and non-opioid systems. *Journal of Psychopharmacology*, **24**, 1561–7.

Hahn RA (1985). A sociocultural model of illness and healing. In L White, B Tursky, and GE Schwartz, eds. *Placebo: theory, research, and mechanisms*, pp. 167–95. Guilford, New York.

Hahn RA (1997). The nocebo phenomenon: concept, evidence, and implications for public health. *Preventive Medicine*, **26**, 607–11.

Hall KT, Lembo AJ, Kirsch I *et al.* (2012) Catechol-O-methyltransferase val158met polymorphism predicts placebo effect in irritable bowel syndrome. *PLoS One*, 7, e48135.

Harrington A (2002). "Seeing" the placebo effect: historical legacies and present opportunities. In HA Guess, A Kleinman, JW Kusek, and LW Engel, eds. *The science of the placebo: toward an interdisciplinary research agenda*, pp. 35–52. British Medical Journal Books, London.

Herrnstein RJ (1962). Placebo effect in the rat. *Science*, **138**, 677–8.

Howick J, Friedemann C, Tsakok M, *et al.* (2013). Are treatments more effective than placebos? A systematic review and meta-analysis. *PLoS One*, **8**, e62599.

Hrobjartsson A and Goetzsche PC (2004). Is the placebo powerless? Update of a systematic review with 52 new randomized trials comparing placebo with no treatment. *Journal of Internal Medicine*, **256**, 91–100.

Hrobjartsson A and Goetzsche PC (2006). Unsubstantiated claims of large effects of placebo on pain. Serious errors in meta-analysis of placebo analgesia mechanism studies. *Journal of Clinical Epidemiology*, **59**, 336–8.

Hrobjartsson A and Goetzsche PC (2007). Powerful spin in the conclusion of Wampold et al.'s re-analysis of placebo versus no-treatment trials despite similar results as in original review. *Journal of Clinical Psychology*, **63**, 373–7.

Hróbjartsson A and Goetzsche PC (2010). Placebo interventions for all clinical conditions. *Cochrane Database of Systematic Reviews*, **1**, CD003974.

Hróbjartsson A and Gøtzsche PC (2001). Is the placebo powerless? An analysis of clinical trials comparing placebo with no treatment. *New England Journal of Medicine*, **344**, 1594–602.

Huber A, Lui F and Porro CA (2013). Hypnotic susceptibility modulates brain activity related to experimental placebo analgesia. *Pain*, **154**, 1509–18.

Humphrey N (2002). Great expectations: the evolutionary psychology of faith-healing and the placebo effect. In C von Hofsten and L Bäckman, eds. *Psychology at the turn of the millennium, vol. 2: social, developmental, and clinical perspectives*, pp. 225–46. Psychology Press, Hove.

Hunsley J and Westmacott R (2007). Interpreting the magnitude of the placebo effect: mountain or molehill? *Journal of Clinical Psychology*, **63**, 391–9.

Jensen KB, Kaptchuk TJ, Kirsch I et al. (2012). Nonconscious activation of placebo and nocebo pain responses. *Proceedings of the National Academy of Science of the United States of America*, **109**, 15959–64.

Kalivas PW, Churchill L and Romanides A (1999). Involvement of the pallidal-thalamocortical circuit in adaptive behavior. *Annals of the New York Academy of Sciences*, **877**, 64–70.

Kamin LJ (1968). "Attention-like" processes in classical conditioning. In MR Jones, ed. *Miami symposium on the prediction of behavior: aversive stimulation*, pp. 9–31. University of Miami Press, Miami, FL.

Kaptchuk TJ (2001). Is the placebo powerless? *New England Journal of Medicine*, **345**, 1277.

Kaptchuk TJ, Kelley JM, Sanchez MN et al. (2010). Placebos without deception: a randomized controlled trial in irritable bowel syndrome. *PLoS One*, **5**, e15591.

Keats AS and Beecher HK (1950). Pain relief with hypnotic doses of barbiturates and a hypothesis. *Journal of Pharmacology and Experimental Therapeutics*, **100**, 1–13.

Keats AS, D'Alessandro GL and Beecher HK (1951). A controlled study of pain relief by intravenous procaine. *Journal of the American Medical Association*, **147**, 1761–3.

Kennedy WP (1961). The nocebo reaction. *Medicina Experimentalis International Journal of Experimental Medicine*, **95**, 203–5.

Kessner S, Sprenger C, Wrobel N, Wiech K and Bingel U (2013). Effect of oxytocin on placebo analgesia: a randomized study. *Journal of the American Medical Association*, **310**, 1733–5.

Kienle GS and Kiene H (1997). The powerful placebo effect: fact or fiction? *Journal of Clinical Epidemiology*, **50**, 1311–18.

Kirsch I (1985). Response expectancy as determinant of experience and behavior. *American Psychologist*, **40**, 1189–202.

Kirsch I (1990). *Changing expectations: a key to effective psychotherapy*. Brooks/Cole, Pacific Grove, CA.

Kirsch I (1999). *How expectancies shape experience*. American Psychological Association, Washington, DC.

Kirsch I, Lynn SJ, Vigorito M and Miller RR (2004). The role of cognition in classical and operant conditioning. *Journal of Clinical Psychology*, **60**, 369–92.

Kirsch I, Moore TJ, Scoboria A and Nicholls SS (2002). The Emperor's new drugs: an analysis of antidepressant medication data submitted to the U.S. Food and Drug Administration. *Prevention & Treatment*, **5**(1).

Kirsch I and Scoboria A (2001). Apples, oranges, and placebos: heterogeneity in a meta-analysis of placebo effects. *Advances in Mind-Body Medicine*, **17**, 307–9.

Kissel P and Barrucand D (1964). *Placebos et effect placebo en medicine*. Masson, Paris.

Kleinman A, Guess HA and Wilentz JS (2002). An overview. In HA Guess, A Kleinman, JW Kusek and LW Engel, eds. *The science of the placebo: toward an interdisciplinary research agenda*, pp. 1–32. British Medical Journal Books, London.

Koban L, Brass M, Lynn MT and Pourtois G (2012). Placebo analgesia affects brain correlates of error processing. *PLoS One*, **7**, e49784.

Koog YH, We SR and Min BI (2011). Three-armed trials including placebo and no-treatment groups may be subject to publication bias: a systematic review. *PLoS One*, **6**, e20679.

Kradin R (2011). The placebo response: an attachment that counteracts the effects of stress-related dysfunction. *Perspectives in Biology and Medicine*, **54**, 438–54.

Kupers R (2001). Is the placebo powerless? *New England Journal of Medicine*, **345**, 1278.

Laska E and Sunshine A (1973). Anticipation of analgesia, a placebo effect. *Headache*, **13**, 1–11.

Last JM (1983). *A dictionary of epidemiology*. Oxford University Press, New York.

Lazarus RS (1991). Cognition and motivation in emotion. *American Psychologist*, **46**, 352–67.

Leuchter AF, Cook IA, Witte EA, Morgan M and Abrams M (2002). Changes in brain function of depressed subjects during treatment with placebo. *American Journal of Psychiatry*, **159**, 122–9.

Leuchter AF, McCracken JT, Hunter AM, Cook IA and Alpert JE (2009) Monoamine oxidase a and catechol-o-methyltransferase functional polymorphisms and the placebo response in major depressive disorder. *Journal of Clinical Psychopharmacology*, **29**, 372–7.

Levesque J, Eugene F, Joanette Y et al. (2003). Neural circuitry underlying voluntary suppression of sadness. *Biological Psychiatry*, **53**, 502–10.

Levine JD, Gordon NC and Fields HL (1978). The mechanisms of placebo analgesia. *Lancet*, **2**, 654–7.

Lichstein J, DeCosta Mayer J and Hauch EW (1955). Efficacy of methantheline (banthine) bromide in therapy of the unstable colon. *Journal of the American Medical Association*, **25**, 634–7.

Lieberman MD, Jarcho JM, Berman S et al. (2004). The neural correlates of placebo effects:a disruption account. *NeuroImage*, **22**, 447– 55.

Lieberman MD, Hariri A, Jarcho JM, Eisenberger NI and Bookheimer SY (2005). An fMRI investigation of race-related amygdala activity in African-American and Caucasian-American individuals. *Nature Neuroscience*, **8**, 720–2.

Lilford RJ and Braunholtz DA (2001). Is the placebo powerful? *New England Journal of Medicine*, **345**, 1277–8.

Lipid Research Clinics Program (1984). The lipid research clinics coronary primary prevention trial results. *Journal of the American Medical Association*, **25**, 351–64.

Lipman JJ, Miller BE, Mays KS et al. (1990). Peak B endorphin concentration in cerebrospinal fluid: reduced in chronic pain patients and increased during the placebo response. *Psychopharmacology*, **102**, 112–16.

Mayberg HS, Silva JA, Brannan SK et al. (2002). The functional neuroanatomy of the placebo effect. *American Journal of Psychiatry*, **159**, 728–37.

McGlashan TH, Evans FJ and Orne MT (1969). The nature of hypnotic analgesia and placebo response to experimental pain. *Psychosomatic Medicine*, **31**, 227–46.

Miller FG (2001). Is the placebo powerless? *New England Journal of Medicine*, **345**, 1277.

Miller EK and Cohen JD (2001). An integrative theory of prefrontal cortex function. *Annual Review of Neuroscience*, **24**, 167–202.

Miller FG and Kaptchuk TJ (2008). The power of context: reconceptualizing the placebo effect. *Journal of the Royal Society of Medicine*, **101**, 222–5.

Moerman DE (2002). *Meaning, medicine and the placebo effect*. Cambridge University Press, Cambridge, MA.

Moerman DE (2003). Doctors and patients: the role of clinicians in the placebo effect. *Advances in Mind-Body Medicine*, **19**, 14–22.

Moerman DE (2013). Against the "placebo effect": a personal point of view. *Complementary Therapies in Medicine*, **21**, 125–30.

Moerman DE and Jonas WB (2002). Deconstructing the placebo effect and finding the meaning response. *Annals of Internal Medicine*, **136**, 471–6.

Mogenson GJ and Yang CA (1991). The contribution of basal forebrain to limbic-motor integration and the mediation of motivation to action. *Advances in Experimental Medicine and Biology*, **295**, 267–90.

Montgomery GH and Kirsch I (1997). Classical conditioning and the placebo effect. *Pain*, **72**, 107–13.

Morton DL, Watson A, El-Deredy W and Jones AK (2009). Reproducibility of placebo analgesia: effect of dispositional optimism. *Pain*, **146**, 194–8.

Nolan TA, Price DD, Caudle R, Murphy NP and Neubert JK (2012). Placebo-induced analgesia in an operant pain model in rats. *Pain*, **153**, 2009–16

Ochsner KN, Bunge SA, Gross JJ and Gabrieli JD (2002). Rethinking feelings: an FMRI study of the cognitive regulation of emotion. *Journal of Cognitive Neuroscience*, **14**, 1215–29.

Ochsner KN, Ray RD, Cooper JC *et al.* (2004). For better or for worse: neural systems supporting the cognitive down- and up-regulation of negative emotion. *NeuroImage*, **23**, 483–99.

Papakostas YG and Daras MD (2001). Placebos, placebo effect, and the response to the healing situation: the evolution of a concept. *Epilepsia*, **42**, 1614–25.

Park LC and Covi L (1965). Nonblind placebo trial. *Archives of General Psychiatry*, **12**, 336–45.

Peciña M, Azhar H, Love TM, *et al.* (2013). Personality trait predictors of placebo analgesia and neurobiological correlates. *Neuropsychopharmacology*, **38**, 639–46.

Pennebaker JW (1997). Writing about emotional experiences as a therapeutic process. *Psychological Science*, **8**, 162–6.

Petrovic P, Dietrich T, Fransson P, Andersson J and Carlsson K (2005). Placebo in emotional processing-induced expectations of anxiety relief activate a generalized modulatory network. *Neuron*, **46**, 957–69.

Petrovic P and Ingvar M (2002). Imaging cognitive modulation of pain processing. *Pain*, **95**, 1–5.

Petrovic P, Kalso E, Petersson KM and Ingvar M (2002). Placebo and opioid analgesia—imaging a shared neuronal network. *Science*, **295**, 1737–40.

Phan KL, Fitzgerald DA, Nathan PJ, Moore GJ, Uhde TW and Tancer ME (2005). Neural substrates for voluntary suppression of negative affect: a functional magnetic resonance imaging study. *Biological Psychiatry*, **57**, 210–9.

Phillips DP, Liu GC, Kwok K, Jarvinen JR, Zhang W and Abramson IS (2001). The Hound of the Baskervilles effect: natural experiment on the influence of psychological stress on timing of death. *British Medical Journal*, **323**, 1443–6.

Pogge RC (1963). The toxic placebo. Part I. Side and toxic effects reported during the administration of placebo medicine. *Medical Times*, **91**, 773–8.

Price DD and Barrell JJ (2000). Mechanisms of analgesia produced by hypnosis and placebo suggestions. *Progress in Brain Research*, **122**, 255–71.

Price DD, Barrell JE and Barrell JJ (1985). A quantitative-experiential analysis of human emotions. *Motivation and Emotion*, **9**, 19–38.

Price DD, Finniss DG and Benedetti F (2008). A comprehensive review of the placebo effect: recent advances and current thought. *Annual Review of Psychology*, **59**, 565–90.

Price DD, Riley J and Barrell JJ (2001). Are lived choices based on emotional processes? *Cognition and Emotion*, **15**, 365–79.

Rainville P, Duncan GH, Price DD, Carrier B and Bushnell MC (1997). Pain affect encoded in human anterior cingulate but not somatosensory cortex. *Science*, **277**, 968–71.

Rausch JL, Johnson ME, Fei YJ et al. (2002) Initial conditions of serotonin transporter kinetics and genotype: influence on SSRI treatment trial outcome. *Biological Psychiatry*, **51**, 723–32.

Reiss S (1980). Pavlovian conditioning and human fear: an expectancy model. *Behavioral Therapy*, **11**, 380–96.

Rescorla RA (1988). Pavlovian conditioning: it's not what you think it is. *American Psychologist*, **43**, 151–60.

Roberts AH (1995). The powerful placebo revisited: the magnitude of non-specific effects. *Mind/Body Medicine*, **3**, 1–10.

Ruck A and Sylvèn C (2006). "Improvement" in the placebo group could be due to regression to the mean as well as to sociobiologic factors. *American Journal of Cardiology*, **97**, 152–3.

Sackett DL (1995). Randomized trials in individual patients. In G Antes, L Edler, R Holle, W Koepcke, R Lorenz and J Windeler, eds. *Biometrie und unkonventionelle Medizine*, pp. 19–33. Landwirtschaftsverlag, Munster-Hiltrup.

Schultz W (2006). Behavioral theories and the neurophysiology of reward. *Annual Review of Psychology*, **57**, 87–115.

Schweinhardt P, Seminowicz DA, Jaeger E, Duncan GH and Bushnell MC (2009). The anatomy of the mesolimbic reward system: a link between personality and the placebo analgesic response. *Journal of Neuroscience*, **29**, 4882–7.

Scott DJ, Stohler CS, Egnatuk CM, Wang H, Koeppe RA and Zubieta J-K (2007). Individual differences in reward responding explain placebo-induced expectations and effects. *Neuron*, **55**, 325–36.

Setlow B, Schoenbaum G and Gallagher M (2003). Neural encoding in ventral striatum during olfactory discrimination learning. *Neuron*, **38**, 625–36.

Shapiro AK and Shapiro E (1997). The placebo: is it much ado about nothing? In A Harrington, ed. *The placebo effect—an interdisciplinary exploration*, pp. 12–36. Harvard University Press, Cambridge, MA.

Shrier I (2001). Is the placebo powerless? *New England Journal of Medicine*, **345**, 1278.

Siegel S (1972). Conditioning of insulin-induced glycemia. *Journal of Comparative Physiology and Psychology*, **78**, 233–41.

Siegel S (1975). Conditioning insulin effects. *Journal of Comparative Physiology and Psychology*, **89**, 189–99.

Siegel S (2002). Explanatory mechanisms for placebo effects: Pavlovian conditioning. In HA Guess, A Kleinman, JW Kusek, LW Engel, eds. *The science of the placebo: toward an interdisciplinary research agenda*, pp 133–57. British Medical Journal Books, London.

Spiegel D, Kraemer H and Carlson RW (2001). Is the placebo powerless? *New England Journal of Medicine*, **345**, 1276.

Stewart-Williams S and Podd J (2004). The placebo effect: dissolving the expectancy versus conditioning debate. *Psychological Bulletin*, **130**, 324–40.

Sunshine A, Laska E, Meisner M and Morgan S (1964). Analgesic studies of indomethacin as analyzed by computer techniques. *Clinical Pharmacology and Therapeutics*, **5**, 699–707.

Swider K and Bąbel P (2013). The effect of the sex of a model in nocebo hyperalgesia induced by social observational learning. *Pain*, **154**, 1312–17.

Thomas KB (1987). General practice consultations: is there any point in being positive? *British Medical Journal*, **294**, 1200–2.

Thompson JJ, Ritenbaugh C and Nichter M (2009). Reconsidering the placebo response from a broad anthropological perspective. *Culture, Medicine and Psychiatry*, **33**, 112–52.

Tobler PN, Fiorillo CD and Schultz W (2005). Adaptive coding of reward value by dopamine neurons. *Science*, **307**, 1642–5.

Tolman EC (1932). *Purposive behavior in animals and men*. Appleton-Century-Crofts, New York.

Tracey I (2010). Getting the pain you expect: mechanisms of placebo, nocebo and reappraisal effects in humans. *Nature Medicine*, **16**, 1277–83.

Travell J, Rinzler SH, Bakst H, Benjamin ZH and Bobb A (1949). Comparison of effects of alpha-tocopherol and a matching placebo on chest pain in patients with heart disease. *Annals of the New York Academy of Sciences*, **52**, 345–53.

Vase L, Riley JL 3rd and Price DD (2002). A comparison of placebo effects in clinical analgesic trials versus studies of placebo analgesia. *Pain*, **99**, 443–52.

Vase L, Robinson ME, Verne GN and Price DD (2005). Increased placebo analgesia over time in irritable bowel syndrome (IBS) patients is associated with desire and expectation but not endogenous opioid mechanisms. *Pain*, **115**, 338–47.

Vögtle E, Barke A and Kröner-Herwig B (2013). Nocebo hyperalgesia induced by social observational learning. *Pain*, **154**, 1427–33.

Voudouris NJ, Peck CL and Coleman G (1989). Conditioned response models of placebo phenomena: further support. *Pain*, **38**, 109–16.

Voudouris NJ, Peck CL and Coleman G (1990). The role of conditioning and verbal expectancy in the placebo response. *Pain*, **43**, 121–8.

Waber RL, Shiv B, Carmon Z and Ariely D (2008). Commercial features of placebo and therapeutic efficacy. *Journal of the American Medical Association*, **299**, 1016–17.

Wager TD, Reading S and Jonides J (2004a). Neuroimaging studies of shifting attention: a meta-analysis. *NeuroImage*, **22**, 1679–93.

Wager TD, Billing JK, Smith EE *et al.* (2004b). Placebo-induced changes in fMRI in the anticipation and experience of pain. *Science*, **303**, 1162–6.

Wager TD and Smith EE (2003). Neuroimaging studies of working memory: a meta-analysis. *Cognitive, Affective & Behavioral Neuroscience*, **3**, 255–74.

Wagner KJ, Willoch F, Kochs EF *et al.* (2001). Dose-dependent regional cerebral blood flow changes during remifentanil infusion in humans: a positron emission tomography study. *Anesthesiology*, **94**, 732–9.

Wall PD (1999). *Pain: the science of suffering.* Weidenfeld & Nicholson, London.

Walsh BT, Seidman SN, Sysko R and Gould M (2002). Placebo response in studies of major depression: variable, substantial, and growing. *Journal of the American Medical Association,* **287**, 1840–7.

Wampold BE, Minami T, Tierney SC, Baskin TW and Bhati KS (2005). The placebo is powerful: estimating placebo effects in medicine and psychotherapy from randomized clinical trials. *Journal of Clinical Psychology,* **61**, 835–54.

Wells RE (1957). Use of reserpine (Serpasil) in the management of chronic alcoholism. *Journal of the American Medical Association,* **163**, 426–9.

Wickramasekera I (2001). The placebo efficacy study: problems with the definition of the placebo and the mechanisms of placebo efficacy. *Advances in Mind-Body Medicine,* **17**, 309–12.

Williams AC (2002). Facial expression of pain: an evolutionary account. *Behavioral and brain Sciences,* **25**, 439–55.

Zhang RR, Zhang WC, Wang JY and Guo JY (2013). The opioid placebo analgesia is mediated exclusively through mu-opioid receptor in rat. *International Journal of Neuropsychopharmacology,* **16**, 849–56.

Chapter 3

Placing placebo effects within the context of the doctor–patient relationship

Summary points

- The doctor–patient relationship is a product of evolution. The big evolutionary step was represented by the fact that animals started grooming others rather than themselves. Social grooming is one of the first examples of social interaction. It represents a very primitive and elementary form of medical care, whereby the groomer takes care of the groomee.

- Placebo responses are tightly linked to the doctor–patient relationship, for they are the result of the psychosocial context around the patient, and the main element of this context is the doctor.

- From a neuroscientific standpoint, the doctor–patient relationship can be subdivided into four steps: feeling sick, seeking relief, meeting the therapist, receiving the therapy.

- The first is the step of "feeling sick," a crucial starting point that triggers the subsequent behavior. It involves sensory systems and brain regions that lead to conscious awareness. For example, the perception of a symptom, like pain, is the product of bottom-up processes and top-down modulation.

- The second step is what makes a patient "seek relief," a kind of motivated behavior which is aimed at suppressing discomfort. This behavioral repertoire is not different from that aimed at suppressing hunger or thirst, and the brain reward mechanisms are crucial in this regard.

- The third step is when the patient "meets the therapist," a special and unique social interaction in which the therapist represents the means to suppress discomfort, thus he himself is a powerful reward. Here many intricate mechanisms are at work, such as trust and hope on the one hand and empathy and compassion on the other.

- Finally, the fourth step is when the patient "receives the therapy," the final act, and surely the most important, of the doctor–patient interaction. The mere ritual of the therapeutic act may generate therapeutic placebo responses through a number of mechanisms, which represent the target of the present book.

3.1 **A closer look into the doctor–patient relationship**

3.1.1 **The doctor–patient relationship has evolved as a special social interaction**

The doctor–patient relationship, or patient–provider interaction, or therapist–patient encounter, has been analyzed by different disciplines such as psychology, sociology, philosophy, and health policy. With the recent advances of neuroscience, today we are in a good position to approach the doctor–patient relationship from a biological perspective and to consider it within the context of social neuroscience. Indeed, in the book *The Patient's Brain: The Neuroscience Behind The Doctor–Patient Relationship* (Benedetti, 2010) this new biological approach has been used to uncover the mechanisms of higher brain functions, such as expectations, beliefs, trust, hope, empathy, and compassion. In addition, since any biological system is a product of evolution which has emerged in animals and humans with a precise purpose, an evolutionary approach of why and how these social mechanisms have emerged and evolved is of paramount importance, for they give us insights into the relationship between the first social interactions in nonhuman primates and early hominids and subsequent medical care.

Many simple behavioral repertoires, like the withdrawal reflex and the scratch reflex, are aimed at protecting the body from possible damage, and they are present in both invertebrates and vertebrates, including man. However, from an evolutionary perspective, these two reflexes differ in at least one important aspect. In the scratch reflex, differently from the withdrawal reflex, the movement is aimed at targeting the potential noxious stimulus and at removing it from the body. This represents an important evolutionary step toward the more complex behavior of grooming, which involves scratching, licking, preening, rubbing, nibbling, and wallowing (Benedetti, 2010). Interestingly, whereas the scratch reflex is triggered by cutaneous stimuli, such as a bug's bite, grooming is a self-directed behavior which does not require the peripheral stimulation of the skin, for its biological function is the care of the body surface (Spruijt et al., 1992). Whereas grooming involves the supraspinal centers, the scratch reflex only requires the spinal cord. Thus the evolutionary step from the peripherally driven scratch reflex to the centrally driven grooming behavior represents an important transition from a simple reflex act to a complex motor pattern for the care of the whole body surface.

Certainly, the big evolutionary jump to social behavior is represented by allogrooming, i.e., taking care of the skin of others. In fact, not only do animals scratch, rub, and lick themselves, but they scratch and rub their companions as well. Social grooming has a function in the regulation of social relationships, and it is not only involved in the care of body surface (Spruijt et al., 1992). It is interesting to note that individuals who are virtually free of parasites, still solicit for and submit themselves to being groomed. Allogrooming time correlates with social group size, which suggests that it has to do with intense social relationships (Dunbar, 2010). Differently from scratch reflexes and self-grooming, which require neuronal circuits in the spinal cord and in the brainstem, respectively, allogrooming is related to the cerebral cortex.

Two actors take part in social grooming: the one being groomed and the groomer. Whereas the former benefits from it in a number of ways, such as pleasure, relaxation, and hygiene, it is less clear what the benefits are for the latter. Since there are no immediate benefits to the groomer, for he spends energies and time to the advantage of others, the act of grooming can be considered an early form of altruistic behavior, the so-called reciprocal altruism. In fact, the role of the groomer and the gromee are related, because any individual can be either a groomer or a groomee. If there is no immediate advantage to the groomer, the service can be returned by the one who is being groomed. Reciprocal altruism explains cases of altruism among nonkin organisms (Trivers, 1971).

Prosocial behavior in early hominids evolved from social grooming in a number of ways. One of these was the care of the individual who needs help, usually the weak, the sick, or the elderly (see Box 3.1). In order to survive in harsh conditions, it was crucial for our ancestors to obtain a daily nutritious diet of meat and other food. However, this daily provision was not guaranteed, because of the high variability of hunting success. Although the first altruistic exchanges were likely to occur among relatives, thus boosting kin selection, subsequently further food exchanges occurred with nonkin that were less lucky on that particular hunting day. According to the reciprocal altruism mechanism, these nonkin recipients eventually returned this favor (van Vugt and Van Lange, 2006).

There are many examples of early forms of compassion, such as a toothless skull dating back 1.7 million years that was found in the site of Dmanisi in the Eurasian republic of Georgia, suggesting that companions might have helped him in finding soft plant food and hammering raw meat with stone tools (Lordkipanidze et al., 2005). Similarly, Neanderthal men have been found to show signs of compassion towards their companions, dating back to about 60,000 years ago. The analysis of undeveloped bone structure indicates that a man at Shanidar caves was a severe cripple from birth. His right upper limb was entirely useless and extensive bone scar tissue indicated that he was blind in his left eye. These extensive lesions suggest that he was apparently cared for by his companions until his death at age 40, which represents a very old age by Neanderthal standards (Wiester, 1983).

Box 3.1 The emergence of consolation and the care of the sick during evolution

Altruistic behavior and sociality are far from being understood in humans. For example, reciprocal altruism is clearly the antithesis of real altruism, as behaving nicely to someone in order to procure return benefits from them in the future is just delayed self-interest. Adoption is a special case whereby reciprocal altruism does not seem to apply to *Homo sapiens*. Biological fitness is reduced in parents who adopt children, for these children are usually unrelated to their adoptive parents. Adoption as well as other human altruistic acts seem to obey neither kin selection nor reciprocal altruism, so they probably need to be treated as real altruistic actions.

All those human altruistic acts that seem to be at odds with the evolutionary theory are clearly related to conscious intentions. In contraposition to biological

Box 3.1 The emergence of consolation and the care of the sick during evolution (continued)

altruism (i.e., kin selection and reciprocal altruism), psychological altruism is used to mean the conscious intention of helping somebody else. Psychological altruism may represent a form of genuine altruism whereby individuals may indeed care about helping others. Many directed altruistic behaviors in humans are based on empathy, that is, the capacity to share the emotional state of another and to adopt his perspective. In this sense, the altruistic act may represent a self-reward, for it is aimed at placating the altruist's internal state.

A possible origin of empathy may be represented by the evolution from emotional contagion, whereby the emotional state of a subject is matched with an object, to sympathetic concern, whereby both concern about another's state and the attempts to ameliorate it are present (de Waal, 2008). In the latter, sympathy consists of feelings of sorrow for a distressed other. The best example of sympathetic concern is consolation, which is widely present in apes and humans but not in monkeys, and which may consist of putting an arm around a companion who has been defeated in a fight (Fig. 3.1). The next evolutionary step occurs when the capacity to take another's perspective has emerged, the so-called empathic perspective-taking (de Waal, 2008). In *Homo*, and particularly in *Homo sapiens*, the members of the same social group, with their sympathetic concern and empathic repertoire, were likely to evolve into those who helped each other in a number of circumstances, including the care of the sick (Benedetti, 2010).

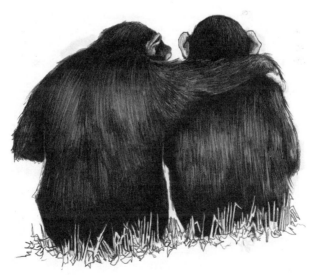

Fig. 3.1 An ape soothing a companion who has been defeated in a fight.

In early hominids these altruistic acts were adopted by different members of the group. However, in the course of evolution a single member of the group assumed the role of the person who takes care of the sick, namely the shaman. Prehistoric shamanism represents the first example of medical care, which is characterized by a good relationship between the sick and the shaman. The sick trust the shaman and believe in his therapeutic capabilities, thus they refer to him for any psychological, spiritual, or physical discomfort. In this way, the shaman acquired a more and more central role and a higher social status in any social group across different cultures. While shamanistic procedures are mainly based on religious beliefs and the supernatural origin of diseases, several rational treatments emerged over the centuries. For example, a broken arm or leg was covered in river clay or mud and the cast allowed to dry hard in the sun; animal skin was used for bandages; and surgical procedures, such as skull trepanning, were carried out. The transition from shamans to modern doctors is recent and depended on the emergence of modern scientific knowledge and methodology (Benedetti, 2010).

3.1.2 The doctor–patient interaction involves four different steps

Following this evolutionary and biological approach, the whole process of the doctor–patient encounter can be subdivided into at least four steps (Benedetti, 2010, 2013) (Fig. 3.2). The first is "feeling sick," the starting point that triggers the subsequent

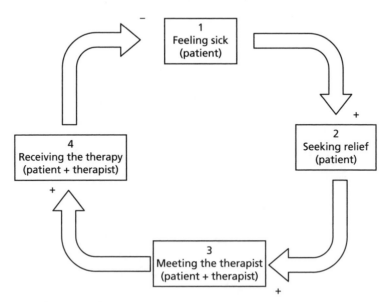

Fig. 3.2 The four steps of the doctor–patient relationship. The interaction between the healer/doctor and his patient can be envisaged as a homeostatic system in which the variable to be controlled is represented by the feeling of sickness (symptoms). The very act of administering a treatment is a psychological and social event that is sometimes capable of inhibiting a symptom such as pain, even though the treatment is fake.

behavior. This involves all those sensory systems that convey different pieces of information related to peripheral organs and apparatuses, as well as brain regions that lead to conscious awareness. Perception of a symptom such as pain is the product of bottom-up processes taking place in the peripheral and central nervous system and of top-down modulation from cognitive/evaluative and emotional/motivational brain areas. The second step is "seeking relief," a kind of motivated behavior which is aimed at suppressing discomfort. This behavioral repertoire is not different from that aimed at suppressing hunger or thirst, and the brain reward mechanisms are crucial in this regard. These first two steps are the key elements that lead the patient to look for a healer/doctor who himself represents a powerful reward (Benedetti, 2010, 2013).

The third step is when the patient "meets the therapist," a special and unique social interaction in which the therapist represents the means to suppress discomfort. Here many intricate mechanisms are at work, such as trust and hope in the patient and empathy and compassion in the doctor. In the patient's brain, expectations, beliefs, trust, and hope are key elements, whereas in the doctor's brain, empathic and compassionate behavior represents an essential factor. Finally, the fourth step is when the patient "receives the therapy," the final and perhaps the most important act of the doctor–patient interaction. The mere ritual of the therapeutic act may generate therapeutic responses (placebo responses), which sometimes may be as powerful as those generated by real medical treatments. Of course, these placebo responses represent the target of the present book.

It can be seen in Fig. 3.2 that these four steps can be conceived as a homeostatic system, in which a variable has to be maintained within a physiological range. The feeling of sickness is the variable to be controlled. It tells a motivational system to seek relief. This is aimed at adopting the appropriate behavioral repertoire to eliminate the feeling of sickness. In a social group, such a behavioral repertoire is represented by the social contact with the healer, whose role is to suppress suffering through a therapeutic agent or procedure. This system is always at work, regardless of whether the healer administers effective or ineffective therapies. Even if the therapy is totally ineffective, the patient's expectation of benefit (the placebo response) may be sufficient to inhibit discomfort. The real difference between shamans and modern doctors is that, whereas shamanic procedures are likely to lack specific effects completely, at least in most circumstances, modern doctors rely on effective procedures and medications with specific mechanisms of action. But this social–neural system is always there, as an ancestral system which is ready to come out, both with shamans and with modern doctors.

3.1.3 Placebo responses are tightly linked to the doctor–patient relationship

Looking at Fig. 2.3 of the previous chapter and Fig. 3.2 in the present chapter, the link between placebo and doctor–patient interaction appears straightforward. The main element in the psychosocial context around the patient that leads to the placebo response is the doctor, and more in general the health professional. Indeed, any element in Fig. 2.3 is related to the figure of the doctor, who uses communication, words, and medical instruments, and administers pills, injections, and medications (Benedetti, 2002). Similarly, the behavioral repertoire that is adopted by the patient when seeking relief in Fig. 3.2 is aimed at looking for a doctor, who represents the means for relieving discomfort. It is not surprising, therefore, that a crucial element that triggers the placebo response comes from the very special social encounter between the patient and his doctor.

Kaptchuk et al. (2008) investigated whether placebo effects can experimentally be separated into three components: (1) assessment and observation, (2) therapeutic ritual, and (3) doctor–patient relationship. They studied patients with irritable bowel syndrome and assessed the relative magnitude of these components. The patients underwent one of the following interventions: waiting list (observation), placebo acupuncture alone, or placebo acupuncture with a patient–practitioner relationship augmented by warmth, attention, and confidence. At 3 weeks, the proportion of patients reporting adequate relief was the following: 28% on waiting list, 44% in acupuncture group, and 62% in acupuncture with augmented patient–practitioner relationship group. The same trend in response existed in symptom severity score and quality of life, and the results were similar at 6-week follow-up. Overall, factors contributing to the placebo effect can be progressively combined in a manner resembling a graded dose escalation of component parts, and the patient–practitioner relationship is the most robust component.

The role of communication between the doctor and the patient has been emphasized many times, both in placebo (Bensing and Verheul, 2010) and nocebo effects (Colloca and Finniss, 2012), and the important role of psychological and social factors in illness stressed by a number of authors (e.g., Engel, 1977) (Box 3.2). A detailed account of the four steps in the doctor–patient relationship is given by Benedetti (2010, 2013). The following sections represent a summary of the first three steps (feeling sick, seeking relief, meeting the therapist). They help place the fourth step (receiving the therapy and generating placebo responses) within the context of the whole doctor–patient interaction.

Box 3.2 The biopsychosocial model

Although many psychological and social aspects have been recognized over the centuries by physicians and psychologists as contributing factors to the emergence of certain diseases, the scientific formulation of such a contribution is relatively recent. Engel (1977) challenged the medical and scientific community by putting forward a new medical model that takes into account biological, psychological, and social factors as important determinants of illness. Engel's biopsychosocial model has had a great impact upon the scientific community, and its scientific foundations have been partly supported by the emergence of modern concepts in psychosomatics, psychoneuroimmunology, and psychoneuroendocrinology.

The basic idea of the biopsychosocial model is not so much to deny biomedical research but rather to criticize its narrow focus on the anatomical, physiological, and molecular mechanisms. There is no doubt that the new acquisitions of anatomy, physiology, and, more recently, molecular biology, have been crucial to

---

Box 3.2 The biopsychosocial model (continued)

the advancement of biomedical research. The detailed knowledge of the origin and possibly the management of a disease has mainly relied on these biological acquisitions and, accordingly, has positively impacted on the medical profession. However, emerging experimental evidence in modern medicine indicates powerful influences of the mind over the body, whereby the patient's psychological state and the social factors impinging onto him are all involved in both the pathophysiology and the treatment outcomes of a given disease.

To recognize that the patient's psychological state may influence biological factors means to pose the patient, with his emotional, cognitive, and motivational experiences, at the center of medical care. In the history of medicine this certainly represents an important step, as it was neglected in many medical cultures over the centuries. This does not mean that it was psychoneuroendocrinoimmunology that led to the patient-centered medical care, but it certainly posed some of the scientific bases for this approach. For example, a doctor-centered approach, whereby the doctor was supposed to have magical powers, was typical of many cultures, such as ancient Egypt and medieval Europe, whereas a more scientific and humanistic approach in the doctor–patient relationship was present in the Greek culture. Here there was a higher degree of humanism in dealing with the needs, well-being, and interests of people, and medical ethics was posed above the self-interests of class and status.

The biopsychosocial approach has to do not only with the pathophysiology of illness, but also with possible management. It gave rise to a series of therapeutic interventions which are called, as a whole, mind–body medicine. Mind–body interventions are aimed at targeting those psychosocial factors that are supposed to be at the very origin of many diseases, although their effectiveness is often questioned. These include hypnosis, meditation, cognitive behavioral therapy, relaxation, and imagery techniques.

3.2 **Feeling sick**

3.2.1 **A symptom is a combination of bottom-up and top-down processes**

The sensory experience giving rise to what we call a symptom, such as pain, is built up from the periphery to the central nervous system according to bottom-up processes that convey many pieces of information to the brain. Simultaneously, the incoming sensory experience is shaped by top-down influences that make a symptom different from patient to patient (Fig. 3.3). Therefore, the symptom experience of each patient is unique and is not comparable to others. Many factors shape it, including psychological, social, and cultural factors, thus the physiological study of the sensory signals that build up a symptom gives us important information on both the mechanisms of the symptom itself and complex brain processes.

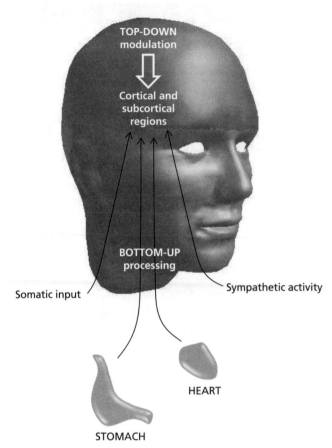

Fig. 3.3 General organization of the sensibility arising from the periphery and its modulation. The afferent pathways from different regions of the body reach a variety of subcortical and cortical areas. Besides this bottom-up processing there is an important top-down modulation by a number of cognitive and affective factors.

Interoceptive sensibility, or interoception, that is, the sensory inputs arising from internal organs, plays a fundamental role in the perception of different symptoms. Brain imaging studies have greatly contributed to the understanding of interoceptive processing in the central nervous system. Many regions have been found to be activated by visceral stimulation. In particular, many studies have been performed by applying different types of stimuli to the gastrointestinal tract. For example, the mechanical stimulation of the esophagus at different intensities, from the mildest stimulus that produces awareness to stronger stimuli, has been found to activate bilaterally the parietal operculum, the insula, and the primary somatosensory cortex (Aziz et al., 1997; Binkofski et al., 1998). The stimulation of the rectum by means of a rectal balloon has been found to increase cerebral blood flow particularly in precentral motor areas, in the primary somatosensory cortex, and in the thalamus, as well as to elicit evoked potentials that are correlated to the amount of distension (Rothstein et al., 1996). In a study of gastric distension, Stephan et al. (2003) found the activation of four key regions: dorsal brainstem, left inferior frontal gyrus, bilateral insula, and right subgenual anterior cingulate cortex. In the cardiovascular and respiratory systems, King et al. (1999) found activations in the insular cortex, medial prefrontal cortex, and thalamus by using maximal inspiration, the Valsalva maneuver, and isometric handgrip to induce changes in heart rate, blood pressure, and respiratory function. Likewise, Critchley et al. (2004) observed enhanced activity in the insula, somatomotor cortex, supplementary motor area, and anterior cingulate cortex when subjects had to judge the timing of their own heartbeats.

Therefore, a common finding across the different studies investigating interoception is represented by the activation of the insular cortex. There is now compelling experimental evidence that the insula plays a crucial role in interoceptive awareness, and more in general in human awareness. This evidence comes from several lines of research in different fields whereby awareness was investigated. For example, insula activation has been found during awareness of body movements, self-recognition, vocalization and music, emotional feelings, like maternal and romantic love, anger, fear, disgust, trust, and empathy. In addition, insula activation is also present during visual-auditory awareness, time perception, attention, perceptual decision-making, and cognitive control (Craig, 2009). Interestingly, in virtually all studies of emotions, there is a co-activation of the insular and anterior cingulate cortex, which is likely to be based on the dual projection of the lamina-1 spinothalamocortical tract to both regions (Craig, 2002, 2009). Whereas the anterior insular cortex is a likely locus of awareness, the anterior cingulate cortex is likely to initiate behaviors.

A peculiar feature of the anterior insular cortex and the anterior cingulate cortex in hominoid primates is the presence of clusters of large spindle-shaped neurons among the pyramidal neurons in layer 5. These are called "von Economo neurons," and Craig (2009) proposed that they are the substrate for fast interconnections between the physically separated anterior insular and anterior cingulate cortices. Interestingly, there is a phylogenetic progression of the von Economo neurons. In fact, they are present in adult humans, but progressively decrease in children, gorillas, and chimpanzees, and are completely lacking in macaque monkeys (Nimchinsky et al., 1999). It is also worth noting that patients with frontotemporal dementia and degeneration of the von Economo neurons in the insula show a loss of emotional awareness (Seeley et al., 2006).

The interoceptive signals arising from the peripheral receptors undergo a top-down modulation by a variety of emotional, motivational, cognitive, and social factors. Different emotional states, such as anxiety and depression, or different cognitive tasks, like attention or distraction, may have profound effects on interoceptive awareness, such that perceptions can be reported in different ways from time to time. Gastrointestinal function is particularly amenable to top-down influences. For example, irritable bowel syndrome and noncardiac chest pain are affected by many psychosocial factors which can modulate the perception of the symptoms (Whitehead et al., 1988; Ho et al., 1998).

Although a few data are available to date, the top-down modulation of interoceptive sensibility is likely to be a complex phenomenon that involves many neural systems and that is associated with specific types of modulation. For example, in a study by Phillips et al. (2003), the brain responses to nonpainful esophageal stimulation were studied in association with emotional stimuli. Either neutral or fearful facial expressions were presented to healthy volunteers while undergoing distension of the esophagus with a balloon and during scanning with functional magnetic resonance imaging. Activation within right insular and bilateral dorsal anterior cingulate gyrus was found to be significantly greater during esophageal stimulation with fearful than with neutral faces. In addition, anxiety and discomfort were measured after presentation of faces depicting either low, moderate, or high intensities of fear. Both anxiety and discomfort, as well as activation within the left dorsal anterior cingulate gyrus and bilateral anterior insulae, were greater with high-intensity compared with low-intensity expressions. Therefore, visceral stimulation occurring in a negative emotional context is associated with altered brain responses in the anterior cingulate gyrus and insula, which indicates a modulatory effect of emotional context upon interoceptive sensibility.

3.2.2 Negative emotions amplify pain perception

Top-down influences upon symptom perception are also well documented for negative emotions such as anger. Anger affects pain more severely when it is directed at oneself than when directed at others, such as healthcare providers (Okifuji et al., 1999). Anger has been found to induce more consistent changes in pain unpleasantness rather than pain intensity (Huynh Bao and Rainville, 2003; Rainville, 2004). In addition, anger activates some regions of the brain that are also involved in pain processing, like the anterior cingulate cortex, the amygdala, and the brainstem (Damasio et al., 2000). There is also some experimental evidence that the endogenous opioid systems are involved in anger-associated changes in pain. In fact, a reduction in endogenous opioid activity has been found during anger (Bruehl et al., 2002, 2003).

There is also a clear-cut link between depression and pain. A high degree of comorbidity between chronic pain and depression is widely recognized (Vimpari et al., 1995; Feinmann, 1999; Korszun, 2002; Mongini et al., 2007), and there is compelling evidence that depressed pain-free individuals are on average two times more likely to develop chronic musculoskeletal pain than nondepressed pain-free individuals (Magni et al., 1994; Carroll et al., 2004; Larson et al., 2004). It should be noted, however, that patients suffering from major depression can show normal or even reduced sensitivity to noxious stimuli applied to the skin (Lautenbacher et al., 1994; Bar et al., 2003, 2006, 2007; Dickens et al., 2003), but they show hyperalgesia for deep somatic pain (Bar et al., 2005), which indicates a high degree of variability in this population of patients. Neuroimaging studies in patients with major depression disorder have shown higher activation levels in left ventrolateral thalamus, the right ventrolateral prefrontal cortex and the dorsolateral prefrontal cortex (Bar et al., 2007), and increased activation in the right amygdala and decreased activation in periaqueductal gray, rostral anterior cingulate, and prefrontal cortices (Strigo et al., 2008). In addition, Giesecke et al. (2005) found that fibromyalgia patients with major depression showed bilateral amygdala activation and a signal increase in the anterior insula following painful stimulation, whereas fibromyalgia patients without depressive symptoms showed no changes. Likewise, Schweinhardt et al. (2008) found an activation cluster in the medial prefrontal cortex of rheumatoid arthritis patients that correlated with the degree of depressive symptoms.

A lack of descending inhibition might be one of the mechanisms which is responsible for these effects (Julien et al., 2005; Klauenberg et al., 2008), but the activation of descending facilitatory pathways may also occur, and indeed studies in animals have identified a descending facilitatory projection from the periaqueductal gray to the rostral ventral medulla inducing pro-nociceptive effects (Carlson et al., 2007). Key regions in this descending pain modulatory network are prefrontal, anterior cingulate and insular cortices, amygdala, hypothalamus, and brainstem structures like the periaqueductal gray, rostral ventromedial medulla, dorsolateral pons/tegmentum, and the descending projections to the spinal dorsal horn, although the prefrontal cortex is likely to play a major role (Tracey and Mantyh, 2007; Wiech and Tracey, 2009). According to this perspective, a negative emotions-induced hyporesponsivity of the prefrontal cortex might provide the basis for the aggravation of pain. In other words, the prefrontal hyporesponsivity might be triggered by negative emotions (Wiech and Tracey, 2009). Interestingly, Wager et al. (2008) found evidence that the activation of the prefrontal cortex leads to a reduction in negative emotion by influencing those structures that are directly involved in emotional experiences.

3.3 Seeking relief

3.3.1 Motivation aims to regulate internal states and to get a reward

Whereas in a simple reflex there is a good correlation between the intensity of the stimulus and the magnitude of the response, in more complex behavioral responses such correlation is lacking. In other words, the same stimulus does not always produce the same response. The concept of motivation emerged from the need to explain this variability of behavioral responses. Motivation is characterized by a set of factors that trigger, maintain, and orient behavior. The concept of motivation can be better explained by considering homeostasis, i.e., the fact that a given system or physiological parameter is in equilibrium in normal circumstances (Hull, 1951). For example, the temperature of the body is within a given homeostatic range in normal conditions (36–37°C in humans). Likewise, liquids and some nutritional substances, such as lipids and glycids, are maintained within a given homeostatic range. Any perturbation of this homeostasis leads to a tension of the organism, which is called drive, or motivation. This drive forces humans and animals to start the appropriate action, like looking for a warmer place, water, or food, so as to restore the normal homeostatic equilibrium. As soon as homeostasis returns to normal, the motivated behavior ends. Cultural factors play a crucial role in humans compared to the natural motivated behaviors. For example, money is a powerful incentive to motivated behavior in most individuals and, similarly, high scores are potent incentives for many students.

The general organization of motivated behavior can be summarized as shown in Fig. 3.4A. Either an increase or decrease in the variable to be controlled, for example, body temperature or food/water intake, is revealed through receptors that send afferent signals to the control system. This in turn compares these changes with a reference value and, accordingly, adjusts the physiological variable. There are at least two

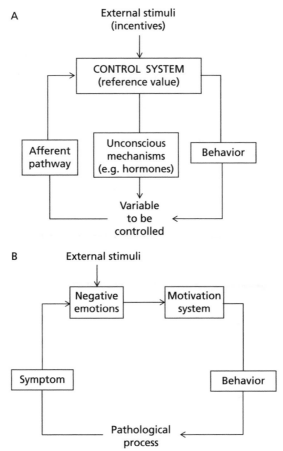

Fig. 3.4 Motivated behavior. (A) General organization of a system aimed at suppressing discomfort. Changes in a variable to be controlled, e.g., body temperature or food/water intake, are detected by some receptors that send afferent signals to the control system. This compares these changes with a reference value and, accordingly, restores the normal value of the variable through both unconscious mechanisms, such as hormone secretion, and the activation of a behavioral act, e.g., looking for some water. External stimuli, or incentives, may trigger motivated behavior even in the absence of changes in the variable to be controlled, e.g., drinking in the absence of liquids depletion. (B) Organization of the system aimed at suppressing sickness. This schema is reframed from the more general model in A. Pathological processes, e.g., tissue damage, is the variable to be controlled. Thence, a symptom, e.g., pain, travels along the afferent pathway and gives rise to negative emotions, e.g., anxiety. The motivational system is activated, with increased motivation to suppress the discomfort. Finally, a specific behavioral repertoire is started that is aimed at seeking relief by suppressing the pathological process (compare with Fig. 3.2). External stimuli, e.g., a negative diagnosis, may induce negative emotions directly, without the presence of any symptom.

mechanisms through which this adjustment takes place. First, some completely unconscious mechanisms, such as hormone secretion, are activated that make the variable return to a normal value. Second, a behavioral repertoire is triggered, e.g., looking for some water, that restores the normal homeostatic range. External stimuli, or incentives, always operate upon the control system and may trigger motivated behavior even in the absence of changes in the variable to be controlled, for example, drinking even though there was no depletion of water in the body.

Motivation and reward are intimately related. Motivated behavior is aimed at getting a reward, be it a cultural reward such as money or the suppression of discomfort such as hunger. A distinction between discomfort suppression and reward search is not straightforward. For example, trying to suppress discomfort involves a reward, because being discomfort-free can be certainly considered a form of reward. Likewise, it turns out that reward search, be it food or money, is certainly aimed at placating a negative internal state.

In the last few decades, there have been substantial advances in the understanding of the neurobiological mechanisms of motivation and reward (Benedetti, 2010). Specific mechanisms have been identified for specific motivated behaviors, for example, the mechanisms that are aimed at suppressing hunger and thus stimulate food intake are very complex, involving both neural and hormonal regulatory factors. Thirst mechanisms are complex as well. There are two types of thirst: hypovolumetric and osmotic. In hypovolumetric thirst, the extracellular volume of liquids decreases and this decrease is detected by pressure receptors. In osmotic thirst, osmolarity is increased, for example, because of an increase of sodium chloride in extracellular fluids. Thirst can be merely hedonistic, without any need to introduce liquids into the organism. For example, water intake can be aimed only at placating the uncomfortable sensation of dry mouth. The homeostatic and motivational model also applies to thermoregulation, whereby the motivated behavior aims to seek either warm or cold places.

The homeostatic/motivational model of Fig. 3.4A can also be applied to pathological processes, as shown in Fig. 3.4B (Benedetti, 2010). Here there are a number of variables to be controlled, e.g., tissue damage, whereas the afferent pathway originates from receptors in the impaired tissue. This is a sensory pathway that gives rise to a symptom, e.g., pain, through interoceptive and/or nociceptive afferents, and to negative emotions such as anxiety (compare with "feeling sick" in Fig. 3.2). It turns out that negative emotions trigger the motivational system, with increased motivation to suppress the discomfort. Finally, a specific behavioral repertoire is started that is aimed at seeking relief (compare with "seeking relief" in Fig. 3.2). It should be noted that a symptom is not always necessary to evoke negative emotions and to trigger the motivational system. External stimuli, for example, the negative diagnosis by a doctor, may induce negative emotions directly, without the presence of any symptom. Therefore, the systems in Fig. 3.2 and Fig. 3.4A,B are similar, all representing homeostatic adjustments.

From an evolutionary perspective, it is interesting to note that motivated behavior that is triggered by sickness is present in animals, with more or less simple behavioral repertoires, as well as in humans, with much more complex behavioral acts, such as going to a doctor's office. In animals, behavior that aims to fight sickness is adaptive in nature, that is, animals may adopt the most appropriate behavioral repertoires that can reduce the severity and shorten the duration of illness (Weary et al., 2009). Many of the behaviors shown by ill animals are part of a coordinated strategy to fight disease (Hart, 1988; Dantzer, 2004). For example, heat conservation during infection is achieved through both physiological responses, like vasoconstriction, and behavioral responses, such as postural changes. These strategies allow energy to be preserved, particularly by considering that sick animals may reduce food intake. In this regard, reduction in appetite helps promote recovery (Johnson, 2002; Weary et al., 2009). Animal behavior that aims to fight sickness may have even more complex meanings. It may signal vigor and/or need (Weary et al., 2009). Where and when possible, sick animals can mask any signs of vulnerability, especially if the illness makes them an easier target for predation. This may be true in early and mild stages of a disease, for it is more difficult to mask signs of vulnerability when the illness is more severe. Conversely, animals may benefit from signaling their infirmity, for example, for soliciting parental care. Therefore, different forms of motivated behavior may take place in different situations. Preys that are continuously exposed to predators are likely to mask their sickness, whilst domestic animals are more likely to signal their infirmity.

As occurs in animals, different motivated behaviors are also present in humans, and these depend mainly on cultural differences. Mainstream medicine and the conventional doctor is the most common means through which this motivated behavior is accomplished in Western societies, but alternative medicines are also common. Conversely, in non-Western societies, traditional practices and shamanism are more usual. It is important to realize that the ability, competence, and skills of the healer do not matter at all. What counts is the patient's behavior, regardless of the healer whom he refers to. It is like a thirsty man who wants to placate his discomfort. In the study of motivation, what matters is his water-seeking behavior, regardless of the place where he goes. He can choose either the right or the wrong place, according to his beliefs and expectations. Therefore, it must be clear that, when studying motivation to suppress sickness, the behavioral repertoire that is adopted does not have to be necessarily the correct choice.

3.3.2 Motivation and reward mechanisms involve the mesolimbic dopaminergic system

The mesolimbic dopaminergic system (see Fig. 2.10 for a simplified schema) has been found to be activated in a number of reward-seeking behaviors, such that today it is better known as the motivation/reward dopaminergic system (Schultz et al., 2000; Schultz, 2002). This holds true for hunger, sex, electrical self-stimulation, and drug self-administration (Box 3.3). Whereas all these behaviors are present in both animals and humans, it is worth noting that there are reward-seeking behaviors that are typical of human beings, in which the very same reward network is activated. For example, monetary reward typically activates the mesolimbic dopaminergic system (Knutson et al., 2001; Scott et al., 2007). The overlap of the observed activations of the mesolimbic dopamine system in response to a variety of motivated behaviors and rewards, such as alimentary stimuli and food intake, sexual arousal and sexual activity, drugs of abuse and euphoria-inducing drugs, and monetary incentives and gamble, is consistent with a contribution of common circuitry to the processing of diverse rewards as well as to the initiation of different motivation-induced behavioral repertoires.

Box 3.3 The experiment by Olds and Milner

In the 1950s, Olds and Milner (1954) paved the road to the understanding of both the anatomy and physiology of the motivation/reward system. In their classical experiment, they implanted an electrode in several regions of the rat brain. The electrode was connected to a stimulator that could be activated by pressing a lever within the cage. Thus the rat, which was free to move around the cage, had the possibility to press the lever and to stimulate himself whenever he wanted (Fig. 3.5). After a first period of wandering in his cage, he randomly pressed the lever, thus self-delivering an electrical stimulation. After a short period of learning, his behavior changed completely. The rat started pressing the lever many times per minute, reducing dramatically the time spent for feeding, drinking, and grooming behavior. This effect is called intracranial electrical self-stimulation. Sometimes its magnitude and efficacy is so big that the health conditions of some rats deteriorate because of the suppression of both feeding and drinking behavior.

The key questions that emerged from this and other experiments were mainly two: why rats stimulate themselves and which brain areas induce the self-stimulation effect. As to the first question, the most plausible explanation is that rats stimulate themselves repeatedly and compulsively because they experience a pleasant sensation. For this reason, the electrical self-stimulation is called positive reinforcement, or otherwise reward. In other words, the activation of these centers by electrical stimulation induces pleasure, thus the animals adopt a motivated behavior that aims to repeatedly seek a reward. In support of the fact that animals feel a pleasant sensation there are several studies in humans. From the early studies in humans by Heath (1963) to more recent human studies (e.g., Benedetti et al., 2004), it has been found that the intraoperative stimulation of several limbic areas may produce pleasant sensations and even compulsive self-stimulation. For example, patients may report a general feeling of pleasure, such as happiness, or more specific pleasurable sensations, like sexual orgasm.

As to the second question, i.e., which regions produce these effects, many sites have been discovered over the past years. Their stimulation elicits the self-stimulation phenomenon, thereby indicating that these regions are involved in

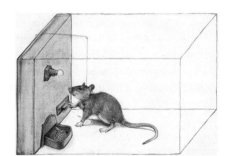

Fig. 3.5 A rat self-stimulating his own brain through a lever.

Box 3.3 The experiment by Olds and Milner (continued)

motivation/reward mechanisms. The most powerful effects can be obtained by stimulating the septal area, some regions of the hypothalamus, like the lateral hypothalamus, the medial forebrain bundle, and the ventral tegmental area. The general organization that has emerged from these and other studies is represented by the ventral tegmental area that sends a dopaminergic projection to the nucleus accumbens as well as to other regions, such as the amygdala. The nucleus accumbens, in turn, projects to the prefrontal cortex.

Motivated behavior that aims to suppress discomfort from sickness and to seek the reward of clinical amelioration can be approached within the context of motivation/reward mechanisms (Benedetti, 2010). There is compelling experimental evidence that the mesolimbic dopaminergic system may be activated when a subject expects clinical improvement. Most, if not all, of this evidence comes from the placebo literature and will be discussed in detail in Part 2, particularly for pain and Parkinson's disease. When a patient seeks relief, he eventually expects the reward of the positive therapeutic outcome, irrespective of whether or not a therapy has been started. In other words, the patient expects that his own seeking behavior will probably lead to a successful outcome.

For example, de la Fuente-Fernandez et al. (2001) assessed the release of endogenous dopamine by using positron emission tomography after placebo administration, and found that dopamine was released in the striatum, corresponding to a change of 200% or more in extracellular dopamine concentration and comparable to the response to amphetamine in subjects with an intact dopamine system. Likewise, Mayberg et al. (2002) measured the changes in brain glucose metabolism by means of positron emission tomography in patients with unipolar depression who were treated with either placebo or fluoxetine for 6 weeks. They found ventral striatal (nucleus accumbens) and orbital frontal changes in both placebo and drug responders at 1 week of treatment, that is, well before clinical benefit. Thus these changes are not associated with the clinical response, but rather to expectation and anticipation of the clinical benefit. This pattern of activation of the nucleus accumbens is in agreement with an involvement of reward mechanisms in antidepressant placebo responses. In another brain imaging study in which both positron emission tomography and functional magnetic resonance imaging were used, Scott et al. (2007) tested the correlation between the responsiveness to placebo and that to monetary reward. These authors found that placebo responsiveness was related to the activation of dopamine in the nucleus accumbens, as assessed by using in vivo receptor binding positron emission tomography. The very same subjects were then tested with functional magnetic resonance imaging for monetary responses in the nucleus accumbens. A correlation between the placebo responses and the monetary responses was found: the larger the nucleus accumbens responses to monetary reward, the stronger the nucleus accumbens responses to placebos. This study indicates common reward mechanisms for placebo responsiveness and monetary responses.

3.4 **Meeting the therapist**

3.4.1 **Trust, admiration, and hope involve both neural and hormonal systems**

The encounter between the patient and the doctor is a complex social interaction that embraces plenty of cognitive and emotional factors, such as trust and hope in the patient and empathy and compassion in the doctor. The study of the underlying psychobiological mechanisms is not a simple one for at least two reasons. First, there is an intricate interplay among different psychological factors and often it is not possible to identify the most important. For example, the doctor's empathic behavior is not always present. Likewise, the patient's trust may be in some circumstances completely lacking. Second, we do not know very much about the neural underpinnings of complex social interactions, like trust and compassion. Nonetheless, it is possible today to have a general idea of what is going on in both the patient's and the doctor's brain when they meet.

For example, usually the patient's trust is likely to play an important role. Trust can be conceptualized as a set of beliefs that the therapist will behave in a certain way (Thom and Campbell, 1997). Patients usually base their trust on the therapist's competence, compassion, confidentiality, reliability, and communication (Pearson and Raeke, 2000). Patients' trust in their physicians has always been considered as an important element that per se may have beneficial effects on the overall health status (Box 3.4). This may occur through a better adherence to treatments as well as the reinforcement of clinical relationship and patient satisfaction (Pearson and Raeke, 2000).

Face exploration is not necessary for trustworthiness judgments, for a time lag of only 100 ms is sufficient for judgments (Willis and Todorov, 2006). Patients with amygdala damage show an impairment in recognizing emotional facial expressions, and patients with bilateral amygdala lesions show a bias to perceive untrustworthy faces as trustworthy (Adolphs et al., 1998). There is accumulating evidence on the role of the amygdala in trustworthiness judgments that comes from imaging studies (Winston et al., 2002). In general, the amygdala response to faces increases as the untrustworthiness of the faces increases (Engell et al., 2007).

Trust behavior has been found to undergo hormonal modulation by oxytocin. An increase in plasma oxytocin was found in subjects who participated in a trust game whereby cooperative behavior can benefit both parties (Zak et al., 2004). In a different study, it was found that in a trust game the intranasal administration of oxytocin was associated to a larger amount of money given by an investor to a trustee (Kosfeld et al., 2005). Interestingly, oxytocin receptors are abundant in the amygdala (Huber et al., 2005). The neural circuitry of trustworthy behavior was studied by combining the intranasal administration of oxytocin with functional magnetic resonance imaging (Baumgartner et al., 2008). The investigators found that oxytocin induced no change in trusting behavior after the subjects learned that their trust had been breached several times, while the control subjects who had not received oxytocin decreased their trust. This difference in trust adaptation was associated with a reduced activation in the amygdala, the midbrain regions, and the dorsal striatum in subjects receiving oxytocin. Taken together, these findings suggest that oxytocin acts on its own receptors in the amygdala by reducing neural activity, thereby restoring an emotion of trustworthiness.

Box 3.4 Scales for the assessment of trust and hope

Trust

Trust in doctors can be measured. The first study that was aimed at measuring the patient's trust was performed by Anderson and Dedrick (1990), who created a 11-item Trust in Physician Scale, as follows:

1 I doubt that my doctor really cares about me as a person.

2 My doctor is usually considerate of my needs and puts them first.

3 I trust my doctor so much that I always try to follow his/her advice.

4 If my doctor tells me something is so, then it must be true.

5 I sometimes distrust my doctor's opinion and would like a second one.

6 I trust my doctor's judgment about my medical care.

7 I feel my doctor does not do everything he/she should for my medical care.

8 I trust my doctor to put my medical needs above all other considerations when treating my medical problems.

9 My doctor is a real expert in taking care of medical problems like mine.

10 I trust my doctor to tell me if a mistake was made about my treatment.

11 I sometimes worry that my doctor may not keep the information we discuss totally private.

The following is another scale, the Patient Trust Scale by Kao et al. (1998a, 1998b). In this psychometric evaluation, patients are asked how much they trust their physician:

1 to put their health and well-being above keeping down health plan costs

2 to keep personally sensitive medical information private

3 to provide them with information on all potential medical options and not just options covered by the health plan

4 to refer them to a specialist when necessary

5 to admit them to the hospital when needed

6 to make appropriate medical decisions regardless of health plan rules and guidelines

7 to judge about their medical care

8 to perform necessary medical tests and procedures regardless of costs

9 to offer them high-quality medical care

10 to perform only medically necessary tests and procedures.

It is interesting to note how much the concerns about health costs are represented in this psychometric evaluation and, in particular, the concerns about the priority of health and well-being over health plan rules, guidelines, and costs. Not surprisingly, this reflects the patient's concerns about receiving appropriate medical care, regardless of health plan rules and costs.

Box 3.4 Scales for the assessment of trust and hope (continued)

Hope

Hope can be measured as well. The first scale assesses trait hope, i.e., hope as a trait of personality (Snyder et al., 1991a). Its items are the following:

1 I can think of many ways to get out of a jam.

2 I energetically pursue my goals.

3 I feel tired most of the time.

4 There are lots of ways around any problem.

5 I am easily downed in an argument.

6 I can think of many ways to get the things in life that are important to me.

7 I worry about my health.

8 Even when others get discouraged, I know I can find a way to solve the problem.

9 My past experiences have prepared me well for my future.

10 I've been pretty successful in life.

11 I usually find myself worrying about something.

12 I meet the goals that I set for myself.

All the key elements in Snyder's theory of hope (Snyder, 2002) are tested, namely, goals, pathways, and planning to meet goals, as well as the motivational components. For example, in items 6 and 8, it is explicitly asked whether individuals are capable of using alternative pathways in order to reach the goals they had set for themselves.

The second scale is about state hope and is not very different from the first one. However, in this case the main emphasis is on how respondents describe themselves as they are "right now" (Snyder et al., 1996). The items are as follows:

1 If I should find myself in a jam, I could think of many ways to get out of it.

2 At the present time, I am energetically pursuing my goals.

3 There are lots of ways around any problem that I am facing now.

4 Right now, I see myself as being pretty successful.

5 I can think of many ways to reach my current goals.

6 At this time, I am meeting the goals that I have set for myself.

Thus, although many elements take part in hope, at least two key factors can be identified: expectation and motivation. The subject expects the future to be better than the present and is strongly motivated to adopt the necessary behavioral repertoire in order to get the goals that he had set for himself.

Trust is related to admiration. If one admires a person, one is likely to trust them. Admiration may represent a very important aspect of the therapist–patient encounter, for it can be elicited either by observing virtuous behavior towards the suffering of others or by displays of virtuosic skill. In the first case, admiration has to do with social/psychological circumstances, i.e., virtue, whereas in the second case it is related to physical circumstances, i.e., skilful abilities. Admiration has been found to engage the posteromedial cortices, i.e., the posterior cingulate cortex, the retrosplenial area, and the precuneus. However, whereas admiration for virtue induces activation in the inferior/posterior portion of the posteromedial cortices, admiration for skills produces a larger activation in the superior/anterior portion of the posteromedial cortices (Immordino-Yang et al., 2009). Thus admiration is mediated by two discrete systems, one for virtue and the other for skills (Fig. 3.6).

Another important element in the patient is hope (Box 3.4). This can be defined as a positive motivational state that is based on a sense of successful goal-directed energy and planning to meet goals (Snyder et al., 1991b; Snyder, 2002). Motivation is central to hope, and actually it interacts with goal-directed behavior. High-hope individuals are capable of using alternative pathways if an impediment of any sort occurs in the planned behavior, so that the same goal can be reached in a different way (Snyder, 2002). Some studies indicate that hope has beneficial effects on health, for example better coping with arthritis and pain (Snyder, 2002). Only a few data exist on the biological underpinnings of hope. For example, a negative correlation between prefrontal binding to serotonin 5-HT2A receptors and levels of hopelessness was found in attempted suicide, according to the rule: the lower the binding to serotonin receptors, the higher the degree of hopelessness (van Heeringen et al., 2003). An activation of the hypothalamus–pituitary–adrenal axis has also been found in a number of studies that used inescapable shocks as a model (Henkel et al., 2002), and indeed adverse experiences might lead to stress sensitivity. This, in turn, would lead to excessive norepinephrine release and its subsequent depletion, with the consequent hopelessness (Mann, 2003).

3.4.2 Nonverbal communication can be crucial during the doctor–patient interaction

Nonverbal communication is critical in any social encounter, including the special situation of the doctor–patient interaction. Nonverbal messages and intentions can be communicated either consciously or unconsciously to others, and indeed gestural communication may have represented a primitive form of language (Rizzolatti and Arbib, 1998). There are a number of sensory inputs that represent the basis of nonverbal communication, most notably vision and touch.

Facial expressions represent an excellent source of information and play a fundamental role in signaling social intentions from which people infer meaning (Frith and Frith, 1999). A number of brain imaging studies in humans support the idea that the lateral side of the right mid-fusiform gyrus, the "fusiform face area" or FFA, is activated robustly and specifically by faces (Kanwisher et al., 1997; Tsao and Livingstone, 2008). It should be noted, however, that the fusiform face area does not respond only to face stimuli but also to nonface object, albeit less robustly. The information that is gained

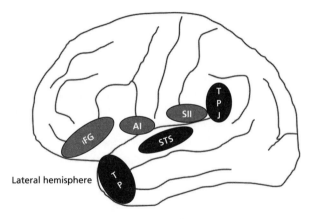

○ Admiration for skills and compassion for physical pain

○ Admiration for virtue and compassion for social pain

● Cognitive perspective taking

● Empathic emotional ability

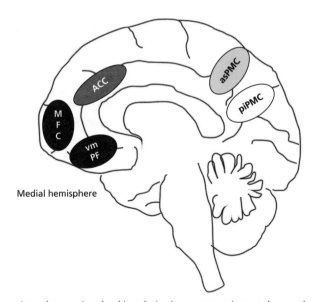

Fig. 3.6 Brain regions that are involved in admiration, compassion, and empathy. During the doctor–patient relationship, several complex brain functions are involved, such as the patient's admiration/trust towards the figure of the doctor, as well as the doctor's empathic and compassionate behavior. ACC, anterior cingulate cortex; AI, anterior insula; asPMC, anterosuperior posteromedial cortex; iFG, inferior frontal gyrus; MFC, medial frontal cortex; piPMC, posteroinferior posteromedial cortex; SII, secondary somatosensory area; STS, superior temporal sulcus; TP, temporal pole; TPJ, temporal parietal junction; vmPF, ventromedial prefrontal cortex. Reproduced from *Physiological Reviews*, 93 (3), Placebo and the New Physiology of the Doctor-Patient Relationship, Fabrizio Benedetti, pp. 1207–1246, figure 4, DOI: 10.1152/physrev.00043.2012 Copyright 2013, The American Physiological Society.

from faces is fundamental for social interaction, including the doctor–patient encounter. Eye contact, i.e., the mutual eye gaze that connects people together, represents another important aspect of social interaction and solicits attention and interest of the interacting persons (Senju and Johnson, 2009). At least five regions have been found to be activated more by direct gaze than by averted gaze: the fusiform gyrus (or fusiform face area), the anterior part of the right superior temporal sulcus, the posterior part of right superior temporal sulcus, the medial prefrontal cortex and orbitofrontal cortex, and the amygdala (Senju and Johnson, 2009).

As for vision, touch may convey strong emotional information in many circumstances. For example, social grooming is an important mediator of social relationships in nonhuman primates (section 3.1.1). In humans, a powerful emotional tactile stimulus is represented by hand-holding, which can be considered a nonverbal supportive social behavior in all respects. Coan et al. (2006) studied married women who were subjected to the threat of electric shock in three different conditions: while holding their husband's hand, while holding the hand of an anonymous male experimenter, or holding no hand at all. Holding the spouse's hand produced a decrease in unpleasantness ratings compared to no hand-holding, whilst holding the stranger's hand did not decrease unpleasantness. Reduced activation was found in the right dorsolateral prefrontal cortex, left caudate–nucleus accumbens, and superior colliculus when the women held their husband's hand. A more limited reduction of activation occurred when they held the hand of a stranger, e.g., in the ventral anterior cingulate cortex, posterior cingulate, and right postcentral gyrus. These effects of spousal hand-holding were related to marital quality: the higher the marital quality, the lesser the activation in the right anterior insula, superior frontal gyrus, and hypothalamus during spouse hand-holding, but not during stranger hand-holding.

3.4.3 Different forms of empathy and compassion are related to different neural networks

Facial expressions are likely to have evolved for eliciting medical attention from others (Williams, 2002). A greater facial expression of pain in the presence of potential caregivers than in their absence is of primary importance, so that the presence of potential caregivers would prompt the release of suppression of pain facial expressions. This, in turn, triggers the caregiver's empathic and compassionate behavior. The social connection between the suffering patient, who expresses his discomfort, and the empathic doctor is at the very heart of the doctor–patient relationship. Jensen et al. (2014) investigated physicians' brain activations during patient–physician interaction while the patient was experiencing pain. They found that physicians activated brain regions implicated in expectancy for pain relief and increased attention during treatment of patients, including the right ventrolateral and dorsolateral prefrontal cortices. The physician's ability to take the patients' perspective was correlated with increased activations in the rostral anterior cingulate cortex. Overall, physician treatment seems to involve neural representations of expectation, reward processing, and empathy, paired with increased activation in attention-related structures.

Empathy refers to an intersubjective process through which the cognitive and emotional experiences of another come to be shared, without losing sight of the original source of the experience (Decety and Jackson, 2004). It is important to note that empathy is distinguished from compassion (Batson et al., 2007; Eisenberg, 2007; Hein and Singer, 2008). Empathy is not necessarily linked to prosocial motivation, namely, the concern about the others' well-being. By contrast, prosocial motivation is involved in compassion. In fact, compassion enables individuals to enter into and maintain relationships of caring and tends to motivate us to help people who are emotionally suffering.

Experimental evidence suggests that there are at least two mechanisms of empathy: emotional contagion and cognitive perspective-taking (de Waal 2008). Whereas the former is thought to support our ability to empathize emotionally, i.e., to share the other person's emotional feelings ("I feel what you feel"), the latter involves complex cognitive components, whereby one infers the state of the other person ("I understand what you feel"). Whereas cognitive perspective taking activates the medial prefrontal regions, the superior temporal sulcus, the temporal pole, and the temporoparietal junction (Frith and Frith, 2006; Saxe, 2006), empathizing with another person has been found to activate somatosensory and insular cortices as well as the anterior cingulate cortex (Hein and Singer, 2008) (Fig. 3.6).

Compassion can be evoked by witnessing situations of personal loss and social deprivation (social pain), or by witnessing bodily injury (physical pain). Whereas the former pertains to social/psychological circumstances, the latter has to do with immediate physical circumstances (Immordino-Yang et al., 2009). Compassion for social and physical pain has been found to engage two different neural circuits (Fig. 3.6). The former is associated with strong activation in the inferior/posterior portion of the posteromedial cortices, whereas the latter produced a larger activation in the superior/anterior portion of the posteromedial cortices (Immordino-Yang et al., 2009). These neural networks, one for the emotions related to someone else's psychological state and the other for the emotions related to someone else's physical state, are engaged by both compassion and admiration (see section 3.4.1).

Interestingly, compassionate concern towards a suffering person is related to the motivation to help and, accordingly, a positive intrinsic reward feeling may occur as a result of experiencing compassion for others (Sprecher and Fehr, 2006). Indeed, Kim et al. (2009) found that compassionate attitude activated a neural network in the midbrain/ventral striatum/septal network region, a key region involved in prosocial/social approach motivation and reward mechanisms. These findings emphasize the differences between empathic behavior, which does not necessarily involve motivational systems, and compassionate behavior, whereby the motivation to alleviate others' suffering represents the central element.

3.4.4 **Pain can be made a positive experience**

The different meaning that is attributed to a symptom can be crucial in its global perception. For example, clinicians have long known that cancer pain can be perceived as more unpleasant than postoperative pain (Ferrell and Dean, 1995; Smith et al., 1998;

Cormie et al., 2008), and this can be due to the different meanings of cancer on the one hand and of surgery on the other. Whereas the former often means death, the latter is associated to healing and recovery. Similarly, different religions attribute different meanings to pain and suffering, and this may lead to different pain experiences (Henderson, 2000; Whitman, 2007; Koffman et al., 2008).

In a study, the meaning of pain was changed from negative to positive in healthy subjects through verbal suggestions (Benedetti et al., 2013). The subjects had to tolerate ischemic arm pain as long as they could. However, whereas one group was informed about the aversive nature of the task, as done in any pain study, a second group was told that the ischemia would be beneficial to the muscles, thus stressing the beneficial nature of the pain endurance task. In this latter group, pain tolerance was significantly higher compared to the first one, an effect that was partially blocked by the opioid antagonist naltrexone alone and by the cannabinoid antagonist rimonabant alone. However, the increased tolerance was antagonized completely by the combined administration of naltrexone and rimonabant, which suggests that a positive approach to pain reduces the global pain experience through the co-activation of the opioid and cannabinoid systems. These findings show that the way patients interpret their own symptoms may have a dramatic effect on their emotional experience.

In a different study, pain perception, skin conductance, and brain activation patterns to moderate pain were investigated in two different contexts (Leknes et al., 2013). In the "control context" participants had a 50% chance of receiving a moderate painful stimulation or a nonpainful warm stimulation, whereas in the "relative relief context" participants had a 50% chance of receiving a moderate or high painful stimulation. Thus, in the control session moderate pain was perceived as the worst possible outcome whereas in the relative relief session, moderate pain was perceived as the best possible outcome and represented relative relief. Moderate pain was perceived as painful and elicited negative feelings in the control context (worst outcome) but it was perceived surprisingly pleasant in the pain relief context (best outcome) and similar in magnitude to the nonpainful warm stimulation in the control context. The measured change in skin conductance during moderate noxious stimulation was significantly lower during moderate pain in the relative relief context compared to the control context. Moreover, when moderate pain was perceived as pleasant, the activity in the insula and dorsal anterior cingulate cortex was significantly attenuated whereas the activity in the reward circuitry, including the medial orbitofrontal and ventromedial prefrontal cortices, significantly enhanced. The fact that pain can acquire a positive meaning within the appropriate context suggests that the manipulation of the context in this direction may be harnessed to the patient's advantage.

3.5 Receiving the therapy

3.5.1 Mechanism-based or disease-based classification of placebo effects?

Placebo responses occur within this very complex sequence of events, from feeling sick and seeking relief to meeting the therapist (Benedetti, 2010, 2013). The final, and perhaps the most important, step in the doctor–patient relationship is represented by the very act of receiving a treatment. The ritual of the therapeutic act and the effects that it may have on the therapeutic outcome are the elements which have received great attention in the past few years and represent the main target of the present book. As described in Chapter 2, and particularly in sections 2.2 and 2.3, the psychosocial context and the therapeutic ritual surrounding the treatment and the patient have been approached by using the placebo response as a model to understand the underlying physiological mechanisms. The doctor, and more in general the healer, is surely the key element in this therapeutic ritual (see section 3.1.3).

One of the main things we have learned over the past years is that there is not a single mechanism of the placebo response, and actually there is not a single placebo response but many, so that different mechanisms are involved in different medical conditions and across different therapeutic interventions. The main challenge in current placebo research is to find out how these different mechanisms should be considered and classified. For example, as we have seen in section 2.3, placebo administration can induce either anxiety reduction or activation of reward mechanisms, depending on different circumstances. Likewise, different forms of learning can take part in placebo responsiveness in different conditions, ranging from classical conditioning to social learning. Or, otherwise, genetic mechanisms may represent the basis for the variability in the magnitude of the placebo response across individuals. Therefore, a first approach to the classification of different placebo responses might be based on the mechanism that is involved, as described in section 2.3.

However, unfortunately today we do not know exactly when and in which conditions these mechanisms take place. For example, anxiety reduction might be important only in some medical conditions but not in others, and learning might be a common mechanism across all medical conditions. Therefore, a second approach to the classification of different placebo responses is a disease-based classification, whereby the biological underpinnings are investigated in different conditions such as pain and motor disorders, and across different systems, like the immune and endocrine system.

To date, it is not clear whether we should differentiate the placebo responses on the basis of the mechanism or rather on the basis of the disease (Benedetti, 2013). This is surely a future challenge in placebo research, and it will be crucial to understand where (in which disease), when (in which circumstance), and how (with which mechanisms) placebos work. Therefore, due to our limited understanding of the relationship between mechanisms and diseases, this book describes the placebo responses across different diseases, namely, with a disease-based classification approach, as will be seen in Parts 2 and 3.

3.6 **Points for further discussion**

1 From an evolutionary perspective, the interplay between altruism, empathy, and the emergence of medical care needs to be investigated in more detail, for it is likely to give us important information on human biology and evolution.

2 Although reciprocal altruism can explain why cases of altruism occur among nonkin organisms, we need to better understand whether there are other human

altruistic acts that obey neither kin selection nor reciprocal altruism. In other words, does genuine altruism exist, in which there is no advantage to the altruistic individual?

3 The doctor–patient relationship is an excellent model to understand complex brain functions mediating trust, hope, empathy, compassion, and altruism. Thus we need to develop better neuroscientific approaches and models in order to investigate these functions.

4 It would be interesting to assess whether replacing the doctor with a machine, e.g., a computer which delivers diagnoses and therapies, makes a difference. In other words, does the human and humane factor matter?

References

Adolphs R, Tranel D and Damasio AR (1998). The human amygdala in social judgment. *Nature*, **393**, 470–4.

Anderson LA and Dedrick RF (1990). Development of the Trust in Physician Scale: a measure to assess interpersonal trust in patient-physician relationships. *Psychological Reports*, **67**, 1091–100.

Aziz Q, Anderson JLR, Valind S *et al.* (1997). Identification of human brain loci processing esophageal sensation using positron emission tomography. *Gastroenterology*, **113**, 50–9.

Bar KJ, Brehm S, Boettger MK, Boettger S, Wagner G and Sauer H (2005). Pain perception in major depression depends on pain modality. *Pain*, **117**, 97–103.

Bar KJ, Brehm S, Boettger MK, Wagner G, Boettger S and Sauer H (2006). Decreased sensitivity to experimental pain in adjustment disorder. *European Journal of Pain*, **10**, 467–71.

Bar KJ, Greiner W, Letsch A, Kobele R and Sauer H (2003). Influence of gender and hemispheric lateralization on heat pain perception in major depression. *Journal of Psychiatric Research*, **37**, 345–53.

Bar KJ, Wagner G, Koschke M *et al.* (2007). Increased prefrontal activation during pain perception in major depression. *Biological Psychiatry*, **62**, 1281–7.

Batson CD, Eklund JH, Chermok VL, Hoyt JL and Ortiz BG (2007). An additional antecedent of empathic concern: valuing the welfare of the person in need. *Journal of Personality and Social Psychology*, **93**, 65–74.

Baumgartner T, Heinrichs M, Vonlanthen A, Fischbacher U and Fehr E (2008). Oxytocin shapes the neural circuitry of trust and trust adaptation in humans. *Neuron*, **58**, 639–50.

Benedetti F (2002). How the doctor's words affect the patient's brain. *Evaluation and the Health Professions*, **25**, 369–86.

Benedetti F (2010). *The patient's brain: the neuroscience behind the doctor–patient relationship*. Oxford University Press, Oxford.

Benedetti F (2013). Placebo and the new physiology of the doctor-patient relationship. *Physiological Reviews*, **93**, 1207–46.

Benedetti F, Colloca L, Lanotte M, Bergamasco B, Torre E and Lopiano L (2004). Autonomic and emotional responses to open and hidden stimulation of the human subthalamic region. *Brain Research Bulletin*, **63**, 203–11.

Benedetti F, Thoen W, Blanchard C, Vighetti S and Arduino C (2013). Pain as a reward: changing the meaning of pain from negative to positive co-activates opioid and cannabinoid systems. *Pain*, **154**, 361–7.

Bensing JM and Verheul W (2010). The silent healer: the role of communication in placebo effects. *Patient Education and Counseling*, **80**, 293–9.

Binkofski F, Schnitzler A, Enck P *et al.* (1998). Somatic and limbic cortex activation: a functional magnetic resonance imaging study. *Annals of Neurology*, **44**, 811–15.

Bruehl S, Burns JW, Chung OY, Ward P and Johnson B (2002). Anger and pain sensitivity in chronic low back pain patients and pain-free controls: the role of endogenous opioids. *Pain*, **99**, 223–33.

Bruehl S, Chung OY, Burns JW and Biridepalli S (2003). The association between anger expression and chronic pain intensity: evidence for partial mediation by endogenous opioid dysfunction. *Pain*, **106**, 317–24.

Carlson JD, Maire JJ, Martenson ME and Heinricher MM (2007). Sensitization of pain-modulating neurons in the rostral ventromedial medulla after peripheral nerve injury. *Journal of Neuroscience*, **27**, 13222–31.

Carroll LJ, Cassidy JD and Cote P (2004). Depression as a risk factor for onset of an episode of troublesome neck and low back pain. *Pain*, **107**, 134–9.

Coan JA, Schaefer HS and Davidson RJ (2006). Lending a hand. Social regulation of the neural response to theat. *Psychological Science*, **17**, 1032–9.

Colloca L and Finniss D (2012). Nocebo effects, patient-clinician communication, and therapeutic outcomes. *Journal of the American Medical Association*, **307**, 567–8.

Cormie PJ, Nairn M, Welsh J and Guideline Development Group (2008). Control of pain in adults with cancer: summary of SIGN guidelines. *British Medical Journal*, **337**, a2154.

Craig AD (2002). How do you feel? Interoception: the sense of the physiological condition of the body. *Nature Reviews Neuroscience*, **3**, 655–66.

Craig AD (2009). How do you feel—now? The anterior insula and human awareness. *Nature Reviews Neuroscience*, **10**, 59–70.

Critchley HD, Wiens S, Rothstein P, Ohman A and Dolan RJ (2004). Neural systems supporting interoceptive awareness. *Nature Neuroscience*, **7**, 189–95.

Damasio AR, Grabowski TJ, Bechara A *et al.* (2000). Subcortical and cortical brain activity during the feeling of self-generated emotions. *Nature Neuroscience*, **3**, 1049–56.

Dantzer R (2004). Cytokine-induced sickness behavior: a neuroimmune response to activation of innate immunity. *European Journal of Pharmacology*, **500**, 399–411.

Decety J and Jackson PL (2004). The functional architecture of human empathy. *Behavioral and Cognitive Neuroscience Reviews*, **3**, 71–100.

de la Fuente-Fernandez R, Ruth TJ, Sossi V, Schulzer M, Calne DB and Stoessl AJ (2001). Expectation and dopamine release: mechanism of the placebo effect in Parkinson's disease. *Science*, **293**, 1164–6.

de Waal FB (2008). Putting the altruism back into altruism: the evolution of empathy. *Annual Review of Psychology*, **59**, 279–300.

Dickens C, McGowan L and Dale S (2003). Impact of depression on experimental pain perception: a systematic review of the literature with meta-analysis. *Psychosomatic Medicine*, **65**, 369–75.

Dunbar RIM (2010). The social role of touch in humans and primates: behavioral function and neurobiological mechanisms. *Neuroscience and Biobehavioral Reviews*, **34**, 260–8.

Eisenberg N (2007). Empathy-related responding and prosocial behavior. *Novartis Foundation Symposia*, **278**, 71–80.

Engel G (1977). The need for a new medical model: a challenge for biomedicine. *Science*, **196**, 129–36.

Engell A D, Haxby J V and Todorov A (2007). Implicit trustworthiness decisions: automatic coding of face properties in human amygdala. *Journal of Cognitive Neuroscience*, **19**, 1508–19.

Feinmann C (1999). *The mouth, the face and the mind*. Oxford University Press, Oxford.

Ferrell BR and Dean G (1995). The meaning of cancer pain. *Seminars in Oncology Nursing*, **11**, 17–22.

Frith CD and Frith U (1999). Interacting minds—a biological basis. *Science*, **286**, 1692–5.

Frith CD and Frith U (2006). The neural basis of mentalizing. *Neuron*, **50**, 531–4.

Giesecke T, Gracely RH, Williams DA, Geisser ME, Petzke FW and Clauw DJ (2005). The relationship between depression, clinical pain, and experimental pain in a chronic pain cohort. *Arthritis and Rheumatism*, **52**, 1577–84.

Hart BL (1988). Biological basis of the behavior of sick animals. *Neuroscience and Biobehavioral Reviews*, **12**, 123–37.

Heath RG (1963). Electrical self-stimulation of the brain in man. *American Journal of Psychiatry*, **120**, 571–7.

Hein G and Singer T (2008). I feel how you feel but not always: the empathic brain and its modulation. *Current Opinion in Neurobiology*, **18**, 153–8.

Henderson SW (2000). The unnatural nature of pain. *Journal of the American Medical Association*, **283**, 117.

Henkel V, Bussfeld P, Moller H-J and Hegerl U (2002). Cognitive-behavioral theories of helplessness/hopelessness: valid models for depression? *European Archives of Psychiatry and Clinical Neuroscience*, **252**, 240–9.

Ho KY, Kang JY, Yeo B and Ng WL (1998). Non-cardiac, non-oesophageal chest pain: the relevance of psychological factors. *Gut*, **43**, 105–10.

Huber D, Veinante P and Stoop R (2005). Vasopressin and oxytocin excite distinct neuronal populations in the central amygdala. *Science*, **308**, 245–8.

Hull CL (1951). *Essentials of behavior*. Yale University Press, New Haven, CT.

Huynh Bao QV and Rainville P (2003). Modulation of experimental pain by emotion induced using hypnosis. *Pain Research and Management*, **Suppl. 8**, 35B.

Immordino-Yang MH, McColl A, Damasio H and Damasio A (2009). Neural correlates of admiration and compassion. *Proceedings of the National Academy of Science of the United States of America*, **106**, 8021–6.

Jensen KB, Petrovic P, Kerr CE et al. (2014). Sharing pain and relief: neural correlates of physicians during treatment of patients. *Molecular Psychiatry*, **19**, 392–8.

Johnson R W (2002). The concept of sickness behavior: a brief chronological account of four key discoveries. *Veterinary Immunology and Immunopathology*, **87**, 443–50.

Julien N, Goffaux P, Arsenault P and Marchand S (2005). Widespread pain in fibromyalgia is related to a deficit of endogenous pain inhibition. *Pain*, **114**, 295–302.

Kanwisher NG, McDermott J and Chun MM (1997). The fusiform face area: a module in human extrastriate cortex specialized for face perception. *Journal of Neuroscience*, **17**, 4302–11.

Kao AC, Green DC, Davis NA, Koplan JP and Cleary PD (1998a). Patients' trust in their physicians: effects of choice, continuity, and payment method. *Journal of General Internal Medicine*, **13**, 681–6.

Kao AC, Green DC, Zaslavsky AM, Koplan JP and Cleary PD (1998b). The relationship between method of physician payment and patient trust. *Journal of the American Medical Association*, **280**, 1708–14.

Kaptchuk TJ, Kelley JM, Conboy LA *et al.* (2008). Components of placebo effect: randomised controlled trial in patients with irritable bowel syndrome. *British Medical Journal*, **336**, 999–1003.

Kim J-W, Kim S-E, Kim J-J *et al.* (2009) Compassionate attitude towards others' suffering activates the mesolimbic neural system. *Neuropsychologia*, **47**, 2073–81.

King AB, Menon RS, Hachinski V and Cechetto DF (1999). Human forebrain activation by visceral stimuli. *Journal of Comparative Neurology*, **41**, 572–82.

Klauenberg S, Maier C, Assion HJ *et al.* (2008). Depression and changed pain perception: hints for a central disinhibition mechanism. *Pain*, **140**, 332–43.

Knutson B, Adams CM, Fong GW and Hommer D (2001). Anticipation of increasing monetary reward selectively recruits nucleus accumbens. *Journal of Neuroscience*, **21**, RC159.

Koffman J, Morgan M, Edmonds P, Speck P and Higginson IJ (2008). Cultural meanings of pain: a qualitative study of black Caribbean and white British patients with advanced cancer. *Palliative Medicine*, **22**, 350–9.

Korszun A (2002). Facial pain, depression and stress—connections and directions. *Journal of Oral Pathology and Medicine*, **31**, 615–19.

Kosfeld M, Heinrichs M, Zak PJ, Fischbacher U and Fehr E (2005). Oxytocin increases trust in humans. *Nature*, **435**, 673–6.

Larson SL, Clark MR and Eaton WW (2004). Depressive disorder as a long-term antecedent risk factor for incident back pain: a 13-year follow-up study from the Baltimore Epidemiological Catchment Area sample. *Psychological Medicine*, **34**, 211–19.

Lautenbacher S, Roscher S, Strian D, Fassbender K, Krumrey K and Krieg JC (1994). Pain perception in depression: relationships to symptomatology and naloxone-sensitive mechanisms. *Psychosomatic Medicine*, **56**, 345–52.

Leknes, S. Berna C, Lee MC, Snyder GD, Biele G and Tracey I (2013). The importance of context: when relative relief renders pain pleasant. *Pain*, **154**, 402–10.

Lordkipanidze D, Vekua A, Ferring R *et al.* (2005). Anthropology: the earliest toothless hominin skull. *Nature*, **434**, 717–18.

Magni G, Moreschi C, Rigatti-Luchini S and Merskey H (1994). Prospective study on the relationship between depressive symptoms and chronic musculoskeletal pain. *Pain*, **56**, 289–97.

Mann JJ (2003). Neurobiology of suicidal behavior. *Nature Reviews Neuroscience*, **4**, 819–28.

Mayberg HS, Silva JA, Brannan SK *et al.* (2002). The functional neuroanatomy of the placebo effect. *American Journal of Psychiatry*, **159**, 728–37.

Mongini F, Ciccone G, Ceccarelli M, Baldi I and Ferrero L (2007). Muscle tenderness in different types of facial pain and its relation to anxiety and depression: a cross-sectional study on 649 patients. *Pain*, **131**, 106–11.

Nimchinsky EA, Gilissen E, Allman JM, Perl DP, Erwin JM, and Hof PR (1999). A neuronal morphologic type unique to humans and great apes. *Proceedings of the National Academy of the United States of America*, **96**, 5268–73.

Okifuji A, Turk DC and Curran SL (1999). Anger in chronic pain: investigations of anger targets and intensity. *Journal of Psychosomatic Research*, **47**, 1–12.

Olds J and Milner P (1954). Positive reinforcement produced by electrical stimulation of the septal area and other regions of the rat brain. *Journal of Comparative Physiological Psychology*, **47**, 419–27.

Pearson SD and Raeke LH (2000). Patients' trust in physicians: many theories, few measures, and little data. *Journal of General Internal Medicine*, **15**, 509–13.

Phillips ML, Gregory LJ, Cullen S *et al.* (2003). The effect of negative emotional context on neural and behavioral responses to oesophageal stimulation. *Brain*, **126**, 669–84.

Rainville P (2004). Pain and emotions. In DD Price and MC Bushnell, eds. *Psychological methods of pain control: basic science and clinical perspectives*, pp. 117–41. IASP Press, Seattle, WA.

Rizzolatti G and Arbib MA (1998). Language within our grasp. *Trends in Neuroscience*, **21**, 188–94.

Rothstein RD, Stecker M, Reivich M *et al.* (1996). Use of positron emission tomography and evoked potentials in the detection of cortical afferents from the gastrointestinal tract. *American Journal of Gastroenterology*, **91**, 2372–6.

Saxe R (2006). Uniquely human social cognition. *Current Opinion in Neurobiology*, **16**, 235–9.

Schultz W (2002). Getting formal with dopamine and reward. *Neuron*, **36**, 241–63.

Schultz W, Tremblay L, and Hollerman JR (2000). Reward processing in primate orbitofrontal cortex and basal ganglia. *Cerebral Cortex*, **10**, 272–8.

Schweinhardt P, Kalk N, Wartolowska K, Chessell I, Wordsworth P and Tracey I (2008). Investigation into the neural correlates of emotional augmentation of clinical pain. *NeuroImage*, **40**, 759–66.

Scott DJ, Stohler CS, Egnatuk CM, Wang H, Koeppe RA and Zubieta JK (2007). Individual differences in reward responding explain placebo-induced expectations and effects. *Neuron*, **55**, 325–36.

Seeley WW, Carlin DA, Allman JM *et al.* (2006). Early frontotemporal dementia targets neurons unique to apes and humans. *Annals of Neurology*, **60**, 660–7.

Senju A and Johnson MH (2009). The eye contact effect: mechanisms and development. *Trends in Cognitive Sciences*, **13**, 127–34.

Smith WB, Gracely RH and Safer MA (1998). The meaning of pain: cancer patients' rating and recall of pain intensity and affect. *Pain*, **78**, 123–9.

Snyder CR (2002). Hope theory: rainbows in the mind. *Psychological Inquiry*, **13**, 249–75.

Snyder CR, Harris C, Anderson JR *et al.* (1991a). The will and the ways: development and validation of an individual-differences measure of hope. *Journal of Personality and Social Psychology*, **60**, 570–85.

Snyder CR, Irving L and Anderson JR (1991b). Hope and health: measuring the will and the ways. In CR Snyder and DR Forsyth, eds. *Handbook of social and clinical psychology: the health perspective*, pp. 285–305. Pergamon Press, Elmsford, NY.

Snyder CR, Sympson SC, Ybasco FC, Borders TF, Babyak MA and Higgins RL (1996). Development and validation of the State Hope Scale. *Journal of Personality and Social Psychology*, **70**, 321–35.

Sprecher S and Fehr B (2006). Enhancement of mood and self-esteem as a result of giving and receiving compassionate love. *Current Research in Social Psychology*, **11**, 227–42.

Spruijt BM, Van Hoof JA and Gispen WH (1992). Ethology and neurobiology of grooming behavior. *Physiological Reviews*, **72**, 825–52.

Stephan E, Pardo JW, Faris PL *et al.* (2003). Functional neuroimaging of gastric distension. *Journal of Gastrointestinal Surgery*, **7**, 740–9.

Strigo A, Simmons AN, Matthews SC, Craig AD and Paulus MP (2008). Association of major depressive disorder with altered functional brain response during anticipation and processing of heat pain. *Archives of General Psychiatry*, **65**, 1275–84.

Thom DH and Campbell B (1997). Patient-physician trust: an exploratory study. *Journal of Family Practice*, **44**, 169–76.

Tracey I and Mantyh PW (2007). The cerebral signature for pain perception and its modulation. *Neuron*, **55**, 377–91.

Trivers RL (1971). The evolution of reciprocal altruism. *Quarterly Review of Biology*, **46**, 35–57.

Tsao DY and Livingstone MS (2008). Mechanisms of face perception. *Annual Review of Neuroscience*, **31**, 411–37.

van Heeringen C, Audenaert K, Van Laere K *et al.* (2003). Prefrontal 5-HT2a receptor binding potential, hopelessness and personality characteristics in attempted suicide. *Journal of Affective Disorders*, **74**, 149–58.

van Vugt M and Van Lange PAM (2006). The altruism puzzle: psychological adaptations for prosocial behavior. In M Schaller, JA Simpson and DT Kenrick, eds. *Evolution and social psychology*, pp. 237–62. Psychology Press, New York.

Vimpari SS, Knuuttila ML, Sakki TK and Kivela SL (1995). Depressive symptoms associated with symptoms of the temporomandibular joint pain and dysfunction syndrome. *Psychosomatic Medicine*, **57**, 439–44.

Wager TD, Davidson ML, Hughes BL, Lindquist MA and Ochsner KN (2008). Prefrontal-subcortical pathways mediating successful emotion regulation. *Neuron*, **59**, 1037–50.

Weary DM, Huzzey JM and von Keyserlingk MAG (2009). Using behavior to predict and identify ill health in animals. *Journal of Animal Sciences*, **87**, 770–7.

Whitehead WE, Bosmajian L, Zonderman AB, Costa PT Jr and Schster MM (1988). Symptoms of psychological distress associated with irritable bowel syndrome. Comparison of community and medical clinic samples. *Gastroenterology*, **95**, 709–14.

Whitman SM (2007). Pain and suffering as viewed by the Hindu religion. *Journal of Pain*, **8**, 607–13.

Wiech K and Tracey I (2009). The influence of negative emotions on pain: behavioral effects and neural mechanisms. *NeuroImage*, **47**, 987–94.

Wiester J (1983). *The genesis connection*. Thomas Nelson Publishers, Nashville, TN.

Williams AC de C (2002). Facial expression of pain: an evolutionary account. *Behavioral and Brain Sciences*, **25**, 439–55.

Willis J and Todorov A (2006). First impressions: making up your mind after 100 ms exposure to a face. *Psychological Science*, **17**, 592–8.

Winston J, Strange B, O'Doherty J and Dolan R (2002). Automatic and intentional brain responses during evaluation of trustworthiness of face. *Nature Neuroscience*, **5**, 277–83.

Zak PJ, Kurzban R and Matzner WT (2004). The neurobiology of trust. *Annals of New York Academy of Science*, **1032**, 224–7.

Part 2

Disease-based classification of placebo effects—most-studied conditions

In contrast to Part 1 (Chapter 2), in which a mechanism-based approach is used, in Part 2, as well as in Part 3, a disease-based approach to the different placebo effects is adopted. In Part 2, the most studied and best understood medical conditions are described. These include pain, some neurological disorders, such as Parkinson's disease, and to a lesser extent some psychiatric disorders. In addition, the immune and the endocrine systems have provided important information on the placebo effect as a model of behavioral conditioning.

Chapter 4

Pain

Summary points

- Most of the knowledge about the neurobiological mechanisms of the placebo effect comes from the field of pain and analgesia.
- Expectation of pain reduction plays a crucial role in placebo analgesia. This is shown by the reduced effectiveness of painkillers when administered covertly (unexpectedly).
- The placebo analgesic effect is mediated by the endogenous opioid systems and antagonized by cholecystokinin in some circumstances. In other conditions, the endocannabinoid system is involved.
- Many brain imaging studies indicate that several areas are involved in placebo analgesia, including the dorsolateral prefrontal cortex and those regions involved in dopaminergic reward mechanisms.
- The prefrontal lobes are fundamental for a placebo response to occur. If there is no prefrontal control, there is no placebo response.
- The nocebo hyperalgesic effect is mediated by anxiety, which activates a cholecystokinin system that, in turn, facilitates pain transmission.
- The endogenous pain modulatory descending circuits represent the biological substrate for the action of placebos on pain.

4.1 Placebo analgesia

4.1.1 Placebo analgesia is the most studied type of placebo effect

Pain is by far the most studied placebo condition, and traditionally a large number of studies on the placebo effect have been performed in experimentally induced pain in healthy subjects or in patients suffering from a kind of painful condition. There are at least two explanations for this. First, pain is a subjective experience which undergoes psychological and social modulation more than any other condition (Boxes 4.1–4.3). The fine tuning of the global pain experience by many psychosocial factors makes pain an excellent model for identifying and understanding the placebo effect; indeed many

Box 4.1 Bottom-up processing of pain

Today we know that there is not a pain center in which the final pain experience emerges, but rather there is a distributed system that is made up of an intricate network of cortical and subcortical areas, each with some specific functions. This network is often referred to as the "pain matrix." The organization of the nociceptive pathways and areas from the spinal cord to the higher centers (bottom-up processing) is quite complex. Part of the spinothalamic tract, the lateral thalamus, and its cortical projections to the first somatosensory area (SI) is usually considered to be crucial for pain perception. The neurons in these regions are somatotopically ordered and have small contralateral receptive fields. This system, which is shown in bold in Fig. 4.1, with its precise somatotopic organization, encodes the sensory-discriminative aspects of pain sensation and is called "lateral system."

Parallel and complementary to this lateral pain system, a "medial system" exists, whose functions deal with the affective-emotional component of pain, i.e., those aspects regarding its unpleasantness, its negative hedonic quality, and the negative emotions associated with it. Without this emotional aspect, which in one word can

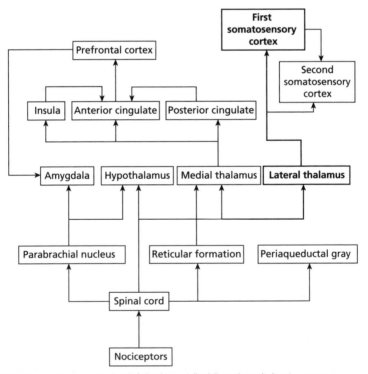

Fig. 4.1 Schematic organization of the lateral (bold) and medial pain systems. Reproduced from Physiological Reviews, 93 (3), Placebo and the New Physiology of the Doctor-Patient Relationship, Fabrizio Benedetti, pp.1207–1246, figure 4, DOI: 10.1152/physrev.00043.2012 Copyright 2013, The American Physiological Society.

Box 4.1 Bottom-up processing of pain (continued)

be called "suffering," the pain experience is incomplete and can hardly be defined as such. In Fig. 4.1 some of the main regions involved in the medial pain system are shown, e.g., the medial thalamus, the insula and the parietal operculum, the prefrontal and orbitofrontal, as well as the anterior and posterior cingulate cortices. Many of these areas are strongly connected with one another and with many other regions of the limbic system. In contrast to the lateral pain system, here the somatotopic organization is generally lacking, suggesting a role in nonspecific arousal rather than its precise spatial and temporal localization.

Therefore, whereas the lateral system is responsible for the discriminative properties of pain perception, that is, how intense pain is, how long it lasts, and where it is localized, the medial pain system is responsible for the affective component, that is, how long pain can be tolerated and how much suffering it produces. This sensory dissociation of pain is also shown by people with brain lesions that involve the medial system (mainly the limbic system). These patients can recognize pain as such and can discriminate its intensity, duration, and localization. However, they can tolerate it for longer times, reporting that the pain does not produce much suffering. The lateral and medial pain systems are affected differently in dementia of the Alzheimer's type (Box 4.2).

---

painful conditions and analgesic responses have always attracted clinicians, clinical scientists, and placebo researchers. The second explanation stems from the influential work by Beecher in the 1950s (Beecher, 1955). Beecher was an anesthesiologist who worked both at the Massachusetts General Hospital and on the battlefield. As an army doctor during the Second World War, his experience with wounded soldiers suffering from acute and severe pain on the battlefield gave an important impetus to placebo research. Basically, Beecher was faced with the problem of a lack of strong analgesics on the battlefield, particularly morphine, so he tried to treat his soldier patients with placebos. Of course, the soldiers were told that the inert substance Beecher had administered was a powerful painkiller. Many of them appeared to respond to the placebo, thus boosting Beecher's curiosity about the phenomenon.

In 1955, Beecher published a seminal paper which influenced placebo research in the following years. He reviewed 15 controlled trials involving 1802 patients (Beecher, 1955). Defining positive outcomes as the "per cent satisfactorily relieved by placebo," Beecher reported effect sizes ranging from 26–58%, with an average of 35%. The notion that about one-third of patients respond to placebo has since permeated medical texts and teachings, even though this work has been criticized on methodological grounds (Wall, 1992; Kienle and Kiene, 1996, 1997).

In a more recent analysis of five studies in which 130 patients received a placebo treatment, 7–37% of patients in the placebo group showed greater than 50% of the maximum possible pain relief (McQuay et al., 1995). These data were obtained in the postoperative setting, and they confirm the variation of the placebo effect in the acute pain setting found by Beecher in 1955. In fact Beecher found, using the dichotomous measure of greater than 50% pain relief, a range of 15–53% in patients who received placebo treatment in five acute pain studies. Therefore, the notion that one-third of patients respond to placebos should be abandoned.

One of the most important flaws in Beecher's conclusion is that no comparisons between placebo groups and natural history groups were considered. As described in detail in section 2.1, without a control condition to assess the natural history of pain, spontaneous remission cannot be ruled out. Therefore it is still debatable whether the studies reviewed by Beecher dealt with real placebo responses.

The best explanation we have today for Beecher's study is that the pain reduction observed in the placebo groups included many factors, such as spontaneous remissions, regression to the mean, and real placebo responses. Despite these methodological limitations, Beecher's view represents a milestone for the placebo effect in medical practice and it was certainly important for boosting the interest of the scientific community. Indeed, today we know that robust placebo responses occur in a number of painful conditions, such as neuropathic pain (Quessy and Rowbotham, 2008; Petersen et al., 2012).

4.1.2 Many factors influence the magnitude of placebo analgesia

In Beecher's study (Beecher, 1955) the figure of 30% of patients who responded to placebo treatment for pain means little, if anything. A real figure is that the magnitude of placebo analgesia may range from no responses to large responses. It has long been known that there are responders and nonresponders, although why this occurs is less clear (see section 2.3.8). In placebo studies, the differences between group averages are usually recorded, rather than observations of individual responses to a placebo intervention. This point is very important because an identical mean change between a placebo group and a no-treatment group might be seen if everyone in the placebo group exhibits a moderate response, or if a relatively small subset exhibits a large response and others show no response at all.

For example, Levine et al. (1979) found that 39% of patients had an analgesic response to placebo treatment, and in a study of ischemic arm pain in normal volunteers, Benedetti (1996) found that 26.9% of them responded to a placebo analgesic, as compared to a no-treatment control group. Another study involving cutaneous heating of the left hand found that 56% of subjects responded to placebo treatment, compared to the no-treatment controls (Petrovic et al., 2002). It can be seen that there are variations across different studies. Indeed, assessing the magnitude of the placebo analgesic effect is not an easy task, as the experimental conditions and the psychological state of the subjects change across different studies. Several studies measured the average change in pain experienced by those receiving placebo and compared this figure to the average change in the no-treatment group; they found that the magnitude of the placebo analgesic effect is about 2 out of 10 units on a visual analogue (VAS) or numerical rating scale (NRS) (Gracely et al., 1983; Levine and Gordon, 1984; Benedetti et al., 1995; Amanzio et al., 2001; Price, 2001).

In studies where the known placebo responders in a group are separated for analysis, the average magnitude of analgesia has been found, not surprisingly, to be significantly greater. For example, when Benedetti (1996) looked only at responders, he found an average placebo analgesia magnitude of 5 units on the 10-unit NRS. This is similar to a postoperative dental study that found a 3.3-cm (out of 10) lower mean post-treatment VAS score for placebo responders compared to nonresponders (Levine et al., 1978).

Today it seems clear that the experimental manipulation used to induce placebo analgesia plays a fundamental role in the magnitude of the response. Among the different manipulations that have been performed, both the type of verbal suggestions and the individual's previous experience have been found to be important.

Verbal suggestions that induce certain expectations of analgesia induce larger placebo analgesic responses than those that induce uncertain expectations. This is illustrated by a study carried out in the clinical setting that investigated the differences between the double-blind and the deceptive paradigm (Pollo et al., 2001). Postoperative patients were treated with buprenorphine, on request, for 3 days consecutively, and with a basal infusion of saline solution. However, the symbolic meaning of this saline basal infusion was varied in three different groups of patients: the first group (natural history or no-treatment group) was told nothing; the second was told the infusion was either a potent analgesic or a placebo (classic double-blind administration); and the third was told that the infusion was a potent painkiller (deceptive administration). The placebo effect of the infusion was measured by recording the doses of buprenorphine requested over the 3-day treatment. It is important to stress once again that the double-blind group received uncertain verbal instructions ("It can be either a placebo or a painkiller. Thus we are not certain that the pain will subside") whereas the deceptive administration group received certain instructions ("It is a painkiller. Thus pain will subside soon"). Compared to the natural history group, a 20.8% decrease in buprenorphine intake was seen with the double-blind administration. An even greater decrease (33.8%) was found in the deceptive administration group. It is important to point out that the time-course of pain was the same in all three groups over the 3-day treatment period. The same analgesic effect was obtained with different doses of buprenorphine, thus subtle differences in the verbal context of the patient may have a significant impact on the magnitude of the response.

In chronic headache pain, a similar effect has been found by using an active treatment (Kam-Hansen et al., 2014). Each patient received either placebo or rizatriptan administered under three information conditions ranging from negative to neutral to positive (told placebo, told rizatriptan or placebo, told rizatriptan). Rizatriptan was superior to placebo for pain relief. When patients were given placebo labeled as (1) placebo, (2) rizatriptan or placebo, and (3) rizatriptan, the placebo effect increased progressively. Rizatriptan had a similar progressive boost when labeled with these three labels. The efficacies of rizatriptan labeled as placebo and placebo labeled as rizatriptan were similar. Therefore, increasing positive information incrementally boosted the efficacy of both placebo and medication in headache, which indicates that the information provided to patients and the ritual of pill taking are important components of care.

Verne et al. (2003) and Vase et al. (2003) conducted two similar studies (Fig. 4.2A,B). Patients with irritable bowel syndrome (IBS) were exposed to rectal distension by

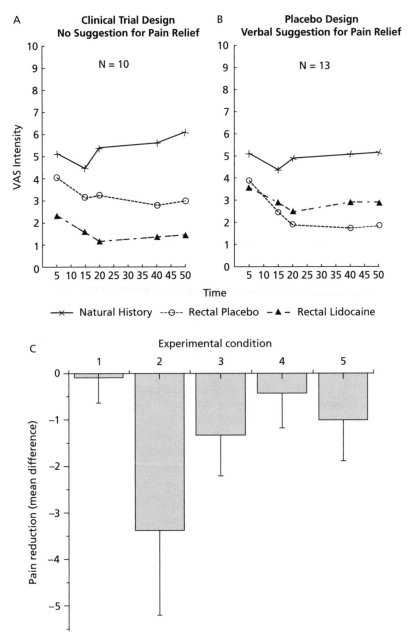

Fig. 4.2 Variability in magnitude of placebo analgesia. (A) A clinical trial design comparing visual analogue scores (VAS) for natural history of visceral pain intensity (crosses), after rectally administered placebo (circles) and after rectally administered lidocaine (triangles), during a 50-minute session. No suggestions for pain relief were given.

means of a balloon barostat, a type of visceral stimulation that simulates their clinical pain. They tested patients under the conditions of untreated natural history (baseline), rectal placebo, and rectal lidocaine. Pain was rated immediately after each stimulus within each condition. The first study was conducted as a double-blind crossover clinical trial, so patients were given an informed consent form stating that they "may receive an active pain-reducing medication or an inert placebo agent" (Verne et al. 2003). In this study, there was a significant pain-relieving effect of rectal lidocaine compared to rectal placebo, and a significant pain relieving effect of rectal placebo (pain in placebo < natural history). In a second study of similar design, at the onset of each treatment condition (rectal placebo, rectal lidocaine), patients were told "The agent you have just been given is known to significantly reduce pain in some patients" (Vase et al. 2003). A much larger placebo analgesic effect was found, which did not significantly differ from that of rectal lidocaine. These two studies show that adding an overt suggestion for pain relief can increase placebo analgesia to a magnitude that matches that of an active agent.

Previous experience can also influence the magnitude of placebo analgesia. In one study, the intensity of painful stimulation was reduced surreptitiously after placebo administration, so leading subjects to believe that an analgesic treatment was effective (Colloca and Benedetti, 2006) (Fig. 4.2C). This procedure induced strong placebo responses after minutes, and these responses, albeit reduced, lasted up to 4–7 days. In a second group of subjects, this procedure was repeated 4–7 days after a totally ineffective analgesic treatment. The placebo responses were markedly reduced compared to the first group. Thus, small and large placebo responses were obtained that depended on several factors, such as previous positive or negative experiences of analgesic treatment and the time lag between the treatment and the placebo responses. These findings indicate that placebo analgesia is finely tuned by prior experience and that these effects may last, albeit reduced, for several days. These results emphasize that the placebo effect may represent a learning phenomenon involving several factors and may explain the large variability in the magnitude of placebo responses among studies.

Fig. 4.2 (continued) The same conditions are tested in (B) but within a placebo design and with verbal suggestions for pain relief; here, placebo is as effective as lidocaine. Reproduced from Lene Vase, Michael E. Robinson, G. Nicholas Verne, Donald D. Price, The contributions of suggestion, desire, and expectation to placebo effects in irritable bowel syndrome patients: An empirical investigation, *Pain*, 105 (1–2), pp. 17–25 Copyright 2003, The International Association for the Study of Pain, with permission. DOI: http://dx.doi.org/10.1016/S0304–3959(03)00073–3 Part (C) shows different degrees of placebo responses (small, medium, and large) elicited in different experimental conditions: 1, natural history; 2, placebo right after conditioning; 3, placebo 1 week after conditioning; 4, placebo after verbal suggestions alone; 5, placebo after conditioning and previous negative therapeutic experience. Reproduced from Luana Colloca and Fabrizio Benedetti, How prior experience shapes placebo analgesia, *Pain*, 124 (1), pp. 126–33 Copyright 2006, The International Association for the Study of Pain, with permission. DOI: http://dx.doi.org/10.1016/j.pain.2006.04.005

Box 4.2 The lateral and medial pain systems in Alzheimer's disease

The lateral and medial pain systems are affected differently in Alzheimer's disease. Both the primary somatosensory cortex and some thalamic nuclei, which belong to the lateral pain system, are relatively unaffected by the histological changes that characterize Alzheimer's disease, thus indicating that a preserved sensory-discriminative function should be expected. By contrast, the intralaminar thalamic nuclei, which represent an important component of the affective/emotional medial pain system, are early and progressively affected by the Alzheimer's disease-related cellular pathology. Therefore, the emotional-affective function should be expected to be affected, as also suggested by the conspicuous neuronal and synaptic loss in the prefrontal and limbic regions. As expected from this pattern of degeneration, a dissociation between the sensory-discriminative component of pain, which is processed in the lateral pain system, and the affective-emotional component, which is processed in the medial system, is present. Benedetti et al. (1999b) tested both pain thresholds and pain tolerance in Alzheimer patients by means of phasic and tonic noxious stimuli. In the first case, electrical stimulation was used, whereas in the second case experimental arm ischemia was studied. By comparing Alzheimer patients with normal subjects of the same age, no difference was found in stimulus detection and pain thresholds, whereas a clear-cut increase in pain tolerance was present in Alzheimer patients. Furthermore, the severity of the disease was assessed by means of the Mini Mental State Examination test (MMSE) and the spectral analysis of the electroencephalogram. The authors found a straightforward correlation between MMSE scores and pain tolerance, such that the more severe the cognitive impairment was, the higher was the tolerance to pain. The analysis of the electroencephalographic power spectra indicated that patients with low alpha and high delta peaks showed an increase in pain tolerance to both electrical stimulation and ischemia. Therefore, whereas the sensory-discriminative component of pain was maintained in Alzheimer patients, pain tolerance was altered and depended on the severity of cognitive impairment.

The strength of previous experience is a crucial factor which contributes to the magnitude of the placebo response. In fact, the number of learning trials that are carried out in a conditioning procedure is related to the subsequent magnitude of the placebo effects. Colloca et al. (2010) tested the effects of either one or four sessions of conditioning on the modulation of both nonpainful and painful stimuli delivered to the dorsum of the foot. Placebo and nocebo manipulations were obtained by pairing green or red light to a series of stimuli that were made lower or higher with respect to a yellow light associated with a series of control stimuli. Subjects were told that the lights would indicate a treatment that would reduce or increase nonpainful and painful stimuli to the foot. They were randomly assigned to two groups: group 1 underwent one session of conditioning whereas group 2 received four sessions of conditioning.

It was found that one session of conditioning induced nocebo responses, but not placebo responses in the no-painful condition. After one session of conditioning, both nocebo and placebo responses to painful stimulation were observed; however, these effects extinguished over time. Conversely, four sessions of conditioning induced robust placebo and nocebo responses to both nonpainful and painful stimuli that persisted over the entire experiment, which suggests that the strength of learning plays a key role. Not only is learning important for psychophysical measurements such as pain rating, but it also affects neurophysiological parameters, like laser evoked potentials (Colloca et al., 2008b). Colloca and Benedetti (2009) showed that social observational learning, whereby placebo responses can be learned by merely observing others, plays an important role as well (see also section 2.3.3).

The strength of learning may have profound implications both in medical practice and in the setting of clinical trials. A representative example is provided by the timing of either placebo administration or repetitive transcranial magnetic stimulation (rTMS) of the motor cortex for neuropathic pain relief. Andrè-Obadia et al. (2011) performed a randomized controlled study including 45 patients, in which they compared the analgesic effects of sham rTMS that either preceded or followed an active rTMS, which could be itself either successful or unsuccessful. Placebo analgesia differed significantly when the sham rTMS session followed a successful or an unsuccessful active rTMS. Placebo sessions induced significant analgesia when they followed a successful rTMS (mean pain decrease of 11%), whereas they tended to worsen pain when following an unsuccessful rTMS (pain increase of 6%). Only when the sham intervention was applied before any active rTMS were placebo scores unchanged from the baseline.

Lui et al. (2010) showed dynamic changes in prefrontal areas during placebo conditioning by means of functional magnetic resonance imaging. Brief laser heat stimuli delivered to one foot, either right or left, were preceded by different visual cues, signaling either painful stimuli alone, or painful stimuli accompanied by a sham analgesic procedure. Cues signaling the analgesic procedure were followed by stimuli of lower intensity in the conditioning session, whereas in the test session both cues were followed by painful stimuli of the same intensity. During the first conditioning trials, progressive signal increases over time were found during anticipation of analgesia compared to anticipation of pain, in a medial prefrontal focus and in bilateral lateral prefrontal foci. These frontal foci were adjacent to, and partially overlapped, those active during anticipation of analgesia in the test session, whose signal changes were related to the magnitude of the placebo behavioral response, and those active during placebo analgesia. This finding suggests that the neural events that lead to learned placebo analgesia are located in both medial and lateral prefrontal regions.

As the magnitude of placebo analgesia depends on many factors, and learning is crucial in several circumstances, the clinical trial setting does not seem to be the best model for studying the placebo analgesic response. In the study by Hrobjartsson and Goetzsche (2001) (section 2.1.7) a meta-analysis was performed of 130 trials in which placebo and no-treatment groups were identified in different pathological conditions. No difference was found between the two groups for many conditions, but a significant placebo effect was found for pain in 29 clinical trials, indicating that pain is one of the best conditions where the placebo effect is present and can be studied.

To further investigate the placebo effect in analgesic studies only, Vase et al. (2002) conducted one meta-analysis that included 23 of the 29 clinical trials included in Hrobjartsson and Goetzsche's meta-analysis (2001); another meta-analysis covered 14 studies that investigated placebo analgesia mechanisms. They found that the magnitudes of placebo analgesic effects were higher in studies that investigated placebo analgesic mechanisms compared with clinical trials in which the placebo was used only as a control condition. Vase et al. (2002) suggest this difference might result from the different placebo instructions and suggestions given in the clinical trial setting compared to the experimental setting. In fact, clinical trial investigators typically avoid giving oral suggestions of analgesia, whereas investigators of the placebo effect typically emphasize analgesic suggestions. Taken together, the two meta-analyses by Hrobjartsson and Goetzsche (2001) and Vase et al. (2002) teach us that placebo analgesia occurs in both the clinical trial setting and the experimental setting, although it is much more pronounced in the latter.

Another factor that may influence the magnitude of placebo analgesia is the experimental or clinical setting wherein the placebo procedure is carried out. For example, Charron et al. (2006) have shown that the placebo analgesic effect is different in experimental and clinical conditions. They studied patients with low back pain after the administration of a placebo for the treatment of their clinical pain and for the treatment of experimentally induced pain by means of the cold pressor test. Ratings of pain intensity, pain unpleasantness, and perceived relief showed larger placebo responses in low back pain compared to cold pressor pain.

4.1.3 **Expectations of improvement may lead to analgesia**

Expectation plays an essential role in placebo analgesia. Modulation of pain perception by placebos depends on expectation, as shown in many studies (Kirsch, 1999; Price et al., 1999, 2008). Montgomery and Kirsch conducted one of the first studies in which expected pain levels were manipulated and directly measured (Montgomery and Kirsch, 1997). They used a design in which subjects were given cutaneous pain via iontophoretic stimuli. Once baseline stimuli were applied, subjects were surreptitiously given stimuli with reduced intensities in the presence of a placebo cream (conditioning procedure). Then the stimulus strength was restored to its original baseline level and several stimuli were then used in placebo test trials to test the effect of conditioning. Subjects rated their expected pain levels just before placebo test trials and were divided into two groups. The first did not know about the stimulus manipulation and their pain ratings during placebo trials were markedly diminished by prior conditioning. However, by performing regression analyses, it was clear this effect was mediated by expected pain levels. Expectancy accounted for 49% of the variance in post-manipulation pain ratings. The second group was informed about the experimental design and learned that the cream was inert. They showed no placebo analgesic effect. Regression analysis and the difference in results across the groups showed that conscious expectation is necessary for placebo analgesia and clarified some previous studies which concluded that conditioning was important in placebo analgesia (Voudouris et al., 1989, 1990).

Using a similar paradigm, Price et al. (1999) applied placebo creams and graded levels of heat stimulation on three adjacent cutaneous regions of the forearm, giving subjects expectations that cream A was a strong analgesic, cream B was a weak analgesic, and cream C was a control agent. Immediately after these conditioning trials, subjects rated their expected pain levels for the placebo test trials wherein the stimulus intensity was the same for all three regions. The conditioning trials led to graded levels of expected pain (C ≥ B ≥ A) for the three creams, as well as graded magnitudes of actual pain (C ≥ B ≥ A) when tested during placebo test trials. Thus, magnitudes of placebo analgesia could be graded across three adjacent skin areas, demonstrating a high degree of somatotopic specificity for placebo analgesia. Expected pain levels accounted for 25–36% of the variance in post-manipulation pain ratings.

In another study (Benedetti et al., 2003b), one group of subjects was pharmacologically preconditioned with ketorolac (a nonopioid analgesic) for 2 days in a row, then the ketorolac was replaced with a placebo on the third day along with verbal suggestions of analgesia. This procedure induced a strong placebo analgesic response. In order to see whether this response was due to the pharmacological preconditioning, a second group of subjects was also preconditioned with ketorolac, but the placebo was given on the third day along with verbal suggestions that the drug was a hyperalgesic agent. These verbal instructions were sufficient not only to completely block placebo analgesia, but also to produce hyperalgesia. This study clearly shows that placebo analgesia depends on expectation of a decrease in pain, even though analgesic preconditioning is performed.

Expectation of analgesia can also make a big difference in clinical trials, so the patient's expectations have to be taken into account whenever a clinical trial is run. In one clinical trial, real acupuncture was compared to sham acupuncture. Patients were asked which group they believed they belonged to (either placebo or real treatment). Patients who believed they belonged to the real treatment group experienced larger clinical improvement than those who believed they belonged to the placebo group (Bausell et al., 2005). In another clinical trial, patients were asked whether they considered acupuncture to be an effective therapy in general and what they personally expected from the treatment. Patients with higher expectations about acupuncture experienced larger clinical benefits than those with lower expectations, regardless of their allocation to real or sham groups (Linde et al., 2007). It did not really matter whether the patients actually received the real or the sham procedure—what mattered was whether they believed in acupuncture and expected a benefit from it.

Kaptchuk et al. (2006) compared two placebo treatments in a clinical trial of 270 patients suffering from arm pain resulting from repetitive use or prolonged static postures. The two placebo treatments were acupuncture with a sham device twice a week for 6 weeks, and a placebo pill once a day for 8 weeks. The investigators found that the sham device had greater effects than the placebo pill on self-reported pain and severity of symptoms over the entire course of treatment. This suggests that placebo effects depend on the behaviors embedded in medical rituals, which, in turn, may induce different expectations. The comparison between two placebos is an interesting experimental approach in order to demonstrate real placebo effects and the involvement of different levels of expectations. In fact, if a placebo is inert and does not produce any psychological effect, two different placebos should not differ from each other. Conversely, if the psychological effect of a placebo treatment is superior to that of another placebo, different outcomes are expected (see also section 8.1.1).

As described in section 2.3.2, expectations may act in association with other factors, such as desire of relief and reduction of anxiety. In other words, placebo phenomena occur within the context of emotional regulation, and symptoms should be influenced by desire, expectation, and intensity of emotional feeling (Price et al., 2008). Desire and expectation interact and underlie common human emotions like sadness, anxiety, and relief (Price et al., 1985, 2001; Price and Barrell, 2000), thus in the context of analgesic studies it is quite plausible that patients and subjects have some degree of desire to avoid, terminate, or reduce evoked or ongoing pain.

By using functional magnetic resonance imaging, Kong et al. (2009b) investigated how expectation can modulate acupuncture treatment. The analysis on two verum acupuncture groups with different expectancy levels showed that expectancy can significantly influence acupuncture analgesia for experimental pain. Positive expectation can amplify acupuncture analgesia as detected by subjective pain sensory rating changes and objective brain changes in response to noxious stimuli. Diminished positive expectation appears to inhibit acupuncture analgesia. This modulation effect was found to be spatially specific, inducing analgesia exclusively in regions of the body where expectation was focused. The same group (Kong et al., 2009a) suggested that the brain network involved in expectation may vary under different treatment situations (verum and sham acupuncture treatment).

4.1.4 Painkillers are much less effective when administered covertly

Some of the best evidence underscoring the crucial role of expectation in the outcome of analgesic treatments is the decreased effectiveness of hidden treatments. As described in section 2.2.4, this involves giving an analgesic covertly (unexpectedly) so the patient is unaware a drug is being injected; the outcome following the hidden (unexpected) administration is compared with that following an open (expected) administration.

In postoperative pain following the extraction of the third molar (Levine et al., 1981; Levine and Gordon, 1984), a hidden intravenous injection of 6–8 mg morphine corresponded to an open intravenous injection of saline solution in full view of the patient (placebo). In other words, telling the patient that a painkiller was being injected (with what was actually a saline solution) is as potent as 6–8 mg of morphine. The investigators concluded that an open injection of morphine in full view of the patient is more effective than a hidden one because in the latter the placebo component is absent.

Careful analysis of the differences between open (expected) and hidden (unexpected) injections in postoperative settings was performed for five widely used painkillers (morphine, buprenorphine, tramadol, ketorolac, metamizole) (Fig. 4.3) (Amanzio et al., 2001; Benedetti et al., 2003a; Colloca et al., 2004). A doctor carried out the open administration, telling the patient (at the bedside) that the injection was a powerful analgesic and that the pain was going to subside in a few minutes. In contrast, hidden injections of the same analgesic at the same dose were performed by an automatic infusion machine that started the painkilling infusion without any doctor or nurse in the room; these patients were completely unaware that analgesic therapy had been started.

One analysis found that the analgesic dose needed to reduce the pain by 50% (AD_{50}) was much higher with hidden infusions than with open ones for all five painkillers, indicating that hidden administration is less effective than open administration (Fig. 4.3A). Another analysis found that the time course of post-surgical pain was significantly different between open and hidden injections. In fact, during the first hour after administration, pain ratings were much higher with a hidden injection than with an open one (Fig. 4.3B).

The difference between open and hidden injections was investigated in a laboratory setting using the experimental model of ischemic arm pain in healthy volunteers (Amanzio et al., 2001). As in the clinical setting, a hidden injection of the nonopioid painkiller, ketorolac, was less effective than an open one. Interestingly, when the opioid antagonist, naloxone, was added to the open injection of ketorolac, the effect was the same as that produced by a hidden injection. This suggests that an open injection in full view of the patient activates endogenous opioids that enhance the effects of the injected painkiller.

Open and hidden administrations have been studied in combination with functional magnetic resonance imaging. Bingel et al. (2011) found that expectation of remifentanil (told remifentanil, gets remifentanil) produced more pronounced analgesic effects compared to no-expectation (told saline, gets remifentanil). Moreover, during a hidden infusion of remifentanil, expectation of interruption (told interruption, gets remifentanil), abolished the analgesic effect of remifentanil. Functional magnetic resonance responses showed that the enhancement of analgesia in the positive expectation condition was associated with activity in the dorsolateral prefrontal cortex and pregenual anterior cingulate cortex, whereas negative expectation of interruption was associated with activity in the hippocampus.

The fact that the hidden administration of a pharmacological agent is less effective than an open one may suggest a different pharmacodynamic action of the drug in the absence of expectations. Although today we do not know whether expectations and therapeutic rituals can indeed modify a receptor, so as to change the drug-receptor binding properties, this mechanism seems unlikely as far as we know today. The global effect of a drug derives from its specific pharmacodynamic action plus the psychological (placebo) effect coming from the very act of its administration. A recent study suggests that these two components operate independently from each other. Atlas et al. (2012) conducted a study to directly examine the relationship between expectations and opioid analgesia. They administered the opioid agonist remifentanil to human subjects during experimental thermal pain and manipulated participants' knowledge of drug delivery using the open–hidden paradigm. Both remifentanil and expectations reduced pain, but drug effects on pain reports and brain activity, as assessed by functional magnetic resonance imaging, did not interact with expectations. Regions associated with pain processing showed no differences in drug effects as a function of expectation in the open and hidden conditions. Instead, expectations modulated activity in frontal cortex, with a separable time course from drug effects. Therefore, drugs and expectations both influence clinically relevant outcomes, yet they seem to operate without mutual interference. This suggests that, although drugs and expectations use the same type of receptors, these receptorial pathways are independent from each other, being located in different areas of the brain.

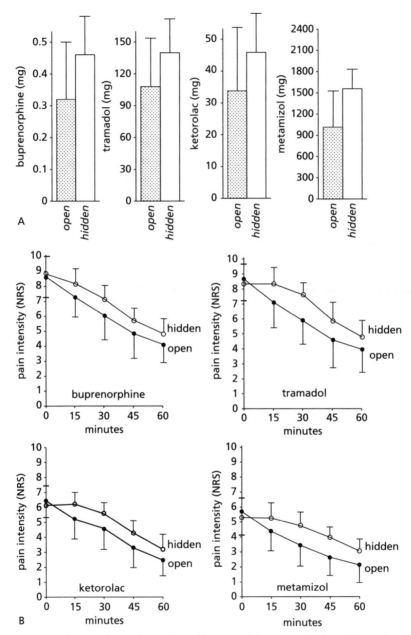

Fig. 4.3 Part (A) shows the analgesic dose of buprenorphine, tramadol, ketorolac, and metamizole needed to reduce pain by 50% (AD_{50}), obtained by means of either open or hidden infusions in postoperative patients. Note that in the hidden conditions, the AD_{50} increased. Reproduced from Martina Amanzio, Antonella Pollo, Giuliano Maggi, and Fabrizio Benedetti, Response variability to analgesics: a role for non-specific activation of endogenous opioids, *Pain*, 90 (3), pp. 205–15 Copyright 2001, The International Association

4.1.5 **Placebo analgesia is today the best model for studying endogenous mechanisms of analgesia**

Placebo administration has been found to activate endogenous mechanisms of analgesia, and today the placebo effect represents one of the most interesting models for understanding when and how these mechanisms are activated (Benedetti, 2007, 2013). As most of our knowledge about placebo analgesia is based on opioid mechanisms, particular attention has been paid to the endogenous opioid systems. However, nonopioid mechanisms are also involved in placebo analgesia (Colloca and Benedetti, 2005; Petrovic et al., 2010), as described in section 4.1.7.

The organization of the endogenous antinociceptive systems is complex (Box 4.3). Thanks to the pioneering work on producing analgesia in the rat by stimulation of the periaqueductal gray (Reynolds, 1969) and the discovery of stereospecific binding sites for opioids (Pert and Snyder, 1973), then endogenous enkephalins (Hughes, 1975) in the central nervous system, we know now that a complex endogenous network exists, which includes both opioid and nonopioid systems (Millan, 2002) (see Box 4.4). Thus, the opioid system is the first step in understanding the intricate mechanisms underlying the placebo analgesic effect.

Opioid receptors can be found throughout the brain, brainstem, and spinal cord (Pfeiffer et al., 1982; Wamsley et al., 1982; Atweh and Kuhar, 1983; Sadzot et al., 1991; Fields and Basbaum, 1999; Fields, 2004). These receptors may exert analgesic effects through different mechanisms (Jensen, 1997), such as modulation at the spinal level and/or control of cortical and brainstem regions. The modulation of the spinal cord is one of the best described (Fields and Basbaum, 1999; Fields, 2004). The opioid system in the brainstem consists of different regions, like the periaqueductal gray, the parabrachial nuclei, and the rostral ventromedial medulla (Fields and Basbaum, 1999; Fields, 2004). Although the opioid receptors are less characterized in the cortex, autoradiographic studies indicate high concentrations of opioid receptors in the cingulate cortex and prefrontal cortex (Pfeiffer et al., 1982; Wamsley et al., 1982; Sadzot et al., 1991) and one of the highest levels of opioid receptor binding has been found in the anterior cingulate cortex (Vogt et al., 1993). Studies performed by means of positron emission tomography and the radioactive opioid 11C-diprenorphine, confirm previous animal and human autoradiographic findings (Jones et al., 1991; Willoch et al., 1999, 2004). In

---

Fig. 4.3 (continued) for the Study of Pain, with permission. DOI: http://dx.doi.org/10.1016/S0304–3959(00)00486–3 Part (B) shows the time course of analgesia for buprenorphine, tramadol, ketorolac, and metamizole. Note that the analgesic response was smaller with hidden injections. In addition, open injections produced an analgesic response as soon as 15 minutes after administration, while hidden injections did not, indicating that this early analgesic response was due, at least in part, to a placebo effect. Reproduced from Martina Amanzio, Antonella Pollo, Giuliano Maggi, and Fabrizio Benedetti, Response variability to analgesics: a role for non-specific activation of endogenous opioids, *Pain*, 90 (3), pp. 205–15 Copyright 2001, The International Association for the Study of Pain, with permission. DOI: http://dx.doi.org/10.1016/S0304–3959(00)00486–3

addition, opioid receptor agonists, such as remifentanil and fentanyl have been shown to act on several regions that are known to be involved in pain processing and contain high concentrations of opioid receptors (Firestone et al. 1996; Adler et al., 1997; Casey et al., 2000; Wagner et al., 2001; Petrovic et al., 2002).

One of the main problems of this endogenous opioid network is understanding when and how it is involved in analgesic effects. For example, it has long been known that fear and stress play an important role in the activation of the endogenous opioid system (Willer and Albe-Fessard, 1980; Fanselow, 1994). It has also been hypothesized that several other contexts are important for activation of the endogenous opioid system (Fields and Basbaum, 1999; Price, 1999). It is likely that the placebo response is now the best-understood mechanism for naturally activating the endogenous opioid network in humans (Colloca and Benedetti, 2005). Placebo research is thus also important for the understanding of the endogenous mechanisms of analgesia.

Box 4.3 Top-down modulation of pain

The organization of the neural circuits that modulate pain is mainly characterized by a hierarchical series of descending pathways (top-down processing) from the cerebral cortex to subcortical regions, like the hypothalamus, amygdala, periaqueductal gray, and nucleus of the solitary tract, down to the parabrachial nucleus, the dorsoreticular nucleus, the rostroventromedial medulla, and the spinal cord (Fig. 4.4). Although the characterization of this descending network mostly relies on

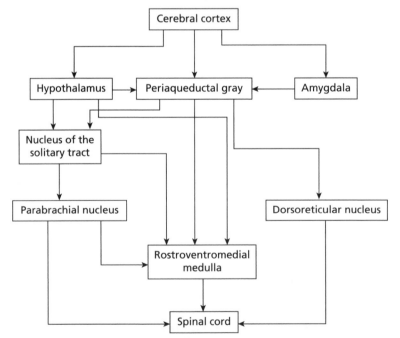

Fig. 4.4 Schematic organization of the descending pain modulating system.

Box 4.3 Top-down modulation of pain (continued)

experiments performed in animals, there are several lines of evidence, both indirect and direct, that the same pain-modulatory system is present in humans.

Many neurotransmitters and neuromodulators have been found to modulate pain through this neuronal network, not only through an inhibitory action but also through a facilitating action. For example, opioid neuropeptides and endocannabinoids inhibit pain whereas cholecystokinin facilitates pain transmission. It is important to point out that sometimes it is difficult to identify a specific action for many neurotransmitters, for they may act as both inhibitory and facilitatory agents. For example, dopaminergic, noradrenergic, and serotoninergic systems may be both inhibitory and facilitatory, depending on at least two factors. First, the receptor that is involved is crucial; different receptors may have opposite action, such as the dopaminergic D1 and D2, the noradrenergic α-1 and α-2, and the serotoninergic 1B and 1A. Second, different combinations of different neurotransmitters may shift the balance from inhibition to facilitation, and vice versa.

A subtle and finely tuned psychosocial modulation is likely to affect these networks in different circumstances and in different individuals. Attention, distraction, social differences across ethnic groups, ages, and sexes, are all factors that may affect these neurochemical systems, and placebo analgesia represents today one of the best models to understand this top-down modulation.

4.1.6 Some types of placebo analgesia are mediated by endogenous opioids

Placebo-induced analgesia activates the endogenous opioid systems in some circumstances. The first study of the biological mechanisms of placebo analgesia used the opioid antagonist naloxone to block opioid receptors (Levine et al., 1978). It was performed in a clinical setting in patients who had undergone extraction of their third molar tooth. The investigators found there was disruption of placebo analgesia after naloxone administration, which indicates the involvement of endogenous opioid systems in the placebo analgesic effect. These findings have been criticized on many grounds (e.g., by Skrabanek, 1978). One of the major criticisms was the lack of adequate control groups, such as a natural history group, as well as the possibility that naloxone per se might have a hyperalgesic effect; from this perspective, the higher pain intensity following naloxone administration would not result from blockade of placebo-induced activation of endogenous opioids, but rather from the hyperalgesic properties of naloxone. This is a fundamental point, because naloxone must not have any hyperalgesic effect in order to be used in studies of the placebo effect. Despite these limitations, Levine et al. (1978) were the first to give scientific credibility to the placebo phenomenon by unraveling the underlying biological mechanisms. In a sense this study represented the passage from the psychological to the biological investigation of the placebo effect.

In the years that followed the publication of the study by Levine et al. (1978) there were attempts to verify and to reproduce the findings. For example, by using the experimental pain model of arm ischemia (the tourniquet technique), Grevert et al. (1983) found partial reversal of placebo analgesia by naloxone, thus confirming those previous findings. Likewise, Levine and Gordon (1984) adopted an elegant experimental design that showed naloxone reversed placebo analgesia in a clinical situation, namely postoperative pain after extraction of the third molar. However, in 1983, Gracely et al. (1983) demonstrated that naloxone may have hyperalgesic effects in postoperative pain, thus shedding some doubt on the opioid hypothesis of placebo analgesia.

Research in this field was rare from 1984–1995, with the exception of a few isolated studies. For example, Lipman et al. (1990) studied chronic pain patients and found that patients who responded to placebo administration showed higher concentrations of endorphins in their cerebrospinal fluid compared with those who did not respond.

From 1995–1999, a long series of experiments with rigorous experimental designs were performed by Benedetti and collaborators. During these years, many unanswered questions were clarified, and the role of endogenous opioids in placebo analgesia was explained. The experimental ischemic arm pain model was used to show that naloxone does not affect this kind of pain; therefore any effect following naloxone administration could be attributed to the blockade of placebo-induced opioid activation (Benedetti, 1996). At the same time, these investigators tested the effects of a cholecystokinin (CCK)-antagonist, proglumide, on placebo analgesia. It was hypothesized, on the basis of the antiopioid action of CCK, that blockade of CCK receptors would enhance the amount of opioids released by the placebo. Indeed, it was found that proglumide potentiated the placebo analgesia, and presented a novel and indirect way to test the opioid hypothesis (Benedetti et al., 1995; Benedetti, 1996). More recently, the activation of the CCK type-2 receptors was performed by means of the agonist pentagastrin, which disrupted placebo responses completely (Benedetti et al., 2011a). Therefore, the activation of the CCK type-2 receptors has the same effect as the μ-opioid receptor antagonist, naloxone, which suggests that the balance between cholecystokinergic and opioidergic systems is crucial in placebo responsiveness in pain. Therefore, one of the most interesting models we have today involves two opposing neurotransmitter systems, opioids and CCK (Fig. 4.5).

In 1984, Fields and Levine (1984) hypothesized that the placebo response can be subdivided into opioid and nonopioid components. In particular, Fields and Levine suggested that different physical, psychological, and environmental situations might affect the endogenous opioid systems differently. This concept was further supported by the finding that the placebo analgesic effect is not always mediated by endogenous opioids (Gracely et al., 1983). Amanzio and Benedetti (1999) partially addressed this issue, showing that both expectation and a conditioning procedure can result in placebo analgesia. The former is capable of activating opioid systems, and the latter activates specific subsystems. In fact, if the placebo response is induced by means of strong expectation cues, it can be blocked by the opioid antagonist naloxone. Similarly, if a placebo is given after repeated administrations of morphine (preconditioning procedure), the placebo response can be blocked by naloxone. Conversely, if the placebo response is induced by means of prior conditioning with a nonopioid drug, it is naloxone-insensitive (Amanzio and Benedetti, 1999).

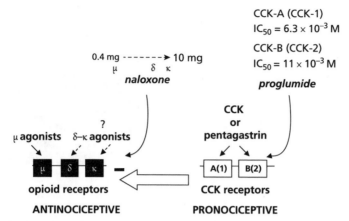

CCK-A (CCK-1)
$IC_{50} = 6.3 \times 10^{-3}$ M

CCK-B (CCK-2)
$IC_{50} = 11 \times 10^{-3}$ M

0.4 mg - - - - - - -► 10 mg
μ   δ   κ
naloxone

proglumide

CCK
or
pentagastrin

?
μ agonists   δ–κ agonists

μ agonists   δ–κ agonists

| μ | δ | κ | — | A(1) | B(2) |

opioid receptors   **CCK receptors**

ANTINOCICEPTIVE   **PRONOCICEPTIVE**

Fig. 4.5 Placebo administration induces activation of μ-opioid receptors. High doses of naloxone are necessary to block the placebo's analgesic effect, meaning that κ and δ receptors may also be involved. This placebo-activated antinociceptive opioid system is antagonized by a CCK-ergic pronociceptive system. In fact, the CCK antagonist, proglumide, is capable of potentiating placebo analgesia. Proglumide is a nonspecific CCK-A (or CCK-1) and CCK-B (or CCK-2) receptor antagonist, as shown by the similar binding affinity, expressed as the concentration required to inhibit by 50% the specific binding of 125I-Bolton-Hunter CCK-8 (IC50), for CCK-A and CCK-B receptors. Reproduced from Fabrizio Benedetti, Mechanisms of placebo and placebo-related effects across diseases and treatments, *Annual Review of Pharmacology and Toxicology*, 48, pp. 33–60 Copyright 2008, Annual Reviews.

Specific placebo analgesic responses can be obtained in different parts of the body (Montgomery and Kirsch, 1996; Price et al., 1999). It was found that these responses are naloxone-reversible (Benedetti et al., 1999a). If four noxious stimuli are applied to the hands and feet and a placebo cream is applied to one hand only, then pain is reduced only on the hand on which the placebo cream had been applied. This highly specific effect is blocked by naloxone, suggesting that the placebo-activated endogenous opioid systems have a precise and somatotopic organization (Benedetti et al., 1999).

A common observation in all these studies is that the naloxone dose needed to block placebo analgesia is as large as 10 mg, which suggests the involvement of different classes of opioid receptors, like the μ, κ, and δ classes of receptors (Fig. 4.5). In fact, the binding affinity of naloxone for κ and δ receptors is about 10–15 times lower than for the μ receptors; thus large doses are supposed to involve κ and δ receptors as well.

In 2002, Petrovic et al. (2002) found that some brain regions in the cerebral cortex and the brainstem are affected by both a placebo and the rapidly acting opioid agonist remifentanil, thus indicating a related mechanism in placebo-induced and opioid-induced analgesia. In particular, administration of a placebo induced the activation of the rostral anterior cingulate cortex and the orbitofrontal cortex. Moreover, there was significant co-variation in activity between the rostral anterior cingulate cortex and the lower pons and medulla, and sub-significant co-variation in activity between the rostral anterior cingulate cortex and the periaqueductal gray. This suggests that the

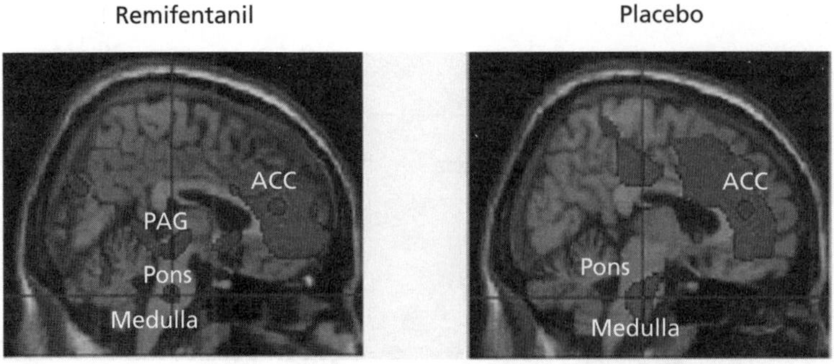

Remifentanil   Placebo

Fig. 4.6 Comparison of the effects of remifentanil, an opioid receptor agonist, and placebo on brain activation. The blue spot indicates the anterior cingulate cortex (ACC) which is activated both by the real drug and the placebo. The red areas are co-activated with the anterior cingulate cortex, suggesting activation of a common neural network by both opioids and placebos, with the exception of periaqueductal gray (PAG), which is co-activated sub-significantly in the placebo condition. Adapted from Predrag Petrovic, Eija Kalso, Karl Magnus Petersson, and Martin Ingvar, Placebo and Opioid Analgesia—Imaging a Shared Neuronal Network, *Science*, 295 (5560), pp. 1737–1740, Copyright 2002, The American Association for the Advancement of Science. Reprinted with permission from AAAS. (See Plate 2.)

pain-modulating circuit of the descending rostral anterior cingulate–periaqueductal gray–rostral ventromedial medulla is involved in placebo analgesia (Fig. 4.6), as previously hypothesized by Fields and Price (1997).

In 2005, the first direct evidence of opioid-mediated placebo analgesia was published (Zubieta et al., 2005). In vivo receptor-binding techniques using the radiotracer carfentanil, a μ-opioid agonist, were used to show that a placebo procedure activates μ-opioid neurotransmission in the dorsolateral prefrontal cortex, the anterior cingulate cortex, the insula, and the nucleus accumbens (Fig. 4.7). A more detailed account of μ-opioid neurotransmission after placebo administration was carried out in another study which used noxious thermal stimulation (Wager et al., 2007). Placebo treatment affected opioid activity in a number of predicted opioid-rich regions that play central roles in pain and affect, including the periaqueductal gray, dorsal raphe and nucleus cuneiformis, amygdala, orbitofrontal cortex, insula, rostral anterior cingulate, and lateral prefrontal cortex. Opioid activity in many of these regions correlated with placebo effects in reported pain. Connectivity analyses on individual differences in opioid binding revealed that placebo treatment increased connectivity between the periaqueductal gray and the rostral anterior cingulate cortex, and increased functional integration among limbic regions and the prefrontal cortex. Overall, the results suggest that endogenous opioid release in core affective brain regions is an integral part of the mechanism whereby expectations regulate affective and nociceptive circuits.

Our knowledge about the involvement of endogenous opioids in placebo analgesia has increased even more in the past few years. For example, it is now clear that a specific descending pain modulating network mediates the analgesic effect that follows

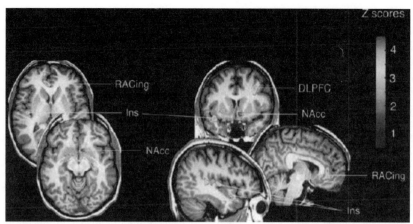

Fig. 4.7 Placebo administration induces the activation of μ-opioid neurotransmission in several brain regions, such as the dorsolateral prefrontal cortex (DLPFC), the anterior cingulate cortex (RACing), the nucleus accumbens (NAcc) and the insula (Ins). Reproduced from Jon-Kar Zubieta, Joshua A. Bueller, Lisa R. Jackson, David J. Scott, Yanjun Xu, Robert A. Koeppe, Thomas E. Nichols, and Christian S. Stohler, Placebo Effects Mediated by Endogenous Opioid Activity on μ-Opioid Receptors, *The Journal of Neuroscience*, 25 (34), pp. 7754–7762 Copyright 2005, The Society for Neuroscience, with permission. (See Plate 3.)

the administration of a placebo. Eippert et al. (2009a) combined naloxone administration with functional magnetic resonance imaging, and found that naloxone reduced both behavioral and neural placebo effects as well as placebo-induced responses in pain-modulatory cortical structures, such as the rostral anterior cingulate cortex. In a brainstem-specific analysis, they also found a similar naloxone modulation of placebo-induced responses in key structures of the descending pain control system, such as the hypothalamus, the periaqueductal gray, and the rostral ventromedial medulla. Interestingly, naloxone abolished placebo-induced coupling between the rostral anterior cingulate cortex and the periaqueductal gray, which predicted both behavioral and neural placebo effects as well as the activation of the rostral ventromedial medulla. The same group found that the activation of this descending system following placebo administration extends to the dorsal horns of the spinal cord, although we do not know whether the spinal effects are mediated by endogenous opioids (Eippert et al., 2009b).

All these opioid-mediated placebo responses have also been investigated in rodents (see section 2.3.7), and similar mechanisms have been described (Guo et al., 2010; Nolan et al., 2012; Zhang et al., 2013). For example, Guo et al. (2010) used the hot-plate test in an attempt to measure the reaction time of mice to a nociceptive stimulus (hot plate) after different types of pharmacological conditioning. This was performed by the combination of the conditioned cue stimulus with the unconditioned drug stimulus, either the opioid morphine or the nonopioid aspirin. If mice were conditioned with morphine, placebo analgesia was completely antagonized by naloxone, whereas if mice were conditioned with aspirin, placebo analgesia was naloxone-insensitive, as already found in humans by Amanzio and Benedetti (1999).

Nolan et al. (2012) used an elegant model of operant conditioning in rats with an affective behavioral endpoint, whereby rodents express their willingness to withstand thermal pain to obtain sweet reward, a kind of conflict-reward assay. This paradigm tests mild noninjurious pain and, unlike other models such as the hot plate, it is likely to incorporate cognitive and affective components of pain, which often represent the most common and debilitating aspects of chronic pain sufferers. In this model, a reward bottle with sweetened milk was positioned such that access to the milk reward was possible contingent on facial contact with a thermode. The rats were conditioned by pairing thermal pain with a subcutaneous injection of morphine. After two conditioning trials, morphine was replaced with saline solution and the analgesic response tested by assessing the ratio of successful licks to lick attempts. This procedure induced a kind of placebo analgesic response that was suppressed by the opioid antagonist naloxone, thus showing that it is mediated by endogenous opioids.

This new approach to the placebo effect by using animal models is promising for future research, for it allows us to investigate those biochemical pathways and neurobiological mechanisms that are not possible to analyze in humans. For example, by using different antagonists of different subtypes of opioid receptors (μ, δ, κ), Zhang et al. (2013) were able to conclude that placebo analgesia is mediated specifically only by the μ-opioid receptors.

Box 4.4 The opioid and cannabinoid systems

The endogenous opioid system is a complex network with many endogenous ligands, receptors as well as with many functions. Endogenous ligands, which come from their respective precursors, show affinity for different receptor subtypes (MOR or μ, DOR or δ, KOR or κ) (Fig. 4.8). The endogenous ligand nociceptin and its ORL receptor are different from the other opioid receptors, for they show antiopioid activity.

The main endogenous ligands of the endocannabinoid system are anandamide and 2-arachidonoylglicerol (2-AG). They are synthetized on demand from membrane phospholipids-related precursors, such as N-arachidonoyl phosphatidylethanolamine

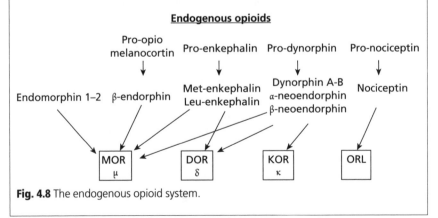

Fig. 4.8 The endogenous opioid system.

Box 4.4 The opioid and cannabinoid systems (continued)

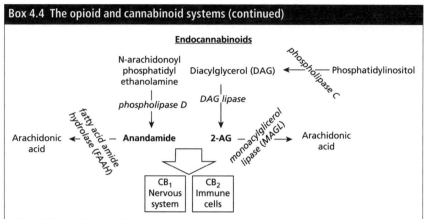

Fig. 4.9 The endocannabinoid system.

and phosphatidylinositol, through different phospholipases, and are quickly degraded to arachidonic acid through the FAAH and MAGL enzymes (Fig. 4.9). They show more affinity for CB_1 cannabinoid receptors, which are located mainly in the nervous system, than for CB_2 receptors, which can be found mainly on the cells of the immune system.

Although Figs. 4.8 and 4.9 are schematic and simplified representations, it is clear that these two systems are very complex, both for their metabolism (synthesis and degradation) and for their multiple action on different receptors. In fact, both the opioids and cannabinoids act at the level of different systems, like the brain and the immune system, as well as the cardiovascular and the gastrointestinal systems.

4.1.7 Some types of placebo analgesia involve the endocannabinoid system

It has long been known that the endogenous opioid systems are not the only mechanisms involved in placebo analgesia. One example of nonopioid-mediated placebo responses is represented by the previous exposure to a nonopioid drug, such as ketorolac (Amanzio and Benedetti, 1999). When ketorolac is administered for 2 days in a row and then replaced with a placebo on the third day, the placebo analgesic response is not reversed by naloxone; this indicates that specific pharmacological mechanisms are involved in a learned placebo response, depending on the previous exposure to opioid or nonopioid substances. Other examples of placebo analgesic effect that are not mediated by opioids have been described in people with IBS (Vase et al., 2005) and in experimental pain in brain imaging studies (Petrovic et al., 2010).

On the basis of these considerations, Benedetti et al. (2011b) induced opioid or non-opioid placebo analgesic responses and assessed the effects of the CB_1 cannabinoid receptor antagonist rimonabant. Differently from naloxone, rimonabant had no effect on opioid-induced placebo analgesia following morphine preconditioning, whereas it completely blocked placebo analgesia following nonopioid preconditioning with the nonsteroid anti-inflammatory drug (NSAID) ketorolac. These findings indicate that those placebo analgesic responses that are elicited by NSAIDs conditioning are mediated by CB_1 cannabinoid receptors. Since the involvement of the CB_1 cannabinoid receptors in placebo analgesia is a recent finding, little is known about their localization and activation. As far as we know today, they are activated following a previous exposure to NSAIDs, which suggests that these drugs, besides the inhibition of cyclooxygenase and prostaglandin synthesis, activate an endocannabinoid pathway (Benedetti et al., 2011b). Indeed, nonopioid drugs, such as metamizole, have been found both to inhibit the enzyme cyclooxygenase and to act on the CB_1 cannabinoid receptors in rodents (Escobar et al. 2012).

On the basis of these considerations, a change in availability of endogenous ligands for CB_1 cannabinoid receptors, such as anandamide, should be expected to modulate placebo analgesia in some circumstances. Indeed, Peciña et al. (2014) investigated the role of the common, functional missense variant Pro129Thr of the gene coding fatty acid amide hydrolase (FAAH), the major degrading enzyme of endocannabinoids, on psychophysical and dopaminergic and opioid responses to pain and placebo-induced analgesia in humans. FAAH Pro129/Pro129 homozygotes reported higher placebo analgesic responses and more positive affective states immediately and 24 hours after placebo administration. Pro129/Pro129 homozygotes also showed greater placebo-induced μ opioid, but not D2/D3 dopaminergic, enhancements in neurotransmission in regions known involved in placebo effects.

Therefore, the endocannabinoid system (Box 4.4) may take part in placebo analgesia in some conditions. Fig. 4.10 shows a simplified schema of the involvement of endocannabinoids in placebo analgesia. The activation of the CB_1 cannabinoid receptors induces placebo analgesic responses (Benedetti et al., 2011b). If the enzyme FAAH does not work properly, anandamide, one of the principal endogenous ligands of CB_1 receptors, is not degraded to arachidonic acid, and thus accumulates within the nervous system (Peciña et al., 2014). This in turn may modulate the CB_1 receptors.

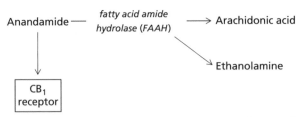

Fig. 4.10 The activation of the CB_1 cannabinoid receptors is a mechanism of placebo analgesia. These receptors can be activated by nonopioid drugs, such as ketorolac, or by anandamide, an endogenous ligand. If FAAH does not work properly, anandamide is not degraded to arachidonic acid and ethanolamine, thus it accumulates in the brain, with the consequent change in the modulation of the CB_1 receptors.

4.1.8 **Placebo analgesia is related to a reward dopaminergic system**

In a brain imaging study in which both positron emission tomography and functional magnetic resonance imaging were used, Scott et al. (2007) tested the correlation between responsiveness to placebo and that to a monetary reward, using a model of experimental pain in healthy subjects. They found that placebo responsiveness was related to the activation of dopamine in the nucleus accumbens, a region involved in reward mechanisms (Ikemoto and Panksepp, 1999; Schultz et al., 2000; Schultz, 2002; Knutson and Cooper, 2005), as assessed by using in vivo receptor-binding positron emission tomography with raclopride, a D2/D3 dopamine receptor antagonist. The very same subjects were then tested with functional magnetic resonance imaging for monetary responses in the nucleus accumbens. What these investigators found was a correlation between the placebo responses and the monetary responses—the larger the nucleus accumbens responses to monetary reward, the stronger the nucleus accumbens responses to placebos.

This study strongly suggests that placebo responsiveness depends on the functioning and efficiency of the reward system. It explains why some individuals respond to placebos and others do not (see also section 2.3.8). Those who have a more efficient dopaminergic reward system would also be good placebo responders. Interestingly, Scott et al. (2007) used an experimental approach that is typical of clinical trials, whereby the subjects know they have a 50% chance of receiving either placebo or active treatment, and whereby no prior conditioning was performed. Thus more powerful placebo responses should have been expected if the subject knew they had a 100% chance of getting active treatment but actually received the placebo (deceptive administration), or if prior pharmacological conditioning had been carried out.

In a different study by the same group, Scott et al. (2008) studied the endogenous opioid and the dopaminergic systems in different brain regions, including those involved in reward and motivational behavior. Subjects underwent a pain challenge, in the absence and presence of a placebo with expected analgesic properties. Positron emission tomography with 11C-labeled raclopride was used for analyzing dopamine and 11C-carfentanil for analyzing opioids. There was placebo-induced activation of opioid neurotransmission in the anterior cingulate, orbitofrontal, and insular cortices, nucleus accumbens, amygdala, and periaqueductal gray matter. Dopaminergic activation was observed in the ventral basal ganglia, including the nucleus accumbens. Both dopaminergic and opioid activity were associated with both anticipation and perceived effectiveness of the placebo, as shown by the reduction in pain ratings. Large placebo responses were associated with greater dopamine and opioid activity in the nucleus accumbens. Interestingly, nocebo responses were associated with a deactivation of dopamine and opioid release. The release of dopamine in the nucleus accumbens accounted for 25% of the variance in placebo analgesic effects. Therefore, placebo and nocebo effects seem to be associated with opposite responses of dopamine and endogenous opioids in a distributed network of regions that form part of the reward and motivation circuit.

4.1.9 **Imaging the brain during placebo-induced expectations of analgesia**

Modern brain imaging techniques have been fundamental in the understanding of placebo analgesia, and many brain imaging studies have been carried out to describe the functional neuroanatomy of the placebo analgesic effect (e.g., Petrovic et al., 2002; Lieberman et al., 2004; Wager et al., 2004, 2007, 2011; Bingel et al., 2005; Zubieta et al., 2005; Kong et al., 2006; Price et al., 2007; Scott et al., 2007, 2008; Eippert et al., 2009a, 2009b; Zubieta and Stohler, 2009; Lui et al., 2010; Tracey, 2010; Meissner et al., 2011; Hashmi et al., 2012).

As described earlier, the first imaging study of placebo analgesia showed that a subset of brain regions is similarly affected by either a placebo or a μ-opioid agonist (Petrovic et al. 2002). In particular, the administration of a placebo induced the activation of the rostral anterior cingulate cortex, the orbitofrontal cortex, and the anterior insula, and there was a significant co-variation in activity between the rostral anterior cingulate cortex and the lower pons/medulla, and a sub-significant co-variation between the rostral anterior cingulate cortex and the periaqueductal gray, suggesting that a descending pain-modulating circuit is involved in placebo analgesia (Fig. 4.6). There is experimental evidence that this modulating descending circuit, as described by Fields and Basbaum (1999), involves the spinal cord, (Matre et al., 2006; Goffaux et al., 2007; Eippert et al., 2009b), and some more details were given in section 4.1.6.

In a functional magnetic resonance imaging study of experimentally induced pain in healthy subjects, Wager et al. (2004) found that placebo analgesia was related to decreased neural activity in pain-processing areas of the brain (Fig. 4.11). Pain-related neural activity was reduced within the thalamus, anterior insular cortex, and anterior cingulate cortex during the placebo condition as compared with the baseline condition. The magnitudes of these decreases were correlated with reductions in pain ratings. Not only did Wager et al. (2004) image the time period of pain but also the time period of the anticipation of pain (Fig. 4.11). They hypothesized increases in neural activity within brain areas involved in expectation, and indeed they found significant positive correlations between increases in brain activity in the anticipatory period and decreases in pain and pain-related neural activity during stimulation within the placebo condition. The brain regions showing positive correlations during the anticipatory phase included the orbitofrontal cortex, dorsolateral prefrontal cortex, rostral anterior cingulate cortex, and midbrain periaqueductal gray. The dorsolateral prefrontal cortex is a region that has been associated with the representation and maintenance of information needed for cognitive control, consistent with a role in expectation (Miller and Cohen, 2001). On the other hand, the orbitofrontal cortex is associated with functioning in the evaluative and reward information relevant to allocation of control, consistent with a role in affective or motivational responses to anticipation of pain (Dias et al., 1996).

The anterior cingulate cortex is often reported to be involved in placebo analgesia, although some discordant results have been obtained. For example, it was found to have increased activity in a study by Petrovic et al. (2002) and decreased activity in a study by Wager et al. (2004), which might be explained on the basis of the different experimental settings.

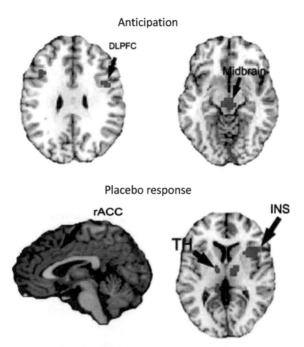

Fig. 4.11 Administration of a placebo following thermal painful stimulation induces anticipatory responses in the dorsolateral prefrontal cortex (DLPFC) and midbrain, which increase their activity. During the placebo analgesic response, some areas decrease their activity, such as the rostral anterior cingulate cortex (rACC), the thalamus (TH), and the insula (INS). Adapted from Tor D. Wager, James K. Rilling, Edward E. Smith, Alex Sokolik, Kenneth L. Casey, Richard J. Davidson, Stephen M. Kosslyn, Robert M. Rose, and Jonathan D. Cohen, Placebo-Induced Changes in fMRI in the Anticipation and Experience of Pain, *Science*, 303 (5661), pp. 1162–1167 Copyright 2004, The American Association for the Advancement of Science. Reprinted with permission from AAAS. (See Plate 4.)

Most of the brain imaging studies aimed at investigating placebo analgesia have been performed in experimental settings in healthy volunteers. By contrast, Price et al. (2007) conducted a functional magnetic resonance imaging study in which brain activity of IBS patients was measured in response to rectal distension by a balloon barostat (see also section 9.1.3 and Fig. 9.2). A large placebo effect was produced by suggestions and accompanied by large reductions in neural activity in the thalamus, the primary and secondary somatosensory cortices, the insula, and the anterior cingulate cortex during the period of stimulation. It was accompanied by increases in neural activity in the rostral anterior cingulate cortex, bilateral amygdala, and periaqueductal gray (Price et al., 2008). This study is quite important and informative, as it shows that placebos act on the brain in a clinically relevant condition in the same way as they do in the experimental setting. Therefore, the involvement of key areas in placebo analgesia, such as the anterior cingulate cortex, is not limited to experimental noxious stimuli but also extends to clinical pain. The study by Price et al. (2007) is also interesting because reductions in brain activity occurred during the stimulus presentation itself, not just when subjects reported pain. In fact it has been argued that the length of the painful stimulation may be critical for the measurement of placebo effects, as most studies used short heat or electric shock as pain stimuli and recorded activity decreases during periods extending after the stimulus offset, thus possibly including a later cognitive reappraisal of the significance of pain and/or late neural activity influenced by report bias.

In order to determine whether expectation of analgesia exerts its psychophysical effect through changes of the perceptual sensitivity of early cortical processes (in the primary and secondary somatosensory areas) or on later cortical elaborations, such as stimulus identification and response selection in the anterior cingulate cortex, Lorenz et al. (2005) used high temporal resolution techniques (magnetoencephalography). They found that activity in the secondary somatosensory cortex was highly correlated to the extent of influence of the subjective pain rating by prestimulus expectation, while anterior cingulate cortex activity seemed to be associated only to stimulus intensity and related attentional engagement. In another study on laser-evoked potentials by Wager et al. (2006), early nociceptive components were found to be affected by placebos. Therefore, later cognitive reappraisal of the significance of pain and/or late neural activity influenced by report bias cannot be responsible for this early modulation. This indicates that the very early sensory components are affected by placebo manipulation.

Overall, all these brain imaging data have been summarized by using a meta-analysis approach with the activation likelihood estimation method (Amanzio et al., 2013). Nine functional magnetic resonance studies and two positron emission tomography studies were selected for the analysis. During the expectation phase of analgesia, areas of activation were found in the left anterior cingulate, right precentral and lateral prefrontal cortex, and in the left periaqueductal gray. In the phase following pain stimulation, activations were found in the anterior cingulate and medial and lateral prefrontal cortices, in the left inferior parietal lobule and postcentral gyrus, anterior insula, thalamus, hypothalamus, periaqueductal gray, and pons. Conversely, deactivations were found in the left mid- and posterior cingulate cortex, superior temporal and precentral gyri, in the left anterior and right posterior insula, in the claustrum and putamen, and in the right thalamus and caudate body. These meta-analytic data summarize all brain imaging studies and give a global figure of the sequence of events following placebo administration: after the activation of a pain modulatory network during the expectation phase and the early pain phase, several deactivations occur in different areas involved in pain processing.

4.1.10 **No prefrontal control, no placebo response**

A common finding across different neuroimaging studies is represented by the involvement of the prefrontal areas in the placebo response, for example, the dorsolateral prefrontal cortex. Since in Alzheimer's disease the frontal lobes are severely affected, with marked neuronal degeneration in the dorsolateral prefrontal cortex, the orbitofrontal cortex, and the anterior cingulate cortex (Thomson et al., 2003), and the prefrontal lobes are responsible for complex mental functions (Box 4.5), it is reasonable to expect a disruption of placebo responsiveness in these patients.

On the basis of these considerations, Benedetti et al. (2006b) studied Alzheimer patients at the initial stage of the disease and after 1 year, in order to see whether the placebo component of the therapy was affected by the disease. The placebo component of the analgesic therapy was found to be correlated with both cognitive status and functional connectivity among different brain regions, according to the rule "the more impaired the prefrontal connectivity, the smaller the placebo response." In a more recent study, Stein et al. (2012) used diffusion tensor magnetic resonance imaging to test the hypothesis of the role of white matter integrity in placebo responsiveness. The individual placebo analgesic effect was found to be correlated with white matter integrity indexed by fractional anisotropy, particularly in the right dorsolateral prefrontal cortex, left rostral anterior cingulate cortex, and the periaqueductal gray. Probabilistic tractography seeded in these regions showed that stronger placebo analgesic responses were associated with increased mean fractional anisotropy values within white matter tracts connecting the periaqueductal gray with the rostral anterior cingulate cortex and the dorsolateral prefrontal cortex. Therefore, both the study on Alzheimer patients (Benedetti et al., 2006b) and on white matter integrity in normal subjects (Stein et al., 2012) demonstrate the importance of prefrontal functioning and connectivity in the placebo response.

Box 4.5 Prefrontal executive control

The set of frontal functions that control purposive behavior are named executive functions, or executive control. Frontal executive functions control volition, planning, programming, anticipation, inhibition of inappropriate behaviors, and monitoring of complex goal-directed, purposeful activities. The impairment of frontal lobes implies the loss of executive control, with the disruption of planning capacity, working memory, attention, stimuli discrimination, abstraction, and capacity of initiating the required behavior. Not only are executive functions related to the functioning of the frontal lobes, but also to subcortical regions that belong to cortical-subcortical loops. For example, dementia affecting the striatum, globus pallidus, thalamus, and white matter may interrupt prefrontal-subcortical loops that are involved in executive control. In addition, it should be noted that these cortical-subcortical loops also involve the limbic system, thereby influencing emotional behavior as well, like uninhibited behaviors and impulsivity.

The Frontal Assessment Battery (FAB) is an easy test that can be performed at the bedside. It was devised to assess executive functions of the frontal lobes by measuring complex functions, like abstract reasoning, mental flexibility, motor programming, sensitivity to interference commands, inhibitory control, and environmental autonomy (Dubois et al. 2000).

The Frontal Assessment Battery

1 Conceptualization

This function can be investigated by card-sorting tasks, proverb interpretation, or similarities. The last task is easier for bedside assessment and scoring. Subjects have

---

Box 4.5 Prefrontal executive control (continued)

to conceptualize the links between two objects from the same category (e.g., an apple and a banana belong to the category "fruit").

2 Mental flexibility

In this task, subjects need to recall as many words as they can beginning with a given letter in a 1-minute trial.

3 Motor programming

In Luria's motor series, such as "fist–palm–edge," less severely impaired patients are unable to execute the series in correct order, whereas the most severely affected are unable to learn the series. Simplification of the task (two gestures instead of three) and perseveration (inappropriate repetition of the same gestures) may be observed.

4 Sensitivity to interference

Tasks in which verbal commands conflict with sensory information, for example, in the Stroop test, in which the subject must name the colors of words while inhibiting the natural tendency to read the words.

5 Inhibitory control

It can be assessed with the go–no-go paradigm, in which the subjects must inhibit a response that was previously given to the same stimulus, for example, not tapping when the examiner taps twice.

6 Environmental autonomy

Assessment of excessive dependency on environmental cues. For example, the patient conceives the sight of a movement as an order to imitate (imitation behavior); the sight of an object implies the order to use it (utilization behavior); and the sight or sensory perception of the examiner's hands compels the patient to take them (prehension behavior).

To support the crucial role of the prefrontal cortex in the occurrence of placebo responses, Krummenacher et al. (2010) used rTMS to inactivate the prefrontal cortex during placebo analgesia. These investigators inactivated the left and right dorsolateral prefrontal cortex during a procedure inducing placebo analgesia, and found that rTMS completely blocked the analgesic placebo response. Therefore, the inactivation of the prefrontal lobes has the same effects as those observed in prefrontal degeneration in Alzheimer's disease and reduced integrity of prefrontal white matter.

Interestingly, Eippert et al. (2009a) found that the opioid antagonist naloxone blocks placebo analgesia, along with a reduction in the activation of the dorsolateral prefrontal cortex, suggesting that a prefrontal opioidergic mechanism is crucial in the placebo analgesic response. Thus, a disruption of prefrontal control is associated to a loss of placebo response (Benedetti, 2010).

Two clinical implications emerge from these findings. First, in order to compensate for the disruption of placebo/expectation-related mechanisms, we need to consider a possible revision of some therapies in Alzheimer patients. Second, we should consider the potential disruption of placebo mechanisms in all those conditions where the prefrontal regions are involved, as occurs in vascular and frontotemporal dementia as well as in any lesion of the prefrontal cortex.

4.2 Nocebo hyperalgesia

4.2.1 Expectations of worsening may lead to hyperalgesia

Although not always studied under strictly controlled conditions, many interesting nocebo and/or nocebo-like effects are present in daily life and in routine clinical practice (Benedetti et al., 2007; Colloca and Benedetti, 2007). For example, negative diagnoses and prognoses can lead to an amplification of pain intensity and, more in general, negative communication within the healing context may have important effects on patients' emotions (Wells and Kaptchuk, 2012; Holloway et al., 2013). Likewise, nocebo and/or nocebo-related effects may occur when distrust towards medical personnel and therapies are present. In this latter case, unwanted effects and side effects may occur as the result of negative expectations (Flaten et al., 1999; Barsky et al., 2002), and these may reduce, or even conceal, the efficacy of some treatments. For example, it has been found that verbal suggestions can change the direction of nitrous oxide action from analgesia to hyperalgesia (Dworkin et al., 1983). Another example is the health reports that are commonly issued in Western societies; negative warnings sent out by the mass media may have an important impact on the perceived symptoms of many people. In a recent study on headaches caused by mobile phone use, no evidence of radiofrequency-induced headache and pain was found, so the authors concluded that the pain increase was likely to be due to a nocebo effect (Oftedal et al., 2007). Diseases with an important psychological component, like IBS, are also affected by nocebo effects (see section 9.1); sedatives and opioids in postoperative pain management have been found to be influenced by supposed nocebo effects as well (Manchikanti et al., 2005; Svedman et al., 2005). Similarly, some negative expectation-inducing procedures, like voodoo magic, may lead to symptom worsening (see section 1.2.4). Finally, the fear–avoidance model of pain can be seen as a sort of nocebo-like effect, whereby the fear of pain may lead to pain worsening (Vlaeyen and Linton, 2000; Leeuw et al., 2007).

The clinical trials setting is also important for nocebo effects. For example, in analgesic clinical trials, adverse events are reported for the painkiller under evaluation and compared with adverse events in the placebo group. Patients who receive the placebo often report a high frequency of adverse events. Amanzio et al. (2009) compared the rates of adverse events reported in the placebo arms of clinical trials for three classes of antimigraine drugs: nonsteroidal anti-inflammatory drugs (NSAIDs), triptans and anticonvulsants. It was found that the rate of adverse events in the placebo arms of trials with antimigraine drugs was high. In addition, and most interestingly, the adverse events in the placebo arms corresponded to those of the antimigraine medication against which the placebo was compared. For example, anorexia and memory difficulties, which are typical adverse events of anticonvulsants, were present only in the placebo arm of these trials. These results suggest that the adverse events in placebo arms of clinical trials of antimigraine medications depend on the adverse events of the active medication against which the placebo is compared. These findings are certainly in keeping with the expectation theory of placebo and nocebo effects. Similar findings were obtained by Mitsikostas et al. (2011) for headache, Mitsikostas et al. (2012) for fibromyalgia, Häuser et al. (2012) for diabetic peripheral neuropathy, and Papadopoulos and Mitsikostas (2012) for neuropathic pain. These authors emphasized how dropouts due to nocebo effects may confound the interpretation of many clinical trials.

Both in experimental and clinical settings, it has long been known that the perceived intensity of a painful stimulus following negative expectation of pain increase is higher than in the absence of negative expectations. For example, expectation of painful stimulation amplifies perceived unpleasantness of innocuous thermal stimulation (Sawamoto et al., 2000), and the level of expected pain intensity alters perceived pain intensity. In fact, by using two visual cues, each conditioned to one of two noxious thermal stimuli (high and low), Keltner et al. (2006) showed that subjects reported higher pain when the noxious stimulus was preceded by the high-intensity visual cue.

By using a real nocebo procedure, whereby an inert substance was administered along with verbal suggestions of hyperalgesia, Benedetti et al. (1997, 2006a) showed expectation-induced hyperalgesia both in the clinical and experimental setting. In the clinical setting, the situation was a post-surgical manipulation that induced expectations of pain increase, so that the patients were given an inert treatment that they expected to be painful (Benedetti et al., 1997). A straightforward increase in pain was found, and this also occurred in the experimental setting using the tourniquet technique, whereby ischemic pain was induced in one arm (Benedetti et al., 2006a). These effects can be quite powerful, and sometimes pain can be generated from a nonpainful stimulus. For example, a study by Colloca et al. (2008a) used a nocebo procedure, in which verbal suggestions of painful stimulation were given to healthy volunteers before administration of either tactile or low-intensity painful electrical stimuli. This study showed that these anxiogenic verbal suggestions were capable of turning tactile stimuli into pain, as well as low-intensity painful stimuli into high-intensity pain. Therefore, by defining hyperalgesia as an increase in pain sensitivity and allodynia as the perception of pain in response to innocuous stimulation, nocebo suggestions of a negative outcome can produce both hyperalgesic and allodynic effects. In general, several studies have shown that negative expectations have a dramatic effect on pain perception. Indeed, many recent works have shown that nocebo effects occur in a variety of painful conditions, ranging from experimental to clinical pain (e.g., Varelmann et al., 2010; Elsenbruch et al., 2012; Sanderson et al., 2013; van den Broeke et al., 2014).

The open–hidden (expected–unexpected) approach has also proven to be useful in understanding the importance of expectations in nocebo-related phenomena. In this case, open and hidden interruptions of treatments have been studied. An "open" interruption is performed by a doctor who tells the patient that the treatment has been discontinued. A "hidden" interruption is carried out by a computer and the patient does not know about the interruption: he or she believes that the therapy is still being administered.

Benedetti and collaborators (Benedetti et al., 2003a; Colloca et al., 2004) studied the effects of open (expected) versus hidden (unexpected) interruptions of morphine in postoperative patients (Fig. 4.12). These patients, after having received morphine for 48

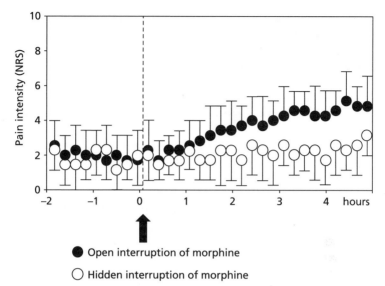

● Open interruption of morphine

○ Hidden interruption of morphine

Fig. 4.12 Open versus hidden interruption of a morphine treatment. The arrow shows the point of morphine interruption. Note the early relapse of pain in the open group (black circles) but not in the hidden one (open circles), indicating that the relapse in the open condition is a psychological effect. NRS, numerical rating scale. Reprinted from The Lancet Neurology, 3 (11), Luana Colloca, Leonardo Lopiano, Michele Lanotte, and Fabrizio Benedetti, Overt versus covert treatment for pain, anxiety, and Parkinson's disease, pp. 679–84 Copyright 2004, with permission from Elsevier.

hours, underwent either open or hidden interruption. In the open condition, they were told that morphine had been stopped; in the hidden condition, morphine was stopped without telling them anything. After interruption of morphine, the pain increase was larger in the open group than in the hidden group. At 10 hours from morphine interruption, more patients of the open group requested further painkillers than those in the hidden group. Therefore, the hidden interruption of morphine prolonged the post-interruption analgesia. This suggests that the open–hidden difference relates to the fact that in the open condition fear and negative expectations of pain relapse (because analgesics are no longer provided) play an important role.

4.2.2 **Learning nocebo effects through observation**

As described in section 2.3.3, placebo effects can be learned through observation, which indicates that social learning plays an important role in placebo responsiveness (Colloca and Benedetti, 2009). The same holds true for nocebo effects. Vögtle et al. (2013) and Swider and Bąbel (2013) studied simultaneously but independently subjects observing a model who simulated more pain in association with either a red light (Swider and Babel, 2013) or the application of an ointment on the skin (Vögtle et al.,

2013). After the observation phase, the experimental subjects showed robust nocebo responses, i.e., hyperalgesic responses, following the presentation of the red light, and this was correlated to empathy scores (Swider and Babel, 2013). Likewise, substantial nocebo responses were found after the observation of the ointment application, and this was correlated to pain catastrophizing (Vögtle et al., 2013). In addition, Swider and Babel (2013) found a gender effect, whereby nocebo hyperalgesia was greater after a male model was observed compared to a female model, regardless of the sex of the experimental subjects.

Therefore, observation and social interaction is important in the overall placebo/nocebo phenomenon, and some personality traits may play a key role, because a correlation was found between the magnitude of the nocebo hyperalgesic responses and empathy and catastrophizing. These findings may have implications both in the clinical trial setting and in medical practice. In the first case, observation of others must be taken into consideration whenever a clinical trial is performed. Patients participating in a clinical trial may be influenced by observing other patients belonging to the same trial. For example, communication among patients enrolled in the same clinical trial is common, and this may influence either positively or negatively the therapeutic outcome. In the second case, doctors and psychologists must consider the possible negative impact that the observation of unsuccessful treatments may have on their patients. This holds true not only in routine medical practice but in daily life as well, whenever others' suffering and negative outcomes are observed, e.g., through the media. Social observational learning can lead to a negative emotional contagion across different individuals, with the consequent activation of nocebo mechanisms.

4.2.3 Nocebo hyperalgesia is mediated by cholecystokinin

Compared with placebo analgesia, much less is known about nocebo hyperalgesia, mainly due to ethical limitations. In fact, whereas the induction of placebo responses is acceptable in many circumstances (Benedetti and Colloca, 2004), the induction of nocebo responses is a stressful and anxiogenic procedure. In fact, to induce nocebo hyperalgesia, an inert treatment is given along with verbal suggestions of pain increase.

In 1997, a trial in postoperative patients was run with the nonspecific cholecystokinin CCK-A/CCK-B (or CCK 1 and 2) receptor antagonist proglumide (Benedetti et al., 1997). The situation was a postsurgical manipulation that induced expectations of pain worsening. It was found that proglumide prevented nocebo hyperalgesia in a dose-dependent manner, even though it is not specifically a painkiller, thus suggesting that the nocebo hyperalgesic effect is mediated by CCK. In fact, a dose as low as 0.05 mg was totally ineffective, while a dose increase to 0.5 mg and 5 mg proved to be effective. As CCK is also involved in anxiety mechanisms, it was hypothesized that proglumide affects anticipatory anxiety (Benedetti et al., 1997; Benedetti and Amanzio, 1997). Importantly, this effect was not antagonized by naloxone. However, due to ethical constraints, these effects were not investigated further in these patients.

In order to better understand the mechanisms underlying nocebo hyperalgesia and to overcome the ethical constraints inherent to the clinical approach, a similar procedure was used in healthy volunteers in whom experimental pain was induced (Benedetti et al., 2006a). It was found that the oral administration of an inert substance, along with verbal suggestions of hyperalgesia, induced both hyperalgesia and hyperactivity of the hypothalamic–pituitary—adrenal (HPA) axis, as assessed by means of adrenocortico-tropic hormone (ACTH) and cortisol plasma concentrations. Both nocebo-induced hyperalgesia and HPA hyperactivity were blocked by the benzodiazepine diazepam, which suggests the involvement of anxiety mechanisms. By contrast, the administra-tion of the mixed CCK-A/CCK-B receptor antagonist, proglumide, blocked nocebo hyperalgesia completely, but had no effect on HPA hyperactivity, suggesting a specific involvement of CCK in the hyperalgesic but not in the anxiety component of the no-cebo effect. Interestingly, neither diazepam nor proglumide showed analgesic proper-ties on baseline pain, as they acted on the nocebo-induced pain increase only. These data suggest that a close relationship between anxiety and nocebo hyperalgesia exists, but also that proglumide does not act by blocking anticipatory anxiety, as previously hypothesized (Benedetti et al., 1997; Benedetti and Amanzio, 1997); rather it inter-rupts a CCK-ergic link between anxiety and pain. Therefore, as shown in Fig. 4.13, in contrast to the anxiolytic action of diazepam, proglumide blocks a CCK-ergic prono-ciceptive system which is activated by anxiety and is responsible for anxiety-induced hyperalgesia. Support for this view comes from a social-defeat model of anxiety in rats, in which CI-988, a selective CCK-B receptor antagonist, prevents anxiety-induced hy-peralgesia (Andre et al., 2005).

Nocebo hyperalgesia is thus an interesting model to better understand when and how the endogenous pronociceptive systems are activated. The pronociceptive and antiopioid action of CCK has been documented in many brain regions (Benedetti, 1997; Hebb et al., 2005; Benedetti et al., 2007). It has been shown that CCK reverses opioid analgesia by acting at the level of the rostral ventromedial medulla (Mitchell et al., 1998; Heinricher et al., 2001) and activates pain-facilitating neurons within the rostral ventromedial medulla (Heinricher and Neubert, 2004). The similarity of the pain-facilitating action of CCK both on brainstem neurons in animals and on nocebo mechanisms in humans may represent an interesting starting point for further research into the neurochemical mechanisms of nocebo-induced hyperalgesia.

It is worth pointing out that the discrepancy between anxiety-induced hyperalgesia and stress-induced analgesia may be only apparent. In fact, stress is known to induce analgesia in a variety of situations, both in animals and in humans. Indeed, when one is under stress, the threshold of pain is increased. However, the nature of the stressor is likely to play a central role. In fact, whereas hyperalgesia may occur when the an-ticipatory anxiety is about the pain itself (Sawamoto et al., 2000; Koyama et al., 2005; Benedetti et al., 2006a; Keltner et al., 2006), analgesia may occur when anxiety is about a stressor that shifts the attention from the pain (Willer and Albe-Fessard, 1980; Ter-man et al., 1986; Flor and Grusser, 1999). We should therefore use these two definitions in two different ways (Colloca and Benedetti, 2007). In the case of anxiety-induced hyperalgesia, we are talking about anticipation of pain, in which attention is focused on the impending pain. We have seen that the biochemical link between this anticipatory anxiety and the pain increase is represented by the CCK-ergic systems. Conversely, we should refer to stress-induced analgesia whenever a general state of arousal stems from a stressful situation in the environment, so that attention is now focused on the

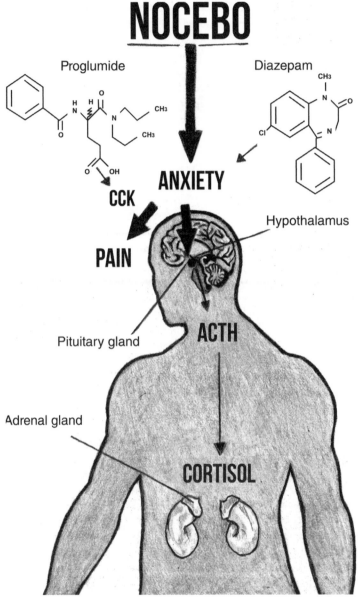

Fig. 4.13 Nocebo administration induces anxiety and this, in turn, activates two different and independent biochemical pathways: a CCK-ergic facilitation of pain and activation of the hypothalamic–pituitary–adrenal (HPA) axis, as assessed by means of increases in plasma adrenocorticotropic hormone (ACTH) and cortisol. The antianxiety drug diazepam blocks anxiety, preventing both hyperalgesia and HPA hyperactivity, but the CCK-antagonist proglumide acts on the CCK-ergic pathway only, inhibiting hyperalgesia but not HPA hyperactivity. CCK, cholecystokinin. From Benedetti F, Lanotte M, Lopiano L and Colloca L (2007). When words are painful—Unraveling the mechanisms of the nocebo effect. *Neuroscience*, **147**, 260–71.

environmental stressor. In this case, there is experimental evidence that analgesia results from the activation of the endogenous opioid systems (Willer and Albe-Fessard,
1980; Terman et al., 1986).

4.2.4 **Imaging the brain when expecting hyperalgesia**

Modern brain imaging techniques have been fundamental to our understanding of
the neurobiology of negative expectations. It should be noted that no inert substance
is given in these studies, and the experimenter typically uses verbal suggestions. Therefore, in this case it is better to talk about nocebo-related effects. Typically, the experimenter tells the subject about the forthcoming pain so as to make the subject expect
a painful stimulation, and both the anticipatory phase and the poststimulus phase are
analyzed.

By using this experimental approach, Sawamoto et al. (2000) found that expectation of painful stimulation amplifies perceived unpleasantness of innocuous thermal
stimulation. These psychophysical findings were correlated to enhanced transient
brain responses to the nonpainful thermal stimulus in the anterior cingulate cortex,
the parietal operculum, and posterior insula. This enhancement consisted in both a
higher intensity signal change (in the anterior cingulate cortex) and a larger volume of
activated voxels (in parietal operculum and posterior insula). Therefore, expecting a
painful stimulus enhances both the subjective unpleasant experience of an innocuous
stimulus and the objective responses in some brain regions.

Overall, negative expectations may result in the amplification of pain (Koyama et al.,
1998; Price, 2000; Dannecker et al., 2003) and several brain regions, like the anterior
cingulate cortex, the prefrontal cortex, and the insula, have been found to be activated
during the anticipation of pain (Chua et al., 1999; Hsieh et al., 1999; Ploghaus et al.,
1999; Porro et al., 2002, 2003; Koyama et al., 2005; Lorenz et al., 2005; Keltner et al.,
2006). These effects are opposite to those elicited by positive expectations, whereby expectations of reduced pain are investigated. In fact, in some studies in which both positive and negative outcomes have been studied with the same experimental approach,
modulation of both subjective experience and brain activation has been found. For example, in a study by Koyama et al. (2005), as the magnitude of expected pain increased,
activation increased in the thalamus, insula, prefrontal cortex and anterior cingulate
cortex. By contrast, expectations of decreased pain reduced activation of pain-related
brain regions, like the primary somatosensory cortex, the insular cortex, and anterior
cingulate cortex. In a different magnetoelectroencephalographic study in which source
localization analysis was performed, Lorenz et al. (2005) found modulation of the
dipole in the secondary somatosensory cortex by nocebo-like and placebo-like suggestions. The dipole was modulated in the same direction as expectations, shrinking
when a decrease in pain was expected and expanding when an increase in pain was
anticipated.

In another study, Keltner et al. (2006) found that the level of expected pain intensity
alters perceived pain intensity, along with the activation of different brain regions (Fig.
4.14). By using two visual cues, each conditioned to one of two noxious thermal stimuli
(high and low), these investigators showed that subjects reported higher pain when

HIGH TEMPERATURE

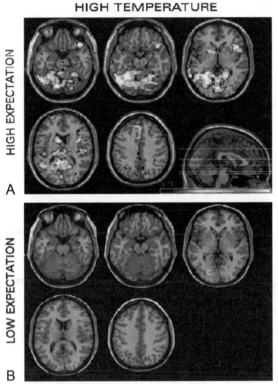

Fig. 4.14 Magnetic resonance imaging showing brain functional responses to a high-temperature stimulus when the subject expects (A) a high-intensity or (B) a low-intensity stimulation. Note that expectation of a high-intensity noxious stimulus activates different areas—the thalamus, insular cortex, somatosensory cortex, anterior cingulate cortex, orbitofrontal cortex, amygdala, ventral striatum, and nucleus cuneiformis in the brainstem—unlike expectation of a low-intensity noxious stimulus. Reproduced from John R. Keltner, Ansgar Furst, Catherine Fan, Rick Redfern, Ben Inglis, and Howard L. Fields, Isolating the Modulatory Effect of Expectation on Pain Transmission: A Functional Magnetic Resonance Imaging Study, *The Journal of Neuroscience*, 26 (16), pp. 4437–4443 doi: 10.1523/JNEUROSCI.4463–05.2006 Copyright 2006, The Society for Neuroscience. (See Plate 5.)

the noxious stimulus was preceded by the high-intensity visual cue. By comparing the brain activation produced by the two visual cues, they found significant differences in the ipsilateral caudal anterior cingulate cortex, the head of the caudate, the cerebellum, and the contralateral nucleus cuneiformis. Interestingly, the imaging results of this study indicate that expectation and noxious stimulus intensity act in an additive manner on afferent pathways activated by cutaneous noxious thermal stimulation.

Somehow differently from the previous studies, Kong et al. (2008) investigated the nocebo responses by administering an inert treatment which the subjects believed to be hyperalgesic. These investigators showed that, after administering the inert treatment along with negative suggestions, subjective pain intensity ratings increased significantly more on nocebo regions compared with the control regions in which no expectation manipulation was performed. Functional magnetic resonance imaging analysis of hyperalgesic nocebo responses to identical calibrated noxious stimuli showed signal increases in brain regions including bilateral dorsal anterior cingulate cortex, insula, superior temporal gyrus, left frontal and parietal operculum, medial frontal gyrus, orbital prefrontal cortex, superior parietal lobule, and hippocampus; right claustrum/putamen, lateral prefrontal gyrus, and middle temporal gyrus. Functional connectivity analysis of spontaneous resting-state showed a correlation between two seed regions (left frontal operculum and hippocampus) and pain network including bilateral insula, operculum, anterior cingulate cortex, and left primary somatosensory and motor cortices. Therefore, nocebo hyperalgesia may be predominantly produced through an affective-cognitive pain pathway (medial pain system), and the left hippocampus may play an important role in this process.

Early enhancement of pain signals in the dorsal horn of the spinal cord has also been found in a study in which nocebo hyperalgesia was investigated in combination with spinal functional magnetic resonance imaging in healthy volunteers (Geuter and Büchel, 2013). The local application of an inert nocebo cream on the forearm increased pain ratings compared with a control cream, and also reduced pain thresholds on the nocebo-treated skin. Pain stimulation induced a strong activation in the spinal cord at the level of the stimulated dermatomes C5/C6, and comparison of the nocebo with the control condition revealed enhanced nocebo-related activity in the ipsilateral dorsal horn of the spinal cord. Therefore, the nocebo hyperalgesic effect envisages a pain-facilitating mechanism at a very early stage of pain processing, that is, in the spinal cord, well before cortical processing.

Taking all these imaging studies together, it appears clear that expectation of either low or high painful stimuli has a strong influence on the perceived pain. As noted earlier, although these studies deal with negative expectations, neither placebos nor nocebos (inert substances) were administered, thus these effects can be better called nocebo-related effects, in which only verbal suggestions were given.

As already described in section 4.1.8, nocebo effects have also been found to be associated with a decrease in dopamine and opioid activity in the nucleus accumbens, thus underscoring the role of the reward and motivational circuits in nocebo effects as well (Scott et al., 2008).

4.3 **Points for further discussion**

1 A better description of the endogenous pain-modulating circuits is needed. It is important to understand when these endogenous systems are activated. For example, are the same endogenous inhibitory systems activated by placebos and by stress? Is there any other circumstance that is capable of activating these systems?

2 The involvement of different neurotransmitters in placebo analgesia needs to be better clarified, particularly their mutual interaction. For example, are there specific circumstances whereby endogenous opioids, endocannabinoids, cholecystokinin, and dopamine are activated?

3   Is it possible to identify those factors that are responsible for the difference between placebo responders and nonresponders? For example, what about the role of learning, genetics, and the efficiency of the dopaminergic reward system?

4   Better-designed brain imaging experiments will hopefully give new insights into placebo analgesia. What we need today is to understand the spatial–temporal relationship between the different regions involved in the placebo analgesic response. For example, where does the first event originate from?

5   These same issues apply to nocebo hyperalgesia. It is important to better understand how anticipatory anxiety induces an amplification of pain intensity.

6   The biochemical pathways that link anxiety to hyperalgesia need to be better identified, in order to see whether neurotransmitters other than cholecystokinin (CCK) are involved. In addition, the CCK pathways need to be better characterized by developing new and specific CCK-antagonists for human use.

7   The deactivation of dopamine and opioids in the nucleus accumbens during the nocebo response needs to be better understood within the context of reward mechanisms.

References

Adler LJ, Gyulai FE, Diehl DJ, Mintun MA, Winter PM and Firestone LL (1997). Regional brain activity changes associated with fentanyl analgesia elucidated by positron emission tomography. *Anesthesiology and Analgesia*, **84**, 120–6.

Amanzio M and Benedetti F (1999). Neuropharmacological dissection of placebo analgesia: expectation-activated opioid systems versus conditioning-activated specific subsystems. *Journal of Neuroscience*, **19**, 484–94.

Amanzio M, Benedetti F, Porro CA, Palermo S and Cauda F (2013). Activation likelihood estimation meta-analysis of brain correlates of placebo analgesia in human experimental pain. *Human Brain Mapping*, **34**, 738–52.

Amanzio M, Corazzini LL, Vase L and Benedetti F (2009). A systematic review of adverse events in placebo groups of anti-migraine clinical trials. *Pain*, **146**, 261–9.

Amanzio M, Pollo A, Maggi G and Benedetti F (2001). Response variability to analgesics: a role for non-specific activation of endogenous opioids. *Pain*, **90**, 205–15.

Andre J, Zeau B, Pohl M, Cesselin F, Benoliel JJ and Becker C (2005). Involvement of cholecystokininergic systems in anxiety-induced hyperalgesia in male rats: behavioral and biochemical studies. *Journal of Neuroscience*, **25**, 7896–904.

André-Obadia N, Magnin M and Garcia-Larrea L (2011). On the importance of placebo timing in rTMS studies for pain relief. *Pain*, **152**, 1233–7.

Atlas LY, Whittington RA, Lindquist MA, Wielgosz J, Sonty N and Wager TD (2012) Dissociable influences of opiates and expectations on pain. *Journal of Neuroscience*, **32**, 8053–64.

Atweh F and Kuhar MJ (1983). Distribution and physiological significance of opioid receptors in the brain. *British Medical Bulletin*, **39**, 47–52.

Barsky AJ, Saintfort R, Rogers MP and Borus JF (2002). Nonspecific medication side effects and the nocebo phenomenon. *Journal of the American Medical Association*, **287**, 622–7.

Bausell RB, Lao L, Bergman S, Lee WL and Berman BM (2005). Is acupuncture analgesia an expectancy effect? Preliminary evidence based on participants' perceived assignments in two placebo-controlled trials. *Evaluation & the Health Professions*, **28**, 9–26.

Beecher HK (1955). The powerful placebo. *Journal of the American Medical Association*, **159**, 1602–6.

Benedetti F (1996). The opposite effects of the opiate antagonist naloxone and the cholecystokinin antagonist proglumide on placebo analgesia. *Pain*, **64**, 535–43.

Benedetti F (1997). Cholecystokinin type-A and type-B receptors and their modulation of opioid analgesia. *News in Physiological Sciences*, **12**, 263–8.

Benedetti F (2007). Placebo and endogenous mechanisms of analgesia. *Handbook of Experimental Pharmacology*, **177**, 393–413.

Benedetti F (2008). Mechanisms of placebo and placebo-related effects across diseases and treatments. *Annual Review of Pharmacology and Toxicology*, **48**, 33–60.

Benedetti F (2010). No prefrontal control, no placebo response. *Pain*, **148**, 357–8.

Benedetti F (2013) Placebo and the new physiology of the doctor-patient relationship. *Physiological Reviews*, **93**, 1207–46.

Benedetti F and Amanzio M (1997). The neurobiology of placebo analgesia: from endogenous opioids to cholecystokinin. *Progress in Neurobiology*, **52**, 109–25.

Benedetti F, Amanzio M, Casadio C, Oliaro A and Maggi G (1997). Blockade of nocebo hyperalgesia by the cholecystokinin antagonist proglumide. *Pain*, **71**, 135–40.

Benedetti F, Amanzio M and Maggi G (1995). Potentiation of placebo analgesia by proglumide. *Lancet*, **346**, 1231.

Benedetti F, Amanzio M, Rosato R and Blanchard C (2011b). Non-opioid placebo analgesia is mediated by CB1 cannabinoid receptors. *Nature Medicine*, **17**, 1228–30.

Benedetti F, Amanzio M and Thoen W (2011a). Disruption of opioid-induced placebo responses by activation of cholecystokinin type-2 receptors. *Psychopharmacology (Berlin)*, **213**, 791–7.

Benedetti F., Amanzio M, Vighetti S and Asteggiano G (2006a). The biochemical and neuroendocrine bases of the hyperalgesic nocebo effect. *Journal of Neuroscience*, **26**, 12014–22.

Benedetti F, Arduino C and Amanzio M (1999a). Somatotopic activation of opioid systems by target-expectations of analgesia. *Journal of Neuroscience*, **9**, 3639–48.

Benedetti F, Arduino C, Costa S *et al.* (2006b). Loss of expectation-related mechanisms in Alzheimer's disease makes analgesic therapies less effective. *Pain*, **121**, 133–44.

Benedetti F and Colloca L (2004). Placebo-induced analgesia: methodology, neurobiology, clinical use, and ethics. *Reviews in Analgesia*, 7, 129–43.

Benedetti F, Lanotte M, Lopiano L and Colloca L (2007). When words are painful—Unraveling the mechanisms of the nocebo effect. *Neuroscience*, **147**, 260–71.

Benedetti F, Maggi G, Lopiano L *et al.* (2003a). Open versus hidden medical treatments: the patient's knowledge about a therapy affects the therapy outcome. *Prevention & Treatment*, **6**(1).

Benedetti F, Pollo A, Lopiano L *et al.* (2003b). Conscious expectation and unconscious conditioning in analgesic; motor and hormonal placebonocebo responses. *Journal of Neuroscience*, **23**, 4315–23.

Benedetti F, Vighetti S, Ricco C *et al.* (1999b). Pain threshold and tolerance in Alzheimer's disease. *Pain*, **80**, 377–82.

Bingel U, Lorenz J, Schoell E, Weiller C and Büchel C (2005). Mechanisms of placebo analgesia: rACC recruitment of a subcortical antinociceptive network. *Pain*, **120**, 8–15.

Bingel U, Wanigasekera V, Wiech K *et al.* (2011). The effect of treatment expectation on drug efficacy: imaging the analgesic benefit of the opioid remifentanil. *Science Translational Medicine*, **3**, 70ra14.

Casey KL, Svensson P, Morrow TJ, Raz J, Jone C and Minoshima S (2000). Selective opiate modulation of nociceptive processing in the human brain. *Journal of Neurophysiology*, **84**, 525–33.

Charron J, Rainville P and Marchand S (2006). Direct comparison of placebo effects on clinical and experimental pain. *Clinical Journal of Pain*, **22**, 204–11.

Chua P, Krams M, Toni I, Passingham R and Dolan R (1999). A functional anatomy of anticipatory anxiety. *NeuroImage*, **9**, 563–71.

Colloca L and Benedetti F (2005). Placebos and painkillers: is mind as real as matter? *Nature Reviews Neuroscience*, **6**, 545–52.

Colloca L and Benedetti F (2006). How prior experience shapes placebo analgesia. *Pain*, **124**, 126–33.

Colloca L and Benedetti F (2007). Nocebo hyperalgesia: how anxiety is turned into pain. *Current Opinion in Anaesthesiology*, **20**, 435–9.

Colloca L and Benedetti F (2009). Placebo analgesia induced by social observational learning. *Pain*, **144**, 28–34.

Colloca L, Lopiano L, Lanotte M and Benedetti F (2004). Overt versus covert treatment for pain, anxiety and Parkinson's disease. *Lancet Neurology*, **3**, 679–84.

Colloca L, Petrovic P, Wager TD, Ingvar M and Benedetti F (2010). How the number of learning trials affects placebo and nocebo responses. *Pain*, **151**, 430–9.

Colloca L, Sigaudo M and Benedetti F (2008a). The role of learning in nocebo and placebo effects. *Pain*, **136**, 211–18.

Colloca L, Tinazzi M, Recchia S *et al.* (2008b). Learning potentiates neurophysiological and behavioral placebo analgesic responses. *Pain*, **139**, 306–14.

Dannecker EA, Price DD and Robinson ME (2003). An examination of the relationships among recalled, expected, and actual intensity and unpleasantness of delayed onset muscle pain. *Journal of Pain*, **4**, 74–81.

Dias R, Robbins TW and Roberts AC (1996). Dissociation in prefrontal cortex of affective and attentional shifts. *Nature*, **380**, 69–72.

Dubois B, Slachevsky A, Litvan I and Pillon B (2000). The FAB. A frontal assessment battery at bedside. *Neurology*, **55**, 1621–6.

Dworkin SF, Chen AC, LeResche L and Clark DW (1983). Cognitive reversal of expected nitrous oxide analgesia for acute pain. *Anesthesia and Analgesia*, **62**, 1073–7.

Eippert F, Bingel U, Schoell ED *et al.* (2009a). Activation of the opioidergic descending pain control system underlies placebo analgesia. *Neuron*, **63**, 533–43.

Eippert F, Finsterbusch J, Bingel U and Büchel C (2009b). Direct evidence for spinal cord involvement in placebo analgesia. *Science*, **326**, 404.

Elsenbruch S, Schmid J, Bäsler M, Cesko E, Schedlowski M and Benson S (2012). How positive and negative expectations shape the experience of visceral pain: an experimental pilot study in healthy women. *Neurogastroenterology and Motility*, **24**, 914–e460.

Escobar W, Ramirez K, Avila C, Limongi R, Vanegas H and Vazquez E (2012). Metamizol, a non-opioid analgesic, acts via endocannabinoids in the PAG-RVM axis during inflammation in rats. *European Journal of Pain*, **16**, 676–89.

Fanselow MS (1994). Neural organization of the defensive behavior system responsible for fear. *Psychonomic Bulletin & Review*, **1**, 429–38.

Fields H (2004). State-dependent opioid control of pain. *Nature Reviews Neuroscience*, **5**, 565–75.

Fields HL and Basbaum AI (1999). Central nervous system mechanisms of pain modulation. In PD Wall and R Melzack, eds. *Textbook of pain*, pp. 309–29. Churchill Livingstone, Edinburgh.

Fields HL and Levine JD (1984). Placebo analgesia—a role for endorphins? *Trends in Neurosciences*, **7**, 271–3.

Fields HL and Price DD (1997). Toward a neurobiology of placebo analgesia. In A Harrington, ed. *The placebo effect: an interdisciplinary exploration*, pp. 93–116. Harvard University Press, Cambridge, MA.

Firestone LL, Gyulai F, Mintun M, Adler LJ, Urso K and Winter PM (1996). Human brain activity response to fentanyl imaged by positron emission tomography. *Anesthesia and Analgesia*, **82**, 1247–51.

Flaten MA, Simonsen T and Olsen H (1999). Drug-related information generates placebo and nocebo responses that modify the drug response. *Psychosomatic Medicine*, **61**, 250–5.

Flor H and Grusser SM (1999). Conditioned stress-induced analgesia in humans. *European Journal of Pain*, **3**, 317–24

Geuter S and Büchel C (2013). Facilitation of pain in the human spinal cord by nocebo treatment. *Journal of Neuroscience*, **33**, 13784–90.

Goffaux P, Redmond WJ, Rainville P and Marchand S (2007). Descending analgesia—when the spine echoes what the brain expects. *Pain*, **130**, 137–43.

Gracely RH, Dubner R, Wolskee PJ and Deeter WR (1983). Placebo and naloxone can alter postsurgical pain by separate mechanisms. *Nature*, **306**, 264–5.

Grevert P, Albert LH, Goldstein A (1983). Partial antagonism of placebo analgesia by naloxone. *Pain*, **16**, 129–43

Guo JY, Wang JY and Luo F (2010). Dissection of placebo analgesia in mice: the conditions for activation of opioid and non-opioid systems. *Journal of Psychopharmacology*, **24**, 1561–7.

Hashmi JA, Baria AT, Baliki MN, Huang L, Schnitzer TJ and Apkarian AV (2012). Brain networks predicting placebo analgesia in a clinical trial for chronic back pain. *Pain*, **153**, 2393–402.

Hebb ALO, Poulin J-F, Roach SP, Zacharko RM and Drolet G (2005). Cholecystokinin and endogenous opioid peptides: interactive influence on pain, cognition, and emotion. *Progress in Neuro-Psychopharmacology & Biological Psychiatry*, **29**, 1225–38.

Heinricher MM, McGaraughty S and Tortorici V (2001). Circuitry underlying antiopioid actions of cholecystokinin within the rostral ventromedial medulla. *Journal of Neurophysiology*, **85**, 280–6.

Heinricher MM and Neubert MJ (2004). Neural basis for the hyperalgesic action of cholecystokinin in the rostral ventromedial medulla. *Journal of Neurophysiology*, **92**, 1982–9.

Holloway RG, Gramling R and Kelly AG (2013). Estimating and communicating prognosis in advanced neurologic disease. *Neurology*, **80**, 764–72.

Hrobjartsson A and Gøtzsche PC (2001). Is the placebo effect powerless? An analysis of clinical trials comparing placebo with no-treatment. *New England Journal of Medicine*, **344**, 1594–602.

Hsieh JC, Stone-Elander S and Ingvar M (1999). Anticipatory coping of pain expressed in the human anterior cingulated cortex: a positron emission tomography study. *Neuroscience Letters*, **26**, 262, 61–4.

Hughes J (1975). Search for the endogenous ligand of the opiate receptor. *Neurosciences Research Program Bulletin*, **13**, 55–8.

Häuser W, Bartram C, Bartram-Wunn E and Tölle T (2012). Adverse events attributable to nocebo in randomized controlled drug trials in fibromyalgia syndrome and painful diabetic peripheral neuropathy: systematic review. *Clinical Journal of Pain*, **28**, 437–51.

Ikemoto S and Panksepp J (1999). The role of nucleus accumbens dopamine in motivated behavior: a unifying interpretation with special reference to reward-seeking. *Brain Research Reviews*, **31**, 6–41.

Jensen TS (1997). Opioids in the brain: supraspinal mechanisms in pain control. *Acta Anaesthesiologica Scandinavica*, **41**, 123–32.

Jones AK, Qi LY, Fujirawa T et al. (1991). In vivo distribution of opioid receptors in man in relation to the cortical projections of the medial and lateral pain systems measured with positron emission tomography. *Neuroscience Letters*, **126**, 25–8.

Kam-Hansen S, Jakubowski M, Kelley JM et al. (2014). Altered placebo and drug labeling changes the outcome of episodic migraine attacks. *Science Translational Medicine*, **6**(218), 218ra5.

Kaptchuk TJ, Stason WB, Davis RB et al. (2006). Sham device vs inert pill: randomised controlled trial of two placebo treatments. *British Medical Journal*, **332**, 391–7.

Keltner, J.R., Furst, A., Fan, C., Redfern, R., Inglis, B and Fields HL (2006). Isolating the modulatory effect of expectation on pain transmission: a functional magnetic imaging study. *Journal of Neuroscience*, **26**, 4437–43.

Kienle GS and Kiene H (1996). Placebo effect and placebo concept: a critical methodological and conceptual analysis of reports on the magnitude of the placebo effect. *Alternative Therapies in Health and Medicine*, **2**, 39–54.

Kienle GS and Kiene H (1997). The powerful placebo effect: fact or fiction? *Journal of Clinical Epidemiology*, **50**, 1311–18.

Kirsch I (1999). *How expectancies shape experience*. American Psychological Association, Washington, DC.

Knutson B and Cooper JC (2005). Functional magnetic resonance imaging of reward prediction. *Current Opinion in Neurology*, **18**, 411–7.

Kong J, Gollub RL, Polich G et al. (2008). A functional magnetic resonance imaging study on the neural mechanisms of hyperalgesic nocebo effect. *Journal of Neuroscience*, **28**, 13354–62.

Kong J, Gollub RL, Rosman I et al. (2006). Brain activity associated with expectancy-enhanced placebo analgesia as measured by functional magnetic resonance imaging. *Journal Neuroscience*, **26**, 381–8.

Kong J, Kaptchuk TJ, Polich G et al. (2009a). Expectancy and treatment interactions: a dissociation between acupuncture analgesia and expectancy evoked placebo analgesia. *NeuroImage*, **45**, 940–9.

Kong J, Kaptchuk TJ, Polich G et al. (2009b). An fMRI study on the interaction and dissociation between expectation of pain relief and acupuncture treatment. *NeuroImage*, **47**, 1066–76.

Koyama T, McHaffie JG, Laurienti PJ and Coghill RC (2005). The subjective experience of pain: where expectations become reality. *Proceedings of the National Academy of Sciences of the United States of America*, **102**, 12950–5.

Koyama T, Tanaka YZ and Mikami A (1998). Nociceptive neurons in the macaque anterior cingulate activate during anticipation of pain. *Neuroreport*, **9**, 2663–7.

Krummenacher P, Candia V, Folkers G, Schedlowski M and Schönbächler G (2010). Prefrontal cortex modulates placebo analgesia. *Pain*, **148**, 368–74.

Leeuw M, Goossens ME, Linton SJ et al. (2007). The fear-avoidance model of musculoskeletal pain: current state of scientific evidence. *Journal of Behavioral Medicine*, **30**, 77–94.

Levine JD and Gordon NC (1984). Influence of the method of drug administration on analgesic response. *Nature*, **312**, 755–6.

Levine JD, Gordon NC, Bornstein JC and Fields HL (1979). Role of pain in placebo analgesia. *Proceedings of the National Academy of Sciences of the United States of America*, **76**, 3528–31.

Levine JD, Gordon NC and Fields HL (1978). The mechanisms of placebo analgesia. *Lancet*, **2**, 654–7.

Levine JD, Gordon NC, Smith R and Fields HL (1981). Analgesic responses to morphine and placebo in individuals with postoperative pain. *Pain*, **10**, 379–89.

Lieberman MD, Jarcho JM, Berman S *et al.* (2004). The neural correlates of placebo effects: a disruption account. *NeuroImage*, **22**, 447–55.

Linde K, Witt CM, Streng A, Weidenhammer W, Wagenpfeil S *et al.* (2007). The impact of patient expectations on outcomes in four randomised controlled trials of acupuncture in patients with chronic pain. *Pain*, **128**, 264–71.

Lipman JJ, Miller BE, Mays KS, Miller MN, North WC *et al.* (1990). Peak B endorphin concentration in cerebrospinal fluid: reduced in chronic pain patients and increased during the placebo response. *Psychopharmacology*, **102**, 112–16.

Lorenz J, Hauck M, Paur RC *et al.* (2005). Cortical correlates of false expectations during pain intensity judgments—a possible manifestation of placebo/nocebo cognitions. *Brain, Behavior and Immunity*, **19**, 283–95.

Lui F, Colloca L, Duzzi D, Anchisi D, Benedetti F and Porro CA (2010). Neural bases of conditioned placebo analgesia. *Pain*, **151**, 816–24.

Manchikanti L, Pampati V and Damron K (2005). The role of placebo and nocebo effects of perioperative administration of sedatives and opioids in interventional pain management. *Pain Physician*, **8**, 349–55.

Matre D, Casey KL and Knardahl S (2006). Placebo-induced changes in spinal cord pain processing. *Journal of Neuroscience*, **26**, 559–63.

McQuay H, Carroll D and Moore A (1995). Variation in the placebo effect in randomized controlled trials of analgesics: all is as blind as it seems. *Pain*, **64**, 331–5.

Meissner K, Bingel U, Colloca L, Wager TD, Watson A and Flaten MA (2011). The placebo effect: advances from different methodological approaches. *Journal of Neuroscience*, **31**, 16117–24.

Millan MJ (2002). Descending control of pain. *Progress in Neurobiology*, **66**, 355–474.

Miller EK and Cohen JD (2001). An integrative theory of prefrontal cortex function. *Annual Review of Neuroscience*, **24**, 167–202.

Mitchell JM, Lowe D and Fields HL (1998). The contribution of the rostral ventromedial medulla to the antinociceptive effects of systemic morphine in restrained and unrestrained rats. *Neuroscience*, **87**, 123–33.

Mitsikostas DD, Chalarakis NG, Mantonakis LI, Delicha EM and Sfikakis PP (2012). Nocebo in fibromyalgia: meta-analysis of placebo-controlled clinical trials and implications for practice. *European Journal of Neurology*, **19**, 672–80.

Mitsikostas DD, Mantonakis LI and Chalarakis NG (2011). Nocebo is the enemy, not placebo. A meta-analysis of reported side effects after placebo treatment in headaches. *Cephalalgia*, **31**, 550–61.

Montgomery GH and Kirsch I (1996). Mechanisms of placebo pain reduction: an empirical investigation. *Psychological Science*, **7**, 174–6.

Montgomery GH and Kirsch I (1997). Classical conditioning and the placebo effect. *Pain*, **72**, 107–13.

Nolan TA, Price DD, Caudle RM, Murphy NP and Neubert JK (2012). Placebo-induced analgesia in an operant pain model in rats. *Pain*, **153**, 2009–16.

Oftedal G, Straume A, Johnsson A and Stovner LJ (2007). Mobile phone headache: a double blind, sham-controlled provocation study. *Cephalalgia*, **27**, 447–55.

Papadopoulos D and Mitsikostas DD (2012). A meta-analytic approach to estimating nocebo effects in neuropathic pain trials. *Journal of Neurology*, **259**, 436–47.

Peciña M, Martínez-Jauand M, Hodgkinson C, Stohler CS, Goldman D and Zubieta JK (2014). FAAH selectively influences placebo effects. *Molecular Psychiatry*, **19**, 385–91.

Pert CB and Snyder SH (1973). Opiate receptor: demonstration in nervous tissue. *Science*, **179**, 1011–13.

Petersen GL, Finnerup NB, Nørskov KN, *et al.* (2012). Placebo manipulations reduce hyperalgesia in neuropathic pain. *Pain*, **153**, 1292–300.

Petrovic P, Kalso E, Petersson KM, Andersson J, Fransson P and Ingvar M (2010). A prefrontal non-opioid mechanism in placebo analgesia. *Pain*, **150**, 59–65.

Petrovic P, Kalso E, Petersson KM and Ingvar M (2002). Placebo and opioid analgesia-imaging a shared neuronal network. *Science*, **295**, 1737–40.

Pfeiffer A, Pasi A, Mehraein P and Herz A (1982) Opiate receptor binding sites in human brain. *Brain Research*, **248**, 87–96.

Ploghaus A, Tracey I, Gati JS *et al.* (1999). Dissociating pain from its anticipation in the human brain. *Science*, **284**, 1979–81.

Pollo A, Amanzio M, Arslanian A *et al.* (2001). Response expectancies in placebo analgesia and their clinical relevance. *Pain*, **93**, 77–84.

Porro CA, Baraldi P, Pagnoni G *et al.* (2002). Does anticipation of pain affect cortical nociceptive systems? *Journal of Neuroscience*, **22**, 3206–14.

Porro CA, Cettolo V, Francescato MP and Baraldi P (2003). Functional activity mapping of the mesial hemispheric wall during anticipation of pain. *NeuroImage*, **19**, 1738–47.

Price DD (1999). *Psychological mechanisms of pain and analgesia*. IASP Press, Seattle, WA.

Price DD (2000). Psychological and neural mechanisms of the affective dimension of pain. *Science*, **288**, 1769–72.

Price DD (2001). Assessing placebo effects without placebo groups: an untapped possibility? *Pain*, **90**, 201–3.

Price DD and Barrell JJ (2000). Mechanisms of analgesia produced by hypnosis and placebo suggestions. *Progress in Brain Research*, **122**, 255–71.

Price DD, Barrell JE and Barrell JJ (1985). A quantitative-experiential analysis of human emotions. *Motivation and Emotion*, **9**, 19–38.

Price DD, Craggs J, Verne GN, Perlstein WM and Robinson ME (2007). Placebo analgesia is accompanied by large reductions in pain-related brain activity in irritable bowel syndrome patients. *Pain*, **127**, 63–72.

Price DD, Finniss DG and Benedetti F (2008). A comprehensive review of the placebo effect: recent advances and current thought. *Annual Review of Psychology*, **59**, 565–90.

Price DD, Milling LS, Kirsch I *et al.* (1999). An analysis of factors that contribute to the magnitude of placebo analgesia in an experimental paradigm. *Pain*, **83**, 147–56.

Price DD, Riley J and Barrell JJ (2001). Are lived choices based on emotional processes? *Cognition & Emotion*, **15**, 365–79.

Quessy SN and Rowbotham MC (2008). Placebo response in neuropathic pain trials. *Pain*, **138**, 479–83.

Reynolds DV (1969). Surgery in the rat during electrical analgesia induced by focal brain stimulation. *Science*, **164**, 444–5.

Sadzot B, Price JC, Mayberg HS *et al.* (1991). Quantification of human opiate receptor concentration and affinity using high and low specific activity and diprenorphine and positron emission tomography. *Journal of Cerebral Blood Flow and Metabolism*, **11**, 204–19.

Sanderson C, Hardy J, Spruyt O and Currow DC (2013). Placebo and nocebo effects in randomized controlled trials: the implications for research and practice. *Journal of Pain and Symptom Management*, **46**, 722–30.

Sawamoto N, Honda M, Okada T *et al.* (2000). Expectation of pain enhances responses to nonpainful somatosensory stimulation in the anterior cingulated cortex and parietal operculum/posterior insula: an event-related functional magnetic resonance imaging study. *Journal of Neuroscience*, **20**, 7438–45.

Schultz W (2002). Getting formal with dopamine and reward. *Neuron*, **36**, 241–63.

Schultz W, Tremblay L and Hollerman JR (2000). Reward processing in primate orbitofrontal cortex and basal ganglia. *Cerebral Cortex*, **10**, 272–8.

Scott DJ, Stohler CS, Egnatuk CM, Wang H, Koeppe RA and Zubieta JK (2007). Individual differences in reward responding explain placebo-induced expectations and effects. *Neuron*, **55**, 325–36.

Scott DJ, Stohler CS, Egnatuk CM, Wang H, Koeppe RA and Zubieta JK (2008). Placebo and nocebo effects are defined by opposite opioid and dopaminergic responses. *Archives of General Psychiatry*, **65**, 220–31.

Skrabanek P (1978). Naloxone and placebo. *Lancet*, **2**, 791.

Stein N, Sprenger C, Scholz J, Wiech K and Bingel U (2012). White matter integrity of the descending pain modulatory system is associated with interindividual differences in placebo analgesia. *Pain*, **153**, 2210–17.

Svedman P, Ingvar M and Gordh T (2005). "Anxiebo," placebo, and postoperative pain. *BMC Anesthesiology*, **5**, 9.

Swider K and Bąbel P (2013). The effect of the sex of a model in nocebo hyperalgesia induced by social observational learning. *Pain*, **154**, 1312–17.

Terman GW, Morgan MJ and Liebeskind JC (1986). Opioid and non-opioid stress analgesia from cold water swim: importance of stress severity. *Brain Research*, **372**, 167–71.

Thompson PM, Hayashi KM, de Zubicaray G *et al.* (2003). Dynamics of gray matter loss in Alzheimer's disease. *Journal of Neuroscience*, **23**, 994–1005.

Tracey I (2010). Getting the pain you expect: mechanisms of placebo, nocebo and reappraisal effects in humans. *Nature Medicine*, **16**, 1277–83.

Varelmann D, Pancaro C, Cappiello EC and Camann WR (2010). Nocebo-induced hyperalgesia during local anesthetic injection. *Anesthesia and Analgesia*, **110**, 868–70.

Vase L, Riley JL III and Price DD (2002). A comparison of placebo effects in clinical analgesic trials versus studies of placebo analgesia. *Pain*, **99**, 443–52.

Vase L, Robinson ME, Verne GN and Price DD (2003). The contributions of suggestion, expectancy and desire to placebo effect in irritable bowel syndrome patients. *Pain*, **105**, 17–25.

Vase L, Robinson ME, Verne GN and Price DD (2005). Increased placebo analgesia over time in irritable bowel syndrome (IBS) patients is associated with desire and expectation but not endogenous opioid mechanisms. *Pain*, **115**, 338–47.

van den Broeke EN, Geene N, van Rijn CM, Wilder-Smith OH and Oosterman J (2013). Negative expectations facilitate mechanical hyperalgesia after high-frequency electrical stimulation of human skin. *European Journal of Pain*, **18**, 86–91.

Verne GN, Robinson ME, Vase L and Price DD (2003). Reversal of visceral and cutaneous hyperalgesia by local rectal anesthesia in irritable bowel syndrome (IBS) patients. *Pain*, **105**, 223–30.

Vlaeyen JW and Linton SJ (2000). Fear-avoidance and its consequences in chronic musculoskeletal pain: a state of the art. *Pain*, **85**, 317–32.

Vogt BA, Sikes RW and Vogt LJ (1993). Anterior cingulate cortex and the medial pain system. In BA Vogt and M Gabriel, eds. *Neurobiology of cingulate cortex and limbic thalamus: a comprehensive handbook*, pp. 313–44. Birkhäuser, Boston, MA.

Voudouris NJ, Peck CL and Coleman G (1989). Conditioned response models of placebo phenomena: further support. *Pain*, **38**, 109–16.

Voudouris NJ, Peck CL and Coleman G (1990). The role of conditioning and verbal expectancy in the placebo response. *Pain*, **43**, 121–8.

Vögtle E, Barke A and Kröner-Herwig B (2013). Nocebo hyperalgesia induced by social observational learning. *Pain*, **154**, 1427–33.

Wager TD, Atlas LY, Leotti LA and Rilling JK (2011). Predicting individual differences in placebo analgesia: contributions of brain activity during anticipation and pain experience. *Journal of Neuroscience*, **31**, 439–52.

Wager TD, Matre D and Casey KL (2006). Placebo effects in laser-evoked pain potentials. *Brain Behavior and Immunity*, **20**, 219–30.

Wager TD, Rilling, JK, Smith EE *et al.* (2004). Placebo-induced changes in fMRI in the anticipation and experience of pain. *Science*, **303**, 1162–6.

Wager TD, Scott DJ and Zubieta JK (2007). Placebo effects on human (micro)-opioid activity during pain. *Proceedings of the National Academy of Sciences of the United States of America*, **104**, 11056–61.

Wagner KJ, Willoch F, Kochs EF, Siessmeier T and Tölle TR (2001). Dose-dependent regional cerebral blood flow changes during remifentanil infusion in humans. A positron emission tomography study. *Anesthesiology*, **94**, 732–9.

Wall PD (1992). The placebo effect: an unpopular topic. *Pain*, **51**, 1–3.

Wamsley JK, Zarbin MA, Young WS and Kuhar MJ (1982). Distribution of opiate receptors in the monkey brain: an autoradiographic study. *Neuroscience*, **7**, 595–613.

Wells RE and Kaptchuk TJ (2012). To tell the truth, the whole truth, may do patients harm: the problem of the nocebo effect for informed consent. *American Journal of Bioethics*, **12**, 22–9.

Willer JC and Albe-Fessard D (1980). Electrophysiological evidence for a release of endogenous opiates in stress-induced "analgesia" in man. *Brain Research*, **198**, 419–26.

Willoch F, Schindler F, Wester HJ *et al.* (2004). Central poststroke pain and reduced opioid receptor binding within pain processing circuitries: a [11C]diprenorphine PET study. *Pain*, **108**, 213–20.

Willoch F, Tolle TR and Wester HJ (1999). Central pain after pontine infarction is associated with changes in opioid receptor binding: a PET study with 11C-diprenorphine. *American Journal of Neuroradiology*, **20**, 686–90.

Zhang RR, Zhang WC, Wang JY and Guo JY (2013). The opioid placebo analgesia is mediated exclusively through mu-opioid receptor in rat. *International Journal of Neuropsychopharmacology*, **16**, 849–56.

Zubieta JK, Bueller JA, Jackson LR *et al.* (2005). Placebo effects mediated by endogenous opioid activity on μ-opioid receptors. *Journal of Neuroscience*, **25**, 7754–62.

Zubieta JK and Stohler CS (2009). Neurobiological mechanisms of placebo responses. *Annals of New York Academy of Science*, **1156**, 198–210.

Chapter 5

Diseases of the nervous system

Summary points

- Besides pain, Parkinson's disease represents an excellent model for studying the neurobiological mechanisms of the placebo effect.

- The placebo effect in Parkinson's disease is mediated by dopamine release in the striatum and is associated with changes in activity of neurons in the subthalamic nucleus, substantia nigra pars reticulata and motor thalamus.

- The therapeutic effects of deep-brain stimulation are powerfully modulated by placebos.

- Although clinical trials on migraine show very high rates of improvement in patients who received placebo, the underlying mechanisms are not known.

- As with migraine, many other neurological diseases, like epilepsy, show improvements in placebo groups, but the mechanisms are not known.

5.1 Parkinson's disease

5.1.1 Parkinson patients who receive placebo show a high rate of improvement

Parkinson's disease is mainly a disorder of movement, although several sensory, cognitive, mood, sleep, and autonomic disturbances may be present as well. There are at least three important motor symptoms: tremor, rigidity, and bradykinesia. Tremor occurs at rest and involves mainly the upper limbs, although other body parts may be subject to tremor, such as the chin. Rigidity involves all the muscles, with a global impairment of movements and gait. Bradykinesia means that movements slow down so that any action is performed very slowly and with difficulty.

Substantial improvements in parkinsonian symptoms are seen in the placebo groups of many clinical trials that assess both pharmacological and surgical treatments for Parkinson's disease. Goetz et al. (2000) reported that 14% of patients enrolled in a 6-month randomized placebo-controlled clinical trial of ropinirole achieved a 50% improvement in motor function while on placebo treatment. All domains of parkinsonism were subject to the placebo effect, but bradykinesia and rigidity were more susceptible than tremor, gait, or balance. In a review of 36 studies, Shetty et al. (1999) found that 12 of them reported a 9–59% improvement in motor symptoms following placebo treatment. In a 24-week-long double-blind trial of pergolide, significant improvements were seen in both the drug-treated group (30%) and the placebo group (23%) (Diamond et al., 1985), and in a trial of deprenyl (selegiline) and tocopherol antioxidative therapy, 21% of patients showed objective improvement in motor function during placebo therapy over 6 months (Goetz et al. 2002).

In a more recent study by Goetz et al. (2008a), placebo data from two studies comparing sarizotan to placebo for the management of dyskinesia were analyzed. Whereas sarizotan did not show any difference compared to placebo, both sarizotan and placebo improved dyskinesia compared to baseline. Older age, lower baseline parkinsonism score, and lower total daily levodopa doses were related to placebo improvement, whereas lower baseline dyskinesia was associated with placebo worsening. In addition, by using a strict definition of placebo-associated improvement, Goetz et al. (2008b) examined rates and timing of placebo responses to identify patient- and study-based characteristics, predicting positive placebo response in several clinical trials. The authors collected individual patient data from the placebo groups of 11 medical and surgical treatment trials involving Parkinson patients with differing disease severities and placebo-assignment likelihoods. A positive placebo response was defined as larger than or equal to 50% improvement in total Unified Parkinson's Disease Rating Scale motor (UPDRSm) score or a decrease by more than or equal to 2 points on at least two UPDRSm items compared to baseline. Positive placebo response rates were calculated at early (3–7 weeks), mid (8–18 weeks), and late (23–35 weeks) stages of follow-up. A total of 858 patients on placebo met inclusion criteria for analysis. The overall placebo response rate was 16% (range: 0–55%). Placebo responses were temporally distributed similarly during early, mid, and late phases of follow-up.

Substantial improvements in patients who receive placebo are also present in surgical treatments of Parkinson's disease. For example, in a study on the effect of intrastriatal implantation of fetal porcine ventral mesencephalic tissue to treat Parkinson's disease (Watts et al. 2001), the degree of motor performance improvement at 18 months was substantial in both the real surgery group and the sham surgery group. In one multicenter, randomized, double-blind, sham-surgery-controlled study of human fetal transplantation (Olanow et al. 2003) there was no difference between the transplant and the sham surgery group, although pilot studies that used an identical technique had demonstrated substantial benefit (Hauser et al., 1999).

As for pain, these trials are aimed at comparing active treatments with placebos, thus in most of them no no-treatment groups are studied. Therefore, the clinical improvements in the placebo groups cannot be attributed to real placebo effects only; spontaneous remission and regression to the mean play a part in the reduction of the symptoms in many cases. Nonetheless, the high rate of placebo effects in clinical trials of Parkinson's disease provided the impetus to investigate placebo responses of parkinsonian patients in more detail.

5.1.2 Expectations modulate parkinsonian symptoms

By studying Parkinson patients under strictly controlled conditions in order to analyze the very nature of the placebo effect, expectation of clinical benefit has been found to play a key role. In a typical placebo procedure in Parkinson patients, a placebo is administered along with verbal suggestions of motor improvement. Therefore, patients expect an improvement of their motor symptoms, such as tremor, muscle rigidity, and bradykinesia (slow movements).

In one study (Pollo et al. 2002), the velocity of movements was analyzed in Parkinson patients who had been implanted with electrodes in the subthalamic nuclei for deep-brain stimulation, a highly effective therapy for Parkinson's disease. They were tested in two opposite conditions. In the first, they expected a good motor performance; in the second, they expected a bad motor performance. The effect of subthalamic stimulation on the velocity of movement of the right hand was analyzed with a movement analyzer (Fig. 5.1A). Patients performed a visual directional-choice task on a rectangular surface, with their right index finger positioned on a central sensor with a green light. After a random interval of a few seconds, a red light turned on randomly in one of three sensors placed 10 cm away from the green light sensor. Patients were instructed to move their hand as quickly as possible in order to reach the target red light sensor. The hand movement was found to be faster when patients expected a good motor performance than when they expected bad performance (Fig. 5.1B). Interestingly, all these effects occurred within minutes, which indicate that expectations induce neural changes very quickly.

In another study by Benedetti et al. (2003), patients implanted for deep-brain stimulation were tested for the velocity of movement of their right hand according to a double-blind experimental design in which neither the patient nor the experimenter knew if the stimulator was turned off. The velocity of hand movement was assessed with a movement analyzer (Fig. 5.1A). The stimulator was turned off several times (at 4 weeks and 2 weeks) before the test session (Fig. 5.1C). Each time, the velocity of movement was measured just before the stimulator was turned off and 30 minutes later. On the day of the experimental session, the stimulator was kept on but patients were told it had been turned off, so as to induce negative expectations of motor performance worsening (nocebo procedure). Although the stimulator was on, motor performance worsened and mimicked the worsening of the previous days (Fig. 5.1C). This nocebo bradykinesia could be prevented completely by verbal suggestions of good motor performance (placebo procedure). Therefore, as with pain, motor performance can be modulated in two opposite directions by placebos and nocebos, and this modulation occurs on the basis of positive and negative expectations about motor performance.

These findings have been reproduced by Mercado et al. (2006) who also found a dissociation of the effects in tremor, rigidity, and bradykinesia. In fact, these authors found significant effects for bradykinesia, but not for tremor and rigidity. On the basis of work done by Pollo et al. (2002), Benedetti et al. (2003), and Mercado et al. (2006), it seems bradykinesia is a symptom that is more sensitive to verbal suggestions than tremor or rigidity. Interestingly, these results are similar to those obtained in the study by Goetz et al. (2000) who reported that all domains of parkinsonism were subject to the placebo effect, but bradykinesia and rigidity were more susceptible than tremor, gait, or balance.

Expectations of motor improvement can also make a big difference in clinical trials. In a clinical trial of human fetal mesencephalic transplantation (a possible treatment

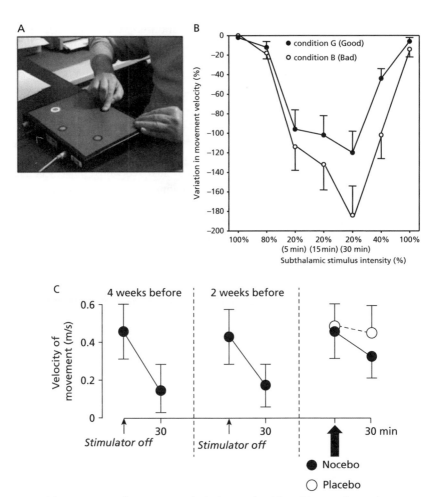

Fig. 5.1 (A) Assessment of movement velocity in people with Parkinson's disease by means of a movement analyzer. Reprinted from *Neuroscience*, 147 (2), F. Benedetti, M. Lanotte, L. Lopiano, and L. Colloca, When words are painful: Unraveling the mechanisms of the nocebo effect, pp. 260–271, Copyright (2007), with permission from Elsevier. (B) Percentage change in movement velocity as a function of the subthalamic stimulus intensity, expressed as percentage of initial stimulation. Condition "bad" refers to expectation of bad performance (open circles) and condition "good" refers to expectation of good performance (black circles). 100% subthalamic stimulation corresponds to the initial stimulus intensity. Note that in condition "bad" the decrease in movement velocity is larger than in condition "good." Reproduced from Antonella Pollo, Elena Torre, Leonardo Lopiano, Mario Rizzone, Michele Lanotte, Andrea Cavanna, Bruno Bergamasco, and Fabrizio Benedetti, Expectation modulates the response to subthalamic nucleus stimulation in parkinsonian patients, *NeuroReport*, 13 (11), pp. 1383–1386 Copyright 2002, Lippincott Williams & Wilkins, with permission. (C) After the stimulator for deep-brain stimulation was turned off at 4 weeks and 2 weeks prior to the experimental session, nocebo suggestions of clinical worsening were given, but the stimulator was kept on. Each time, the velocity of movement was measured just before the stimulator was turned off and 30 minutes

for Parkinson's disease currently under assessment) investigators studied the effect of this treatment compared with placebo treatment for 12 months. They also assessed the patient's perceived assignment to either the active (fetal tissue implant) or placebo treatment (sham surgery). There were no differences between the transplant and sham surgery groups on several outcome measures, such as physical and quality of life scores. However, the perceived assignment of treatment group had a beneficial impact on the overall outcome and this difference was still present 12 months after surgery. Patients who believed they received transplanted tissue had significant improvements in both their quality of life and motor outcomes, regardless of whether they received sham surgery or fetal tissue implantations (McRae et al., 2004) (see also section 10.2.2).

Expectations have been found to change cortical excitability in parkinsonian patients. Lou et al. (2013) randomized 26 Parkinson patients to one of three groups: 0%, 50%, and 100% expectation of receiving levodopa. All subjects received placebo regardless of expectation group. Cortical excitability was measured by the amplitude of motor-evoked potential evoked by transcranial magnetic stimulation. The degree of expectation had a significant effect on motor-evoked potential response: subjects in the 50% and 100% expectation groups responded with a decrease in motor-evoked potentials, whereas those in the 0% expectation group responded with an increase. ·

Besides motor functioning, including tremor (Keitel et al., 2013a), expectation affects cognitive functions as well. Keitel et al. (2013b) investigated how expectation modulates the pattern of motor improvement in deep-brain stimulation of the subthalamic nucleus and its interaction with verbal fluency. Expectations of 24 hypokinetic-rigid parkinsonian patients about the impact of deep-brain stimulation on motor symptoms was manipulated by positive (placebo), negative (nocebo), and neutral (control) verbal suggestions. It was found that expectations significantly affected proximal but not distal movements resulting in better performance in the placebo than in the nocebo condition. Placebo responders with improvement larger than or equal to 25% were characterized by a trend for impaired lexical verbal fluency. Therefore, in this study positive motor expectations exerted both motor placebo and cognitive nocebo responses.

5.1.3 Dopamine depletion in the striatum is the cause of Parkinson's disease

The disruption of dopamine function in the neural pathway from the substantia nigra pars compacta to the striatum (putamen and caudate nucleus) represents the pathophysiological substrate of Parkinson's disease. The primary deficit involves selective

---

Fig. 5.1 (continued) later. Thus the measurement at 30 minutes reflects the worsening of motor performance. Even though the stimulator was still on, the nocebo induced worsening (black circles). Placebo suggestions of improvement antagonized this nocebo effect completely (open circles). The black arrow shows the time of either nocebo or placebo administration. Reproduced from Fabrizio Benedetti, Antonella Pollo, Leonardo Lopiano, Michele Lanotte, Sergio Vighetti, and Innocenzo Rainero, Conscious Expectation and Unconscious Conditioning in Analgesic, Motor, and Hormonal Placebo/Nocebo Responses, *The Journal of Neuroscience*, 23 (10), pp. 4315–4323, Copyright 2003, The Society for Neuroscience.

degeneration of the nigrostriatal dopamine-producing neurons, although at later stages of the disease, other dopamine projections and other neurotransmitters may also be affected. There are in fact different dopaminergic pathways in the brain, such as the mesocortical, the mesolimbic, and the tuberoinfundibular. These pathways are associated with volition and emotional responsiveness, desire, reward, sensory processes, and maternal behavior. The neuropsychiatric pathology associated with Parkinson's disease is attributable to the loss of dopamine along the nonstriatal pathways. As far as the motor system is concerned, dopamine has a critical role in modulation of the functioning of the basal ganglia (Alexander et al., 1986; Haber, 2003) and its depletion results in difficulties initiating movement (akinesia), bradykinesia (slowness of movement), rigidity, tremor at rest, and postural instability.

There are different mechanisms that may explain the disruption of the nigrostriatal neurons. For example, an abnormal accumulation of the protein alpha-synuclein bound to ubiquitin in the damaged cells has been found. The alpha-synuclein–ubiquitin complex forms cytoplasmic inclusions called Lewy bodies. The death of dopaminergic neurons by alpha-synuclein is due to a defect in the transport between the endoplasmic reticulum and the Golgi apparatus. Certain proteins, such as Rab1, may reverse the defect caused by alpha-synuclein in animal models (Cooper et al., 2006). Accumulation of iron is also typically observed in conjunction with the protein inclusions, and iron induces aggregation of synuclein by oxidative mechanisms (Kaur and Andersen, 2002).

The pharmacological treatment of Parkinson's disease is aimed at replacing the lost dopamine by either dopamine precursors or synthetic agonists acting at dopamine receptors. The most widely used form of treatment is L-dopa (levodopa) in various forms. L-dopa is transformed into dopamine in the dopaminergic neurons by DOPA-decarboxylase. However, only a small amount of L-dopa enters the dopaminergic neurons (less than 5%). The remainder is often metabolized to dopamine elsewhere, causing a number of side effects (e.g., Box 5.1). The surgical treatment of Parkinson's disease is represented by deep-brain stimulation, whereby mainly the subthalamic nuclei are chronically stimulated (see section 5.1.5).

Box 5.1 Parkinson's disease and pathological gambling

Since the pathophysiology responsible for Parkinson's disease is represented by the degeneration of dopaminergic neurons in the central nervous system, dopaminergic therapy with dopamine agonists or precursors is the gold standard treatment for Parkinson's disease. However, dopamine is the main neurotransmitter that is involved in reward and motivational mechanisms, and the mesolimbic dopaminergic system is involved in a variety of reward-related behaviors. Therefore, it is not surprising that a long-lasting stimulation of the dopamine receptors in the brain of parkinsonian patients may cause a number of impulse control disorders. Impulsivity can be defined as a lack of behavioral inhibition, and has multiple manifestations, including motor response inhibition, rapid decisions, impulsive action or premature responding, and impulsive choice. In general, the behavioral repertoire

---

Box 5.1 Parkinson's disease and pathological gambling (continued)

is characterized by a preference for small and immediate rewards, instead of larger and delayed rewards. Impulse control disorders include a number of pathological behaviors such as gambling and compulsive shopping. Indeed, in an Italian study (Avanzi et al., 2006), treated Parkinson patients were 25 times more likely to have pathological gambling than general-hospital controls, and this was associated to the treatment with dopamine agonists. Interestingly, dopamine enhances altruistic punishment in parkinsonian patients with impulse control disorders, where violators of social norms are punished when there is a personal cost association with their behavior. Dopamine replacement therapy may influence physiological function either by exogenous tonic dopaminergic stimulation or interference with the endogenous, physiological, phasic striatal dopamine release. Patients and caregivers should be warned about the risk of development of impulse control disorders at treatment onset and actively questioned on follow-up. In particular, patients with a premorbid history of substance or behavioral addictions may be at greater risk for the development of these disorders (Voon et al., 2011).

5.1.4 Placebo administration induces dopamine release in the striatum

In 2001, de la Fuente-Fernández et al. (2001) conducted the first brain imaging study of the placebo effect by means of positron emission tomography (Fig. 5.2). These researchers assessed the release of endogenous dopamine by using raclopride, a radiotracer

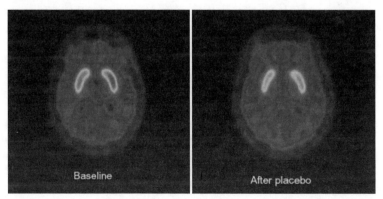

Fig. 5.2 Positron emission tomography image showing the binding of raclopride in the striatum (red areas). Raclopride is an antagonist of dopamine receptors that competes with endogenous dopamine at the D2–D3 receptors. Note the decrease in raclopride binding after placebo administration, meaning that endogenous dopamine has been released. Reprinted from *The Lancet Neurology*, 1 (2), Raúl de la Fuente-Fernández, Michael Schulzer, and A. Jon Stoessl, The placebo effect in neurological disorders, pp. 85–91, Copyright (2002), with permission from Elsevier. (See Plate 6.)

which binds to dopamine D2 and D3 receptors and competes with endogenous dopamine. In this study, patients were aware that they would be receiving an injection of either active drug (apomorphine, a dopamine receptor agonist) or placebo, according to classical clinical trial methodology. After placebo administration (that is, an inert substance that the patient believed to be apomorphine) it was found that dopamine was released in the striatum, corresponding to a change of 200% or more in extracellular dopamine concentration and comparable to the response to amphetamine in subjects with an intact dopamine system. The release of dopamine in the motor striatum (putamen and dorsal caudate) was greater in those patients who reported clinical improvement.

In the studies by de la Fuente-Fernández et al. (2001, 2002a) all patients showed dopamine placebo responses, yet only half the patients reported motor improvement. These patients also released larger amounts of dopamine in the dorsal motor striatum, suggesting a relationship between the amount of dorsal striatal dopamine release and clinical benefit. This relationship was not present in the ventral striatum, in which all patients showed increased dopamine release, irrespective of whether they perceived any improvement. Compared to the dorsal motor striatum, the ventral striatum (nucleus accumbens) is involved in motivation and reward anticipation (Ikemoto and Panksepp, 1999; Schultz et al., 2000; Schultz, 2002; Knutson and Cooper, 2005). Accordingly, the investigators proposed that the dopamine released in the ventral striatum was associated with patient expectation of improvement in symptoms, which could in turn be considered a form of reward (Fig. 5.3). Although we have seen that reward mechanisms are also involved in placebo analgesia (Scott et al., 2007) (section 4.1.8), the studies by de la Fuente-Fernández et al. (2001, 2002a) were the first to relate the placebo effect to reward mechanisms and dopamine release in the nucleus accumbens.

Strafella et al. (2006) confirmed these findings using sham transcranial magnetic stimulation as a placebo. Patients were told they had a 50% chance of receiving either a real or sham treatment, but in all cases they received the sham treatment. These authors found that changes in 11C-raclopride binding were greater in the hemisphere contralateral to the more affected side, particularly in the putamen. Although the patients who perceived clinical benefit had a slightly higher amount of dopamine release in the dorsal and ventral striatum, this difference failed to reach statistical significance.

In order to determine how the strength of expectation of clinical improvement influences the degree of striatal dopamine release in response to placebo in patients with Parkinson's disease, Lidstone et al. (2010) manipulated patients' expectations by telling them that they had a probability of 25%, 50%, 75%, or 100% of receiving active medication when they in fact received placebo. Significant dopamine release occurred when the declared probability of receiving active medication was 75%, but not at other probabilities. Placebo-induced dopamine release in all regions of the striatum was also highly correlated with the dopaminergic response to open administration of active medication. Whereas response to prior medication was the major determinant of placebo-induced dopamine release in the motor striatum, expectation of clinical improvement was additionally required to drive dopamine release in the ventral striatum. Therefore, the strength of belief of improvement can directly modulate dopamine release in parkinsonian patients, and this emphasizes the importance of uncertainty and/or salience both in clinical practice and in the design of clinical trials.

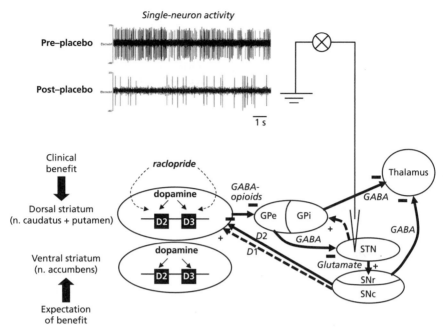

Fig. 5.3 The basal ganglia circuitry involved in Parkinson's disease. By using raclopride, which competes with endogenous dopamine for D2 and D3 receptors, release of dopamine in both the ventral and dorsal striatum is demonstrated (de la Fuente-Fernández et al., 2001.) The former is associated with expectation of clinical benefit, whereas the latter is associated with the benefit itself. In a different study, the neurons of the subthalamic nucleus (STN) were found both to decrease in firing rate and to change from bursting to nonbursting activity (Benedetti et al., 2004b). The dashed lines show excitatory connections between the different nuclei whereas the solid lines show inhibitory connections. D1/D2/D3 dopamine receptors; GABA, gamma-aminobutyric acid; GPe, external globus pallidus; GPi, internal globus pallidus; SNr, substantia nigra pars reticulata; SNc, substantia nigra pars compacta. Reproduced from Fabrizio Benedetti, Mechanisms of placebo and placebo-related effects across diseases and treatments, *Annual Review of Pharmacology and Toxicology*, 48, pp. 33–60 Copyright 2008, Annual Reviews.

5.1.5 The subthalamic nucleus neurons of Parkinson patients show abnormal activity

The subthalamic nucleus is now the major target in the surgical therapy of Parkinson's disease and its identification can require the recording of electrical activity in the subthalamic nucleus. Therefore, during implantation of electrodes for deep-brain stimulation there are at least two criteria for identification of the subthalamic nucleus: one is anatomical, the other electrophysiological. In fact, before surgery, a brain magnetic resonance image (MRI) is obtained for each patient, and at surgery, after positioning a stereotactic frame, a stereotactic computed tomography (CT) scan is performed. Then, the data from the MRI and the CT slices are fused, to obtain in a single image the spatial precision of CT and the high tissue definition of MRI. In this way, the coordinates of the anterior and posterior commissure and the length of the intercommissural line can be assessed. The subthalamic nucleus is anatomically localized 2.5 mm posterior and 4 mm inferior with respect to the mid-commissural point and 12 mm from the midline.

Although this anatomical localization is quite precise, usually it is not sufficient for correct placement of the electrodes in the subthalamic nucleus. Therefore, microrecordings of electrical activity are performed. These have a characteristic pattern which is very useful for identifying the subthalamic nucleus. In fact, after a low background activity that corresponds to a region encompassing the zona incerta (just above the subthalamic nucleus), the subthalamic nucleus is identified by background noise with a sustained and irregular pattern of discharge at a frequency of about 25–45 Hz (Hutchinson et al., 1998), but also higher frequencies can be considered. In addition, single units responsive to contralateral proprioceptive stimuli are usually identified and, in some cases, "tremor neurons" are recorded with an oscillatory discharge of 4–6 Hz (parkinsonian tremor).When the microelectrode exits the subthalamic nucleus, a low background noise is followed by a regular and high-frequency discharge of units belonging to the substantia nigra pars reticulata.

Therefore, by following this anatomical and electrophysiological approach, the activity of single neurons in the subthalamic nucleus, as well as in the surrounding regions, can be recorded in different conditions, for example, after pharmacological challenge. Indeed, several studies have reported that the antiparkinsonian agent, apomorphine, induces changes in the subthalamic nucleus firing pattern of patients with Parkinson's disease (Lozano et al., 2000; Levy et al., 2001; Stefani et al., 2002). Levy et al. (2001) found a certain variability on the firing rates of single neurons under the effect of apomorphine, but Stefani et al. (2002) reported that the administration of apomorphine is invariably followed by a reduction of firing rate from about 40 Hz to about 27 Hz.

According to the classic pathophysiological view of Parkinson's disease, the dopamine depletion in the striatum induces both hyperactivity (high firing rate) (Blandini et al., 2000) and bursting activity (Bergman et al., 1994; Levy et al., 2001) of subthalamic nucleus neurons. This might be due to a lower activity of the external globus pallidus which sends inhibitory projections to the subthalamic nucleus. Therefore, the external globus pallidus hypoactivity would result in decreased inhibition of the neurons of the subthalamic nucleus. High-frequency therapeutic stimulation of the subthalamic nucleus would modify this abnormal activity (Limousin et al., 1998); this might be achieved through stimulation of the inhibitory afferents from the external globus pallidus to the subthalamic nucleus. Other mechanisms have also been hypothesized.

5.1.6 **Placebos restore the normal activity of subthalamic nucleus neurons**

In 2004, the first study of the placebo effect at the single-neuron level was performed by Benedetti and collaborators (Benedetti et al., 2004b) (Fig. 5.3). The subthalamic nucleus plays an essential role in basal ganglia functioning and is a major target in the surgical therapy of Parkinson's disease (Limousin et al., 1998); furthermore, its identification requires the recording of intranuclear electrical activity in awake Parkinson

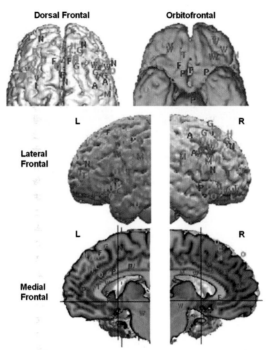

Plate 1 Regions of the frontal lobes showing increased activity in recent studies of self-regulation. Increases are shown for delivery of opiate analgesics compared with resting nondrug control states (blue letters), downregulation of aversive emotional experience (green letters) through emotional reappraisal, and placebo effects on pain or emotional processing (red letters). Some peaks reflect regions for which increases in activity are correlated with reductions in negative emotional experience or pain. One exception is the study by Bishop et al. (2004) in which frontal activation was correlated with a reduced state of anxiety. Peak locations from the same study within 12 mm were averaged together for clarity of presentation. Reproduced from Fabrizio Benedetti, Helen S. Mayberg, Tor D. Wager, Christian S. Stohler, and Jon-Kar Zubieta, Neurobiological mechanisms of the placebo effect, *Journal of Neuroscience*, 25 (45), pp. 10390–402 Copyright 2005, The Society for Neuroscience. (See Fig. 2.13.)

Studies on opioid increases:

F—Firestone et al. 1996
A—Adler et al. 1997
N—Wagner et al. 2001
P—Petrovic and Ingvar 2002

Studies on placebo:

W—Wager et al. 2004b (anticipation)
G—Wager et al. 2004b (pain)
I—Lieberman et al. 2004
V—Petrovic et al. 2002
T—Petrovic et al. 2005
M—Mayberg et al. 2002

Studies on emotion regulation:

L—Levesque et al. 2003
C—Ochsner et al. 2002
O—Ochsner et al. 2004
H—Phan et al. 2005
B—Bishop et al. 2004

Remifentanil   Placebo

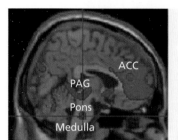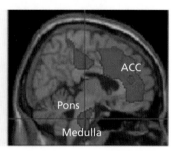

Plate 2 Comparison of the effects of remifentanil, an opioid receptor agonist, and placebo on brain activation. The blue spot indicates the anterior cingulate cortex (ACC) which is activated both by the real drug and the placebo. The red areas are co-activated with the anterior cingulate cortex, suggesting activation of a common neural network by both opioids and placebos, with the exception of periaqueductal gray (PAG), which is co-activated sub-significantly in the placebo condition. Adapted from Predrag Petrovic, Eija Kalso, Karl Magnus Petersson, and Martin Ingvar, Placebo and Opioid Analgesia—Imaging a Shared Neuronal Network, *Science*, 295 (5560), pp. 1737–1740, Copyright 2002, The American Association for the Advancement of Science. Reprinted with permission from AAAS. (See Fig. 4.6.)

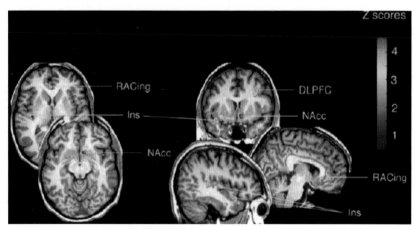

Plate 3 Placebo administration induces the activation of μ-opioid neurotransmission in several brain regions, such as the dorsolateral prefrontal cortex (DLPFC), the anterior cingulate cortex (RACing), the nucleus accumbens (NAcc) and the insula (Ins). Reproduced from Jon-Kar Zubieta, Joshua A. Bueller, Lisa R. Jackson, David J. Scott, Yanjun Xu, Robert A. Koeppe, Thomas E. Nichols, and Christian S. Stohler, Placebo Effects Mediated by Endogenous Opioid Activity on μ-Opioid Receptors, *The Journal of Neuroscience*, 25 (34), pp. 7754–7762 Copyright 2005, The Society for Neuroscience, with permission. (See Fig. 4.7.)

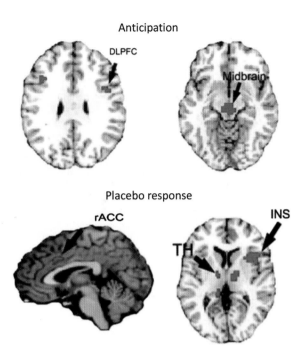

Anticipation

DLPFC

Midbrain

Placebo response

rACC

INS

TH

Plate 4 Administration of a placebo following thermal painful stimulation induces anticipatory responses in the dorsolateral prefrontal cortex (DLPFC) and midbrain, which increase their activity. During the placebo analgesic response, some areas decrease their activity, such as the rostral anterior cingulate cortex (rACC), the thalamus (TH), and the insula (INS). Adapted from Tor D. Wager, James K. Rilling, Edward E. Smith, Alex Sokolik, Kenneth L. Casey, Richard J. Davidson, Stephen M. Kosslyn, Robert M. Rose, and Jonathan D. Cohen, Placebo-Induced Changes in fMRI in the Anticipation and Experience of Pain, *Science*, 303 (5661), pp. 1162–1167 Copyright 2004, The American Association for the Advancement of Science. Reprinted with permission from AAAS. (See Fig. 4.11.)

HIGH TEMPERATURE

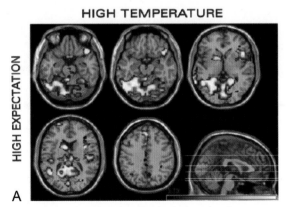

HIGH EXPECTATION

A

Plate 5 Magnetic resonance imaging showing brain functional responses to a high-temperature stimulus when the subject expects (A) a high-intensity or (B) a low-intensity stimulation. Note that expectation of a high-intensity noxious stimulus activates different areas—the thalamus, insular cortex, somatosensory cortex, anterior cingulate cortex, orbitofrontal cortex, amygdala, ventral striatum, and nucleus cuneiformis in the

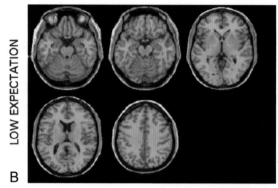

Plate 5 (continued) brainstem—unlike expectation of a low-intensity noxious stimulus. Reproduced from John R. Keltner, Ansgar Furst, Catherine Fan, Rick Redfern, Ben Inglis, and Howard L. Fields, Isolating the Modulatory Effect of Expectation on Pain Transmission: A Functional Magnetic Resonance Imaging Study, *The Journal of Neuroscience*, 26 (16), pp. 4437–4443 doi: 10.1523/JNEUROSCI.4463–05.2006 Copyright 2006, The Society for Neuroscience. (See Fig. 4.14.)

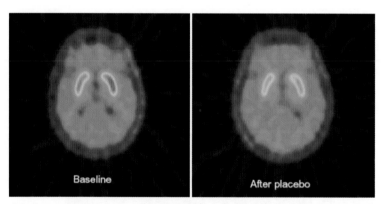

Plate 6 Positron emission tomography image showing the binding of raclopride in the striatum (red areas). Raclopride is an antagonist of dopamine receptors that competes with endogenous dopamine at the D2–D3 receptors. Note the decrease in raclopride binding after placebo administration, meaning that endogenous dopamine has been released. Reprinted from *The Lancet Neurology*, 1 (2), Raúl de la Fuente-Fernández, Michael Schulzer, and A. Jon Stoessl, The placebo effect in neurological disorders, pp. 85–91, Copyright (2002), with permission from Elsevier. (See Fig. 5.2.)

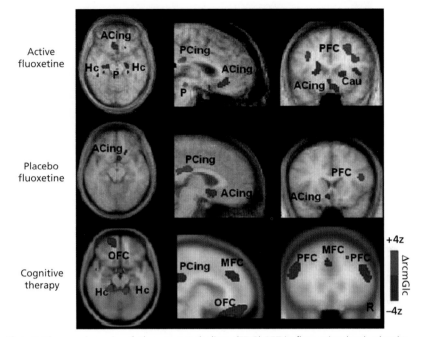

Labels in figure: Active fluoxetine, Placebo fluoxetine, Cognitive therapy; ACing, Hc, P, PCing, PFC, Cau, OFC, MFC, PFC, R; +4z, −4z, ΔrcmGlc

Plate 7 Changes in regional glucose metabolism. (FDG) PET in fluoxetine (top), placebo (middle), and cognitive (bottom) therapy responders measured before and after a standard course of each respective treatment. Axial (left), sagittal (middle), and coronal (right) views show increases in red and decreases in blue. The fluoxetine and placebo group were studied as part of the same double-blind controlled experiment. A common pattern of cortical increases and limbic–paralimbic decreases is seen in both groups, with the active fluoxetine group showing additional changes in the brainstem, hippocampus, insula and caudate nucleus. In contrast, responses to cognitive therapy are associated with a distinctly different pattern—dorsolateral and medial frontal decreases and hippocampal increases. ACing, subgenual anterior cingulate; Cau, caudate nucleus; Hc, hippocampus; MFC, medial frontal cortex; OFC, orbital frontal cortex; P, pons; PCing, posterior cingulate; PFC, prefrontal cortex. Reproduced from Fabrizio Benedetti, Helen S. Mayberg, Tor D. Wager, Christian S. Stohler, and Jon-Kar Zubieta, Neurobiological mechanisms of the placebo effect, *Journal of Neuroscience*, 25 (45), pp. 10390–402 Copyright 2005, The Society for Neuroscience. doi: 10.1523/JNEUROSCI.3458–05.2005 and from Helen S. Mayberg, J. Arturo Silva, Steven K. Brannan, Janet L. Tekell, Roderick K. Mahurin, Scott McGinnis, and Paul A. Jerabek, The Functional Neuroanatomy of the Placebo Effect, *The American Journal of Psychiatry*, 159 (5), pp. 728–737 Copyright 2002, American Psychiatric Association. doi: 10.1176/appi.ajp.159.5.728 (See Fig. 6.1.)

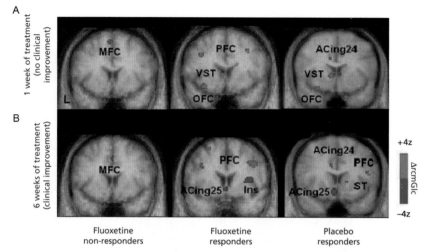

Plate 8 Time course of regional metabolic changes in fluoxetine nonresponders (left), fluoxetine responders (middle), and placebo responders (right). The top panel (A) represents 1 week of treatment (no clinical improvement) and the lower panel (B) represents 6 weeks of treatment (clinical improvement). Ventral striatal and orbital frontal increases are seen uniquely at 1 week in (A) (middle and right) of both active and sham treatment in patients that go on to show clinical response at 6 weeks (B). Such changes are not seen in patients who failed to respond and are no longer present in either group of responders once clinical remission has been achieved (6-week time-point in B). In contrast, response-specific changes in the prefrontal cortex and subgenual cingulate are seen only at 6 weeks (B) and not at the 1-week (A) time-point. ACing24, anterior cingulate Brodmann area 24; ACing25, subgenual anterior cingulate Brodmann area 25; Ins, anterior insula; MFC, medial frontal cortex; OFC, orbital frontal cortex; PFC, prefrontal cortex; VST, ventral striatum. Reproduced from Fabrizio Benedetti, Helen S. Mayberg, Tor D. Wager, Christian S. Stohler, and Jon-Kar Zubieta, Neurobiological mechanisms of the placebo effect, *Journal of Neuroscience*, 25 (45), pp. 10390–402 Copyright 2005, The Society for Neuroscience doi: 10.1523/JNEUROSCI.3458–05.2005 and from Helen S. Mayberg, J. Arturo Silva, Steven K. Brannan, Janet L. Tekell, Roderick K. Mahurin, Scott McGinnis, and Paul A. Jerabek, The Functional Neuroanatomy of the Placebo Effect, *The American Journal of Psychiatry*, 159 (5), pp. 728–737 Copyright 2002, American Psychiatric Association. doi: 10.1176/appi.ajp.159.5.728 (See Fig. 6.2.)

Plate 9 (A) Emotional network and placebo-dependent attenuation of the same network. In the upper panel, the emotional network in the extrastriatal cortex (ExtC) activated by unpleasant pictures can be seen. In the lower panel, some regions in the ExtC show attenuated activation after placebo administration (Amy, amygdala). The t values of the activations are given by the color bars. (B) The amygdala is activated bilaterally by unpleasant emotions (left), and the placebo attenuates the activation of the amygdala/para-amygdaloid complex bilaterally (right).

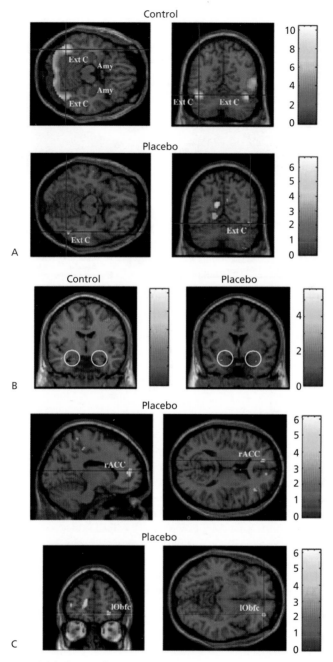

Plate 9 (continued) (C) The rostral anterior cingulate cortex (rACC) (upper) and the right lateral orbitofrontal cortex (lObfc) (lower) are activated by the placebo, as occurs in pain (see sections 4.1.6 and 4.1.9). Reprinted from *Neuron*, 46 (6), Predrag Petrovic, Thomas Dietrich, Peter Fransson, Jesper Andersson, Katrina Carlsson, and Martin Ingvar, Placebo in Emotional Processing—Induced Expectations of Anxiety Relief Activate a Generalized Modulatory Network, pp. 957–969, Copyright (2005), with permission from Elsevier. (See Fig. 6.5.)

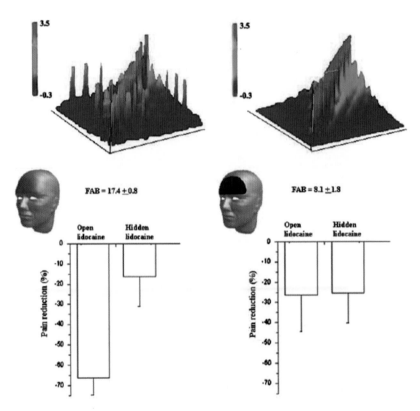

Plate 10 Correlation between electroencephalographic connectivity analysis (assessed by means of mutual information: top panel), cognitive status (assessed by means of Frontal Assessment Battery or FAB) and the placebo component of open and hidden application of local analgesic lidocaine. Note the differences between normal subjects (on the left) and Alzheimer patients (on the right). Alzheimer patients show reduced electroencephalographic connectivity, as shown by the disappearance of the orange peaks (top panel), reduced FAB scores, and reduced effects of open lidocaine. Reproduced from Fabrizio Benedetti, Claudia Arduino, Sara Costa, Sergio Vighetti, Luisella Tarenzi, Innocenzo Rainero, and Giovanni Asteggiano, Loss of expectation-related mechanisms in Alzheimer's disease makes analgesic therapies less effective, *Pain*, 121 (1), pp 133–44 Copyright 2006, The International Association for the Study of Pain, with permission and from *European Journal of Applied Physiology*, 102 (4) pp. 371–380, Experimental designs and brain mapping approaches for studying the placebo analgesic effect, Luana Colloca, Fabrizio Benedetti, Carlo Adolfo Porro, Copyright 2008, Springer Science and Business Media. With kind permission from Springer Science and Business Media. (See Fig. 6.6.)

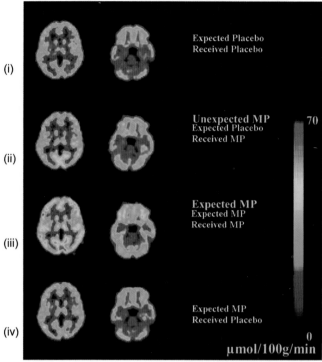

Plate 11 Brain metabolic images at the thalamic and cerebellar levels in cocaine abusers in four conditions: (i) expected placebo, received placebo; (ii) expected placebo, received methylphenidate (MP); (iii) expected methylphenidate, received methylphenidate; and (iv) expected methylphenidate, received placebo. Note the larger increases in metabolism when methylphenidate was expected (iii) than when it was not (ii). Reproduced from Nora D. Volkow, Gene-Jack Wang, Yemin Ma, Joanna S. Fowler, Wei Zhu, Laurence Maynard, Frank Telang, Paul Vaska, Yu-Shin Ding, Christopher Wong, and James M. Swanson Expectation Enhances the Regional Brain Metabolic and the Reinforcing Effects of Stimulants in Cocaine Abusers, *The Journal of Neuroscience*, 23 (36), pp. 11461–11468 Copyright 2003, The Society for Neuroscience, with permission. (See Fig. 6.7.)

NATURAL HISTORY　　　**PLACEBO**

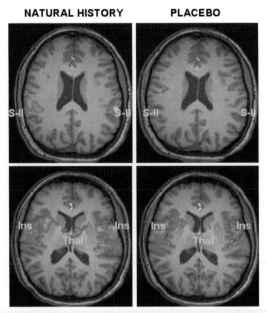

Plate 12 Brain regions showing large reductions in pain-related brain activity during the placebo condition compared with untreated natural history or baseline condition in patients with irritable bowel syndrome. The thalamus (Thal), second somatosensory area (S-II) and insular cortical regions (Ins) show reduced activity. Reproduced from Donald D. Price, Damien G. Finniss, and Fabrizio Benedetti, A Comprehensive Review of the Placebo Effect: Recent Advances and Current Thought, Annual Review of Psychology, 59 (1), pp. 565–590 Copyright 2008, Annual Reviews. DOI: 10.1146/annurev. psych.59.113006.095941. Reproduced with permission of Annual Review http://www.annualreviews.org. (See Fig. 9.2.)

Expectation

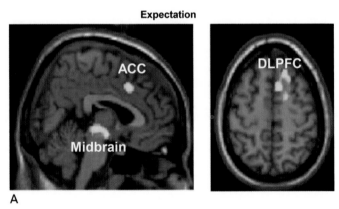

A

Plate 13 Acupuncture has a placebo component in the dorsolateral prefrontal cortex (DLPFC), the anterior cingulate cortex (ACC) and the midbrain, activated by expectation of analgesia (A) and a specific effect in the insula (Ins), which is activated by real acupuncture (B). Reprinted from *NeuroImage*, 4 (7), Jérémie Pariente, Peter White, Richard SJ Frackowiak, and George Lewith, Expectancy and belief modulate the neuronal substrates of pain treated by acupuncture, pp. 1161–67, Copyright (2005), with permission from Elsevier. (See Fig. 10.3.)

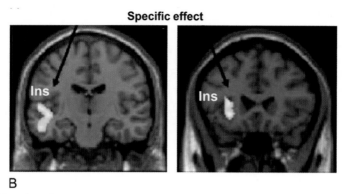

Specific effect

B

Plate 13 (continued)

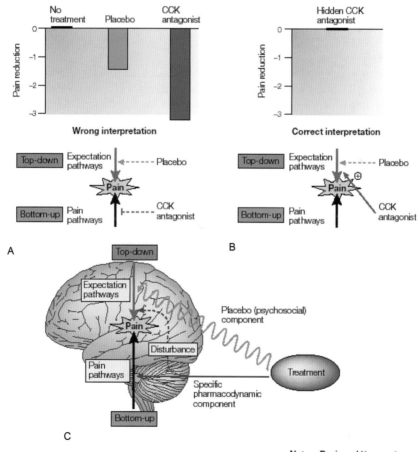

Wrong interpretation

Correct interpretation

A

B

C

Nature Reviews | Neuroscience

Plate 14 An emerging uncertainty principle imposes limitations on our understanding of the effects of a therapeutic agent. (A) A clinical trial with three arms shows that a placebo

Plate 14 (continued) is better than no treatment and that the cholecystokinin (CCK) antagonist, proglumide, is better than a placebo in relieving pain. According to the interpretation of a classical clinical trial, this leads to the erroneous belief that the CCK antagonist acts specifically on pain pathways (the bottom-up action) whereas the placebo acts on expectation pathways (the top-down control). (B) The interpretation in (A) is incorrect because if the same CCK antagonist is given by hidden injection, so that the patient is completely unaware that a drug is being administered and thus has no expectations, the drug is completely ineffective. As the drug has analgesic effects only in association with a placebo procedure, its action is not directed specifically to the pain pathways, but rather to the expectation pathways, which enhances the placebo analgesic response. (C) Any analgesic treatment consists of two components—the specific pharmacodynamic component and the placebo component. The latter is induced by the psychosocial context in which the treatment is given and elicits expectations of improvement. The uncertainty principle in a clinical trial is represented by the fact that a drug might act on expectation pathways (broken arrows) rather than pain pathways, which makes it extremely difficult to conclude whether or not a pharmacological substance is a real painkiller. The only way in which this uncertainty can be partially resolved, and the real pharmacodynamic effect of a painkiller established, is through the elimination of the placebo component, and, therefore, of the expectation pathways, by hidden treatments. Reprinted by permission from Macmillan Publishers Ltd: *Nature Reviews Neuroscience*, 6 (7), Luana Colloca & Fabrizio Benedetti, Placebos and painkillers: is mind as real as matter?, pp. 545–552 Copyright 2005, Nature Publishing Group. Data in (A) and (B) from Benedetti F, Amanzio M and Maggi G, Potentiation of placebo analgesia by proglumide, *Lancet*, 346, page 1231. (See Fig. 11.5.)

patients. Therefore these authors performed a double-blind study in which the activity from single neurons in the subthalamic nucleus before and after placebo administration was recorded to see whether neuronal changes were associated with the clinical placebo response. In order to make the placebo response stronger, the placebo was administered in the operating room after several preoperative administrations of the antiparkinsonian drug apomorphine (pharmacological preconditioning procedure).

Before placebo administration, the activity of neurons was recorded from one subthalamic nucleus prior to implantation of the first electrode and used as a control. After the placebo, which consisted of a subcutaneous injection of saline solution along with the verbal suggestion of motor improvement, neuronal activity was recorded from neurons prior to implanting the second electrode into the other subthalamic nucleus. A placebo response was defined as the decrease of arm rigidity of at least 1 point on the clinical evaluation scale. Patients who showed a straightforward clinical placebo response, assessed by means of arm rigidity and subjective report of well-being, also showed a significantly decreased firing rate compared to the pre-placebo subthalamic nucleus. In order to rule out the possibility that the difference in firing rate between the pre- and post-placebo subthalamic nucleus was independent of the placebo treatment itself, a no-treatment group (natural history) was studied. The patients of this no-treatment group did not undergo any placebo treatment between the implantation of the first and second electrode. All these patients showed no significant differences between the neuronal firing rates of the two subthalamic nuclei, which indicates that the difference between the first and second side of implantation in the placebo group was due to the placebo intervention per se.

Although the mean firing rate of the subthalamic nucleus neurons is a good parameter for assessing activity of the subthalamic nucleus, bursting and oscillatory patterns have also been described in Parkinson's disease and related to motor symptoms and to apomorphine effects (Bergman et al., 1994; Levy et al., 2001). Therefore, in the single-neuron analysis by Benedetti et al. (2004b) the bursting activity of the subthalamic nucleus neurons before and after placebo administration was also investigated, in order to see whether, beside the frequency decrease, there was also a change in the pattern of discharge. They found that the subthalamic nucleus neurons of all placebo responders shifted significantly from a pattern of bursting activity to a pattern of nonbursting discharge. None of the placebo nonresponders showed any difference in the number of bursting neurons before and after placebo administration. Likewise, the no-treatment group showed no significant difference in bursting activity between the first-side and second-side subthalamic nucleus.

In the study by Benedetti et al. (2004b) there was a clear correlation between subjective reports of the patients' clinical responses and neurophysiological responses (Fig. 5.4). In fact, a decrease in firing rate as well as a change from bursting to nonbursting activity of subthalamic nucleus neurons were correlated with both the patients' subjective reports of well-being and the muscle rigidity reduction at the wrist, as assessed by a blinded neurologist. Although it is tempting to speculate that these neuronal changes represent a downstream effect of dopamine release in the striatum, the dopamine release in the striatum (de la Fuente-Fernández et al., 2001) and the single-neuron changes (Benedetti et al., 2004b) were observed in two different studies, thus no

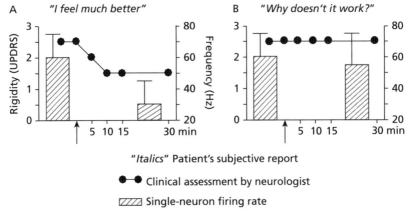

"*Italics*" Patient's subjective report

●—● Clinical assessment by neurologist

▨ Single-neuron firing rate

Fig. 5.4 Correlation between subjective report (italics), arm rigidity (black circles) as assessed by a neurologist, and subthalamic nucleus (STN) single-neuron discharge frequency (bars) in two representative Parkinson's disease patients. The black arrows on the horizontal axes indicate placebo administration. Note the subjective sensation of well-being, along with decrease in arm rigidity and reduced neuronal firing rate in the placebo responder (A) but not in the nonresponder (B). UPDRS Unified Parkinson's Disease Rating Scale. Reproduced from Fabrizio Benedetti, Luana Colloca, Elena Torre, Michele Lanotte, Antonio Melcarne, Marina Pesare, Bruno Bergamasco, and Leonardo Lopiano, *Nature Neuroscience*, 7 (6), pp. 587–88, Copyright 2004, Nature Publishing Group, with permission.

definitive conclusion can be drawn. Nonetheless, on the basis of our knowledge about the basal ganglia circuitry, it is plausible that placebo-induced release of dopamine acting on the inhibitory D2 receptors disinhibits the GABA (gamma-aminobutyric acid) neurons of the external globus pallidus which, in turn, increase their inhibition onto the subthalamic nucleus (Fig. 5.3).

In a subsequent study, Benedetti et al. (2009) extended the previous results on single-neuron recording in the subthalamic nucleus to two thalamic nuclei (VA, ventral anterior and VLa anterior ventral lateral) and the substantia nigra pars reticulata. It is worth remembering that the subthalamic nucleus receives inputs from both the cortex and the external globus pallidus and sends excitatory output pathways to both internal globus pallidus and substantia nigra pars reticulata (Fig. 5.3). Considering the effect of placebo administration on this nucleus (Benedetti et al., 2004b), a significant placebo effect should also be expected in the subthalamic nucleus output regions. Indeed, in parkinsonian patients who exhibited a clinical placebo response, the decrease in firing rate in the subthalamic nucleus was associated with a decrease in the substantia nigra pars reticulata and an increase in the thalamic nuclei. Conversely, placebo nonresponders showed either no changes or partial changes in the subthalamic nucleus only. Thus, the whole subthalamic–nigral–thalamic circuit appears to be important for a clinical placebo response to occur (Fig. 5.5) (see also Frisaldi et al., 2013).

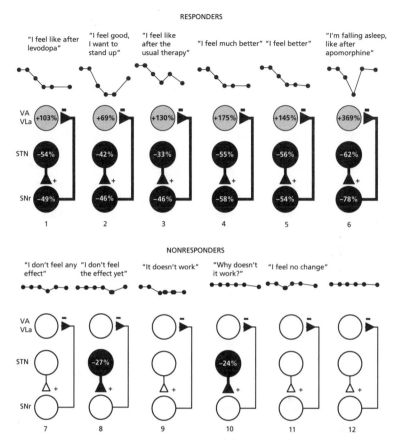

Fig. 5.5 Deactivation (black) and activation (gray) pattern of the STN (subthalamic nucleus)-SNr (substantia nigra pars reticulata)-VA (ventral anterior thalamus)/VLa (anterior ventral lateral thalamus) circuit in placebo responders (subjects 1–6) and nonresponders (subjects 7–12). The percentage decrease or increase in neuronal activity after placebo administration is shown. The decrease in muscle rigidity after placebo (clinical placebo response) is shown with black lines and circles, where the first black circle represents the baseline condition in each patient before placebo administration. The feelings reported by the patients are also shown, with the exception of patient 12. Note that STN and SNr are deactivated and VA/VLa is activated only in those subjects with a large reduction in muscle rigidity and with positive feelings of well-being (placebo responders). By contrast, no neuronal changes are present (white neurons) in those subjects with mild or no muscle rigidity reduction and with no positive subjective sensations (placebo nonresponders). Also note that clinical nonresponders 8 and 10 showed only partial changes, with a significant deactivation of STN but no changes in SNr and VA/VLa. Reproduced from Fabrizio Benedetti, Michele Lanotte, Luana Colloca, Alessandro Ducati, Maurizio Zibetti, and Leonardo Lopiano, Electrophysiological properties of thalamic, subthalamic and nigral neurons during the anti-parkinsonian placebo response, Journal of Physiology, 587 (15), pp. 3869–83, DOI: 10.1113/jphysiol.2009.169425, Copyright 2009, John Wiley and Sons, Inc.

5.2 **Deep-brain stimulation and emotional processing**

5.2.1 **Expectations enhance the excitability of some limbic regions**

During the implantation of the electrodes for deep-brain stimulation, both recording (see sections 5.1.5 and 5.1.6) and stimulation can be performed. In fact, after the definition of the extension of the subthalamic nucleus recording area, with its dorsal and ventral borders, several microstimulations can be carried out. For example, confirmation of good positioning of the electrode tip in the subthalamic nucleus can be obtained by means of microstimulation for the assessment of both clinical effects, such as reduction of rigidity, disappearance of tremor, and side effects, like dyskinesias, muscle contractions, or tingling sensations. Usually, high-frequency stimulation of 130 Hz is used.

Besides the motor responses to deep-brain stimulation described in section 5.1.2, autonomic and emotional responses have also been tested. For example, open and hidden stimulations have been performed to assess the role of expectation in heart rate and emotional responses (Benedetti et al., 2004a; Lanotte et al., 2005). It should be noted that, from an experimental point of view, it is not easy to perform hidden administrations of drugs and then compare them to open ones. In fact, it is necessary to have a computer-controlled infusion pump that is concealed from the patient's view, and special attention must be paid to keep patients completely unaware of the treatment being given. Working with a stimulator that can be switched on and off covertly (out of the patient's view) is much easier and poses fewer methodological problems.

Stimulation of the subthalamic nucleus, and more in general of the subthalamic region, has been shown to produce not only motor-related responses, but also autonomic responses. Both electrical (Van del Plas et al., 1995) and glutamate (Spencer et al., 1988) stimulation of the zona incerta induce cardiovascular responses in rats, and electrical stimulation of the subthalamic nucleus induces conspicuous increases in heart rate, blood pressure and respiratory rate in freely moving cats (Angyan and Angyan, 1999). Similar effects are present in parkinsonian patients who are implanted with electrodes in the subthalamic nuclei (Priori et al., 2001; Kaufmann et al., 2002; Thornton et al., 2002).

A detailed analysis of autonomic responses to intraoperative stimulation of different brain regions has been carried out in Parkinson's patients during the surgical implantation of the electrodes (Benedetti et al., 2004a; Lanotte et al., 2005) (Fig. 5.6). The stimulation of the most dorsal part of the subthalamic region, which includes the zona incerta, produced autonomic responses that did not differ in the hidden and the open conditions. In contrast, stimulation of the most ventral region (which includes the substantia nigra pars reticulata) produced autonomic responses that varied according to open or hidden stimulation. In fact, the hidden (unexpected) stimulation was less effective, so that an increase of stimulus intensity was required to induce an autonomic response, both in heart rate and sympathetic activity, as assessed by means of heart-rate variability analysis. Stimulus–response curves in the dorsal and ventral subthalamic region are shown in Fig. 5.6A. The curves differ for hidden and open conditions only in the ventral part, the region that is involved in associative-limbic functions. This suggests that expectation may change neuronal excitability in limbic structures (Lanotte et al., 2005).

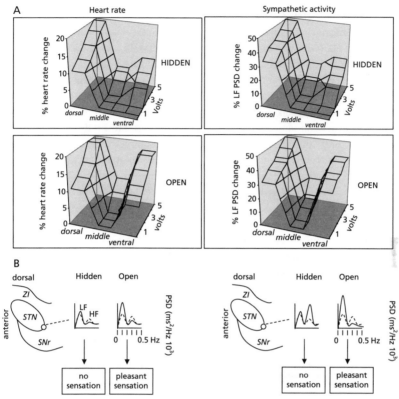

Fig. 5.6 (A) Stimulus–response curves for changes in heart rate and for sympathetic low-frequency (LF) power spectrum density (PSD) changes in the dorsal, middle, and ventral subthalamic regions with both open and hidden stimulation. Note that the stimulus–response relationship, and thus the threshold for eliciting a response, changes only in the ventral (limbic) subthalamic region. Reprinted from *Brain, Behavior, and Immunity*, 19 (6), Michele Lanotte, Leonardo Lopiano, Elena Torre, Bruno Bergamasco, Luana Colloca, and Fabrizio Benedetti, Expectation enhances autonomic responses to stimulation of the human subthalamic limbic region, pp. 500–509, Copyright (2005), with permission from Elsevier. (B) Autonomic and emotional responses in two subjects. In the subject on the left, 4 volts of stimulation of the ventral subthalamic nucleus (STN) elicited a pleasant sensation only during open stimulation, together with LF increase; in the hidden condition, no sensation was reported and no change of LF occurred. In the subject on the right, 4 volts of stimulation of the ventral STN elicited no sensation and a parasympathetic high frequency (HF) increase in the hidden condition; in the open condition, a pleasant sensation was reported, accompanied by sympathetic LF increase. The dashed curves show the baseline before stimulation, and the solid lines show the responses to stimulation. SNr, substantia nigra pars reticulata; ZI, zona incerta. Reprinted from *Brain Research Bulletin*, 63 (3), Fabrizio Benedetti, Luana Colloca, Michele Lanotte, Bruno Bergamasco, Elena Torre, and Leonardo Lopiano, Autonomic and emotional responses to open and hidden stimulations of the human subthalamic region, pp. 203–211, Copyright (2004), with permission from Elsevier.

5.2.2 **Expecting an emotion may change its intensity**

The subthalamic nucleus is also known to be related to associative and limbic functions (Alexander et al., 1986, 1990; Parent and Hazrati, 1995). In fact, the stimulation of the human subthalamic nucleus has been reported to produce emotional-related responses such as euphoria and hypomania (Ghika et al., 1999) and mirthful laughter (Krack et al., 2001), and the stimulation of the substantia nigra pars reticulata has been found to induce acute depression (Bejjani et al., 1999; Kumar et al., 1999). The subthalamic nucleus is known to be connected to the ventral pallidum, a major limbic output region (Turner et al., 2001), and the temporal lobe is an output target of the basal ganglia (Middleton and Strick, 1996). In addition, the activity of the cingulate cortex is modified by high-frequency subthalamic nucleus stimulation (Limousin et al., 1997). Therefore, the subthalamic region, which includes the zona incerta, the subthalamic nucleus, and the substantia nigra pars reticulata, is a complex area that has motor, associative, limbic, cardiovascular, and autonomic functions.

It has long been known that responses evoked by the stimulation of the limbic system (Box 5.2) are not related to specific electrode locations, but rather to the subject's psychological traits and concerns. In other words, limbic stimulation appears to produce effects that are dependent on the ongoing context (Halgren, 1982).

Box 5.2 **Electrical stimulation of the human limbic system**

By probing and stimulating the whole limbic system with electrodes during neurosurgery it is possible to evoke a big range of emotional states. The following is an example of what a patient said during the stimulation of different points of the limbic system by means of two electrodes.

The first stimulation begins.

"What do you feel?" he is asked.

"A pleasant sensation! I feel relaxed, calm, at peace with myself and others, creative, it feels like flying . . . a wonderful sensation . . ."

The stimulation is interrupted. The electrode is moved a little backward, then it is activated again.

"What do you feel now?"

"A really unpleasant sensation!" he answers with anxiety.

He asks to stop. The stimulation is interrupted. The electrode is moved backward further. Another stimulation begins.

"And now what do you feel?"

"I feel like I'm being watched . . . it's acutely embarrassing . . ."

And he adds that the sensation is not well defined. At this point, the second electrode is activated.

Box 5.2 Electrical stimulation of the human limbic system (continued)

"What do you feel?"

"I feel exhausted, sad . . . I don't feel like fighting back"

He asks to stop the stimulation. The electrode is moved back by 1 millimeter. The stimulation starts again.

"What do you feel?"

"You make me anxious . . . I loathe everybody. I'm going to burst into tears . . ."

He asks to stop.

In this patient, both positive and negative emotions are induced in the span of a few minutes: from sensations of well-being and peace to unpleasant and ill-defined sensations, from excitement to anxiety, from embarrassment to loathing, from sadness to tears. If the electrode is placed in a pleasure center, the subject reports sensations of elation, peace and tranquility and sometimes sexual orgasm. Therefore, some individuals adopt a compulsive behavior, and stimulate themselves incessantly in search of pleasure. Some patients would like to keep that electrode implanted in their brain and a button in one hand to press. The stimulation of the limbic system of a woman produced such a pleasant sensation as to make her start to woo the surgeon. A boy who was stimulated in the same way cried out "I like this a lot, you can keep me here as long as you like."

In an open–hidden paradigm study (Benedetti et al., 2004a), three stimulation sites in the subthalamic nucleus ventral pole in three different subjects elicited sensations with an emotional component. Interestingly, the emotional experiences evoked by the subthalamic nucleus ventral pole varied across the two different experimental conditions. Fig. 5.6B shows the data from a subject (left) who reported no sensations with hidden stimulation (stimulus intensity = 4 volts) in the ventral subthalamic nucleus and no autonomic responses occurred. However, a pleasant sensation was reported during open 4-volt stimulation of the same site along with an increase of sympathetic activity. Fig. 5.6B shows another response in another subject (right) whereby hidden 4-volt stimulation induced no sensation along with an increase of parasympathetic activity, whereas open 4-volt stimulation induced a pleasant sensation along with sympathetic hyperactivity.

In this regard, it is important to consider a study by Gospic et al. (2008) who found that pharmacological modulation of emotions was possible with the cholecystokinin (CCK) agonist, pentagastrin, and the opioid agonist, remifentanil. Standardized pictures with either neutral or unpleasant content were presented to healthy volunteers after administering either pentagastrin or remifentanil. Subjects then had to rate their own emotional experience of the pictures. Pentagastrin was found to increase the intensity of unpleasantness for both neutral and unpleasant pictures, whereas it reduced the intensity of pleasantness for the neutral pictures. By contrast, remifentanil increased the pleasantness of neutral pictures. These findings are in keeping with the modulation of placebo analgesia by opioids and CCK (section 4.1.6) as well as with the modulation of nocebo hyperalgesia by CCK (see section 4.2.3), and extend our knowledge about the opposite modulatory effects of opioids and CCK from pain and analgesia to the emotional perception of visual stimuli.

5.3 **Migraine**

5.3.1 **Subcutaneous placebos are better than oral placebos**

Migraine is a painful condition with complex pathophysiological mechanisms (Box 5.3), which is why a discussion about placebo effects in migraine is not included in Chapter 4 on pain. Although the placebo effect has been widely analyzed in clinical trials of antimigraine agents, no information is available about the underlying mechanisms. In other words, there is no study that can discriminate between real placebo responses and other factors, like spontaneous remission. In addition, no neurobiological mechanism is known and the possibility that the same mechanisms of placebo analgesia are also involved in placebo responses in migraine is only speculative. There are, however, some observations that deserve to be taken into consideration. For example, it is interesting to note that the route of administration of placebos can make a difference. In a meta-analysis of 22 clinical trials, de Craen et al. (2000) found that in the oral regimen 25.7% of patients reported no headache or mild headache 2 hours after placebo administration; in the subcutaneous regimen the percentage was 32.4%. The two conditions were statistically significant.

Because adequate controls groups (to rule out spontaneous remissions) are lacking in antimigraine clinical trials, the data of de Craen et al. (2000) are quite important. They suggest that the symbolic meaning of oral versus subcutaneous administration plays an important role. In other words, if the pain reduction was due to spontaneous remission only, no difference should be found between different routes of administration.

5.3.2 **Substantial clinical improvements occur in placebo groups in clinical trials of antimigraine agents**

Pain reduction in placebo groups of clinical trials for the acute treatment of migraine attacks is large. In studies by Henry et al. (1995), Tfelt-Hansen et al. (1995), and Diener (1999) the reduction of pain in the placebo group was between 24% and 26%, whereas in the review by Bendtsen et al. (2003), which compared 11 placebo-controlled studies of treatment of migraine attacks with analgesics, the reduction of pain in the group that received the placebo was on average 30%, with a 95% confidence interval between 23% and 36%. These authors found no difference in the response to placebo for oral compared to parenteral application of the analgesic. The reduction of pain in the placebo group in triptan trials has been analyzed by Ferrari et al. (2001). They found a response rate in the placebo group of 30%. The response was lower in studies comparing eletriptan and sumatriptan to placebo (24%), and higher in studies using almotriptan (35%). In another meta-analysis that included 30,981 patients from 98 studies of treatment of acute migraine attacks, 28.6% of patients improved after 2 hours with placebo (Macedo et al., 2006).

Box 5.3 International Headache Society classification of headache

Although headache is a painful condition, its complex pathophysiology forces clinicians and clinician scientists to differentiate it from other types of pain. The different types of headache are an interesting model to better understand the mechanisms of the placebo effect, thus further research into this condition is necessary. The International Headache Society (IHS) classification of different types of headache is reported here (ICHD-II). However, it should be noted that this classification is a simplification of the complete ICHD-II, for each of these 14 types is further subdivided into different subtypes.

Primary headaches

1 Migraine

2 Tension-type headache

3 Cluster headache and other trigeminal autonomic cephalalgias

4 Other primary headaches

Secondary headaches

5 Headache attributed to head and/or neck trauma

6 Headache attributed to cranial or cervical vascular disorder

7 Headache attributed to nonvascular intracranial disorder

8 Headache attributed to a substance or its withdrawal

9 Headache attributed to infection

10 Headache attributed to disorder of homoeostasis

11 Headache or facial pain attributed to disorder of cranium, neck, eyes, ears, nose, sinuses, teeth, mouth or other facial or cranial structures

12 Headache attributed to psychiatric disorder

Cranial neuralgias, central and primary facial pain, and other headaches

13 Cranial neuralgias and central causes of facial pain

14 Other headache, cranial neuralgia, central or primary facial pain

As far as the prophylactic treatment of migraine is concerned, in a meta-analysis of all placebo-controlled studies of propranolol, the response rate in the placebo group was 14.3% (Holroyd et al., 1991). Other studies on migraine prophylaxis showed placebo rates of 14–21% (Mathew et al., 1995; Klapper, 1997), 16% (Peikert et al., 1996), 22% (van de Ven et al., 1997), and 31% (Diener et al., 2001). Nonpharmacological prophylactic treatments of migraine, like acupuncture, have also been investigated. In two studies, after 8–12 weeks, a response rate as large as 50% was found in placebo groups (Linde et al., 2005; Diener et al., 2006). In general, the placebo response rates in the treatment of acute headache episodes are higher than in headache prophylaxis (Diener, 2010).

As already described in section 4.2.1, nocebo responses are frequent in clinical trials of analgesic drugs, including headache. For example, Amanzio et al. (2009) compared the rates of adverse events reported in the placebo arms of clinical trials for three classes of antimigraine drugs: nonsteroidal anti-inflammatory drugs (NSAIDs), triptans, and anticonvulsants. The adverse events in the placebo arms corresponded to those of the antimigraine medication against which the placebo was compared, such as anorexia and memory difficulties (typical of anticonvulsants), which were present only in the placebo arm of these trials. Thus, the adverse events in placebo arms of clinical trials of antimigraine medications depend on the adverse events of the active medication against which the placebo is compared. Mitsikostas et al. (2011) and Mitsikostas (2012) obtained similar results. In a study on the relationship between headache and mobile phones radiofrequency fields, nocebo has been found to be an important trigger of headache attacks (Stovner et al., 2008).

Most of these studies cannot distinguish between real placebo responses and spontaneous remissions, thus the presence of a real psychobiological placebo phenomenon in migraine is not definitive. However, as already described in section 4.1.3, studies by Linde et al. (2005, 2007) showed that patients with higher expectations about acupuncture treatment experienced larger clinical benefits than those with lower expectations, regardless of their allocation to real or sham acupuncture. In other words, it did not matter whether the patients actually received the real or the sham procedure. What mattered was whether they believed in acupuncture and expected a benefit from it.

In this regard, one particular study is worth mentioning here, even though the small number of subjects in the study precludes any definitive conclusions. Clayton et al. (2005) subdivided women who suffered from menstrual migraine who were treated with sumatriptan into sumatriptan responders and nonresponders, and into placebo responders and nonresponders. They found that placebo responders showed higher plasma concentration of serotonin compared to the other groups, and this increased during the first 10 minutes after the injection. By contrast, placebo nonresponders showed a lower baseline plasma level of serotonin that decreased in the first 10 minutes, suggesting that those patients who have higher levels of serotonin may be biologically predisposed to react to placebos.

Another study tried to investigate the placebo response in headache by using a neurobiological approach. In fact, de Tommaso et al. (2012) evaluated the effect of visual and verbal suggestion on both subjective pain sensation and cortical responses evoked by CO_2 painful laser stimuli in patients with migraine without aura and in healthy controls. The right hand and the right supraorbital zone were stimulated in the interictal phase during a not conditioned and a conditioned task, where laser stimuli were delivered after verbal and visual cues of decreased, increased, or basal intensity. In control subjects pain rating changed, according to the announced intensity, while in migraine patients the basal hyperalgesia remained unmodified. The N1 and N2 amplitudes of the laser-evoked potentials tended to change coherently with the stimulus cue in controls, while an opposite paradoxical increase in decreasing condition was present in migraine. The altered pattern of pain rating and N2 amplitude modulation were related to the frequency of migraine, disability, and allodynia. Therefore, this study is an interesting attempt to characterize the neurophysiological changes in migraine patients following the manipulation of expectations.

Recently, high altitude headache has been investigated as a model to understand the biological underpinnings related to vasodilation-induced pain (Benedetti et al., 2014). In this study, an experimental nocebo group received negative information about the risk of headache at high altitude, whereas the control group did not know about the possible occurrence of headache. A significant increase in headache and salivary prostaglandins and thromboxane in the nocebo group was found compared to the control group, suggesting that negative expectations enhance cyclooxygenase activity. In addition, placebo administration to headache sufferers at high altitude inhibited the nocebo-related component of pain and prostaglandins synthesis, which indicates that the cyclooxygenase pathway can be modulated by both nocebos and placebos.

5.4 **Sleep**

5.4.1 **Placebos for insomnia may induce behavioral and physiological changes**

Little is known about placebo and placebo-related effects in sleep disorders. Recent evidence suggests that placebo administration, along with verbal suggestions that it is a hypnotic agent, may induce both behavioral and neurophysiological changes. A significant effect of a placebo pill was found in an 8-week study, in which a positive trend for better sleep in the placebo group was observed (Walsh et al., 2000). In a meta-analysis by McCall et al. (2003) a dissociation between subjective and objective outcome measures was found in five clinical trials, whereby only subjective measures showed a significant effect after placebo administration. By contrast, Hrobjartsson and Gotzsche (2001) found no beneficial effect of placebo in five clinical trials.

To resolve the issue of subjective versus objective measurements, Fratello et al. (2005) compared subjective, behavioral, polysomnographic, and quantitative electro-encephalographic measurements after administration of a placebo (two 50 mg lactose pills along with the verbal suggestion that they were hypnotics). This study was designed to compare no-treatment and placebo within the same individual. These investigators found that their nights were self-rated as more restful, and the number of nocturnal awakenings decreased. In addition, there was an improvement in behavioral tests (e.g., reaction times) on the morning following the placebo night. This study also showed specific electroencephalographic changes following placebo administration. In particular, there was an increase of 0.5–4 Hz power during non-REM sleep and a decrease in the beta-frequency band during REM sleep. These changes occurred only at central sites.

Placebo administration in subjects with sleep difficulty has also been found to induce side effects. Colagiuri et al. (2012) showed that placebo treatment significantly improves sleep difficulty relative to a no-treatment control group, and that subjects tend to report experiencing a side effect they had been warned about.

In a more recent study, Laverdure-Dupont et al. (2009) examined the possibility that sleep might contribute to the consolidation of new expectations and consequently influence the generation of expectation-mediated placebo effects. Strong expectations of analgesia were generated before sleep by conditioning manipulations wherein the intensity of thermal pain stimulation was surreptitiously reduced after the application of a topical placebo cream. Expectations and placebo analgesic effects were measured the following morning and compared with those of a control daytime group without sleep. Placebo effects were observed in both groups, but correlation analysis showed that the mediating effect of expectations on placebo responses was more robust in the overnight group. Moreover, the relative duration of REM sleep decreased in subjects showing higher analgesic expectations and placebo responses the next morning. These findings suggest that sleep-related processes may influence the association between expectations and placebo analgesia and that REM sleep can predict placebo-induced expectations of pain relief.

Substantial placebo responses may also occur with mechanical interventions, as shown in a study on continuous positive airway pressure for the treatment of obstructive sleep apnea (Stepnowsky et al., 2012). A total of 25 subjects were studied with polysomnography at baseline and after treatment with placebo continuous positive airway pressure. Baseline emotional distress predicted the improvement in response to placebo; highly distressed patients showed greater placebo response.

5.4.2 Restless legs syndrome shows improvements in placebo groups

Another interesting condition is the restless legs syndrome, a sensory-motor disorder of sleep–wake motor regulation that causes disturbed sleep and significantly impaired quality of life. It is characterized by the imperative desire to move the lower limbs associated with paresthesias, motor restlessness, and worsening of symptoms at rest in the evening or at night. Interestingly, restless legs symptoms are relieved by levodopa and dopamine agonists, which are the first choice for the treatment of this disorder, as well as by opioids. As noted by Fulda and Wetter (2008), this unique responsiveness to both dopaminergic agents and opioids places it at the crossroads of the two systems implicated in the placebo response. Reasoning in this way, Fulda and Wetter (2008) performed a meta-analysis from which the following outcome measures were extracted: severity, subjective sleep parameters, sleep parameters derived from nocturnal polysomnography, periodic leg movements during sleep, and daytime functioning. In 24 trials, the pooled placebo response rate was 40%. The placebo effect was large for the primary outcome measure in most studies, which is the International Restless Legs Severity Scale, smaller for other severity scales, moderate for daytime functioning, small to moderate for subjective and objective sleep parameters, very small for periodic legs movements during sleep, and absent for sleep efficiency. Although it is difficult to infer any biological mechanism, restless legs syndrome is certainly an interesting model for investigation of both dopaminergic and opioidergic mechanisms.

De la Fuente-Fernández (2012) investigated whether dopaminergic pretreatment alters placebo and dopamine agonist responses in restless legs syndrome. He found that patients pretreated with dopaminergic medications tended to have blunted responses after placebo administration compared with drug-naïve patients. Dopaminergic pretreatment tended to increase the apparent effect of new dopaminergic drugs by decreasing the placebo effect in the placebo arm without substantially modifying the placebo effect in the active treatment arm. Although no clear mechanism can be inferred, this study highlights a possible interaction between placebo response and dopamine in the restless leg syndrome.

5.5 **Neurological disorders with few or no available data**

A few examples are given here to show that many clinical trials have been performed in different neurological conditions together with analysis of placebo groups, however, few or no data are available that lead to a better understanding of the underlying mechanisms.

A very common neurological condition, often the subject of clinical pharmacological trials, is epilepsy. In epilepsy, the improvement in placebo groups is substantial. In a review of different meta-analyses of anticonvulsant agents for epilepsy (Burneo et al., 2002) 9.3–16.6% of patients in the placebo arm had a reduction in seizure frequency greater than 50%. This represents 20–50% of the effect observed with active agents. Unfortunately, despite this large benefit of placebos, no conclusions can be drawn about the possible mechanisms, and spontaneous remissions and other factors cannot be ruled out completely (Bae et al., 2011; Schmidt et al., 2013; Tachibana and Narukawa, 2013).

Another example is chronic fatigue syndrome, a condition whereby the placebo effect has always been considered large, mainly due to the subjective nature of the disease. Cho et al. (2005) undertook a systematic review of the improvement in placebo groups and found that the pooled placebo response in 29 trials was 19.6%—lower than predicted and lower than in some other medical conditions. The type of intervention significantly contributed to the heterogeneity of the placebo response. Again, although the authors call this a placebo response, there is no way of knowing the mechanisms, including the possibility of spontaneous remission.

These are only a couple of examples of many neurological conditions in which placebo treatments have been found to induce improvements. As control groups are not included in these neurological trials, real placebo effects are not guaranteed; certainly many improvements can be attributable to the natural history of the disease and/or to selection biases (regression to the mean).

Interestingly, Papadopoulos and Mistikostas (2010) found a high rate of nocebo responses in multiple sclerosis. They conducted a systematic search for all randomized, placebo-controlled multiple sclerosis trials published between 1989 and 2009, and found that nocebo responses are substantial and appear to have increased significantly in recent years. In addition, nocebo responses were found to exhibit an association with medication and trial-related factors.

5.6 **Points for further discussion**

1 Nothing is known about the placebo effect in many important neurological disorders, thus we should devise experimental approaches to investigate the placebo effect in other neurological conditions, such as migraine, epilepsy, and multiple sclerosis.

2 Parkinson's disease has emerged as an interesting model for understanding the neurobiology of the placebo effect. The same experimental approach should be extended to other motor disorders as well, for example, by recording from different regions during implantation of electrodes for deep-brain stimulation.

3 Deep-brain stimulation allows recordings to be made from single neurons in awake patients. Thus it is an excellent approach for studying the biophysical properties of neurons during a placebo response.

4 Placebo effects in migraine should be investigated in more detail by using brain imaging techniques. In fact, migraine represents an excellent clinical model for comparison with existing studies on experimental pain.

5 Some sleep-related disorders, like restless legs syndrome, show good therapeutic responses to both dopamine and opioids, thus it would be interesting to understand whether these two neurotransmitters are involved in the placebo effect in these conditions.

References

Alexander GE, Crutcher MD and DeLong MR (1990). Basal ganglia-thalamocortical circuits: parallel substrates for motor, oculomotor, "prefrontal" and "limbic" functions. *Progress in Brain Research*, **85**, 119–46.

Alexander GE, DeLong MR, and Strick PL (1986). Parallel organization of functionally segregated circuits linking basal ganglia and cortex. *Annual Review of Neuroscience*, **9**, 357–81.

Amanzio M, Corazzini LL, Vase L and Benedetti F (2009). A systematic review of adverse events in placebo groups of anti-migraine clinical trials. *Pain*, **146**, 261–9.

Angyàn L and Angyàn Z (1999). Subthalamic influences on the cardiorespiratory functions in the cat. *Brain Research*, **847**, 130–3.

Avanzi M, Baratti M, Cabrini S, Uber E, Brighetti G and Bonfa F (2006). Prevalence of pathological gambling in patients with Parkinson's disease. *Movement Disorders*, **21**, 2068–72.

Bae EH, Theodore WH, Fregni F, Cantello R, Pascual-Leone A and Rotenberg A (2011). An estimate of placebo effect of repetitive transcranial magnetic stimulation in epilepsy. *Epilepsy Behavior*, **20**, 355–9.

Bejjani BP, Damier P, Arnulf I *et al.* (1999). Transient acute depression induced by high-frequency deep-brain stimulation. *New England Journal of Medicine*, **340**, 1476–80.

Bendtsen L, Mattsson P, Zwart JA and Lipton RB (2003). Placebo response in clinical randomized trials of analgesics in migraine. *Cephalalgia*, **23**, 487–90.

Benedetti F, Colloca L, Lanotte M, Bergamasco B, Torre E and Lopiano L (2004a). Autonomic and emotional responses to open and hidden stimulations of the human subthalamic region. *Brain Research Bulletin*, **63**, 203–11.

Benedetti F, Colloca L, Torre E, Lanotte M, Melcarne A *et al.* (2004b). Placebo-responsive Parkinson patients show decreased activity in single neurons of subthalamic nucleus. *Nature Neuroscience*, **7**, 587–8.

Benedetti F, Durando J and Vighetti S (2014). Nocebo and placebo modulation of hypobaric hypoxia headache involves the cyclooxygenase-prostaglandins pathway. *Pain*, **155**, 921–8.

Benedetti F, Lanotte M, Colloca L, Ducati A, Zibetti M and Lopiano L (2009). Electrophysiological properties of thalamic, subthalamic and nigral neurons during the anti-parkinsonian placebo response. *Journal of Physiology*, **587**, 3869–83.

Benedetti F, Lanotte M, Lopiano L and Colloca L (2007). When words are painful—unraveling the mechanisms of the nocebo effect. *Neuroscience*, **147**, 260–71.

Benedetti F, Pollo A, Lopiano L *et al.* (2003). Conscious expectation and unconscious conditioning in analgesic; motor and hormonal placebo/nocebo responses. *Journal of Neuroscience*, **23**, 4315–23.

Bergman H, Wichmann T, Karmon B and DeLong MR (1994). The primate subthalamic nucleus. II. Neuronal activity in the MPTP model of parkinsonism. *Journal of Neurophysiology*, **72**, 507–20.

Blandini F, Nappi G, Tassorelli C and Martignoni E (2000). Functional changes of the basal ganglia circuitry in Parkinson's disease. *Progress in Neurobiology*, **62**, 63–88.

Burneo JG, Montori VM and Faught E (2002). Magnitude of the placebo effect in randomized trials of antiepileptic agents. *Epilepsy & Behavior*, **3**, 532–4.

Cho HJ, Hotopf M and Wessely S (2005). The placebo response in the treatment of chronic fatigue syndrome: a systematic review and meta-analysis. *Psychosomatic Medicine*, **67**, 301–13.

Clayton AH, West SG, McGarvey E, Leslie C and Keller A (2005). Biochemical evidence of the placebo effect during the treatment of menstrual migraines. *Journal of Clinical Psychopharmacology*, **25**, 400–1.

Colagiuri B, McGuinness K, Boakes RA and Butow PN (2012). Warning about side effects can increase their occurrence: an experimental model using placebo treatment for sleep difficulty. *Journal of Psychopharmacology*, **26**, 1540–7.

Cooper AA, Gitler AD, Cashikar A *et al.* (2006). Alpha-synuclein blocks ER-Golgi traffic and Rab1 rescues neuron loss in Parkinson's models. *Science*, **313**, 324–8.

De Craen AJM, Tijssen JGP, de Gans J and Kleijnen J (2000). Placebo effect in the acute treatment of migraine: subcutaneous placebos are better than oral placebos. *Journal of Neurology*, **247**, 183–8.

de la Fuente-Fernández R (2012). The powerful pre-treatment effect: placebo responses in restless legs syndrome trials. *European Journal of Neurology*, **19**, 1305–10.

de la Fuente-Fernández R, Phillips AG, Zamburlini M *et al.* (2002a). Dopamine release in human ventral striatum and expectation of reward. *Behavioral Brain Research*, **136**, 359–63.

de la Fuente-Fernández R, Ruth TJ, Sossi V, Schulzer M, Calne DB and Stoessl AJ (2001). Expectation and dopamine release: mechanism of the placebo effect in Parkinson's disease. *Science*, **293**, 1164–6.

de la Fuente-Fernández R, Schulzer M and Stoessl AJ (2002). The placebo effect in neurological disorders. *Lancet Neurology*, **1**, 85–91.

de Tommaso M, Federici A, Franco G *et al.* (2012). Suggestion and pain in migraine: a study by laser evoked potentials. *CNS and Neurological Disorders—Drug Targets*, **11**, 110–26

Diamond SG, Markham CH and Treciokas LJ (1985). Double-blind trial of pergolide for Parkinson's disease. *Neurology*, **35**, 291–5.

Diener HC (1999). Efficacy and safety of intravenous acetylsalicylic acid lysinate compared to subcutaneous sumatriptan and parenteral placebo in the acute treatment of migraine.

A double-blind, double dummy, randomized, multicenter, parallel group study. The ASA-SUMAMIG Study Group. *Cephalalgia*, **19**, 581–8.

Diener HC (2010). Placebo effects in treating migraine and other headaches. *Current Opinion in Investigational Drugs*, **11**, 735–9.

Diener H, Kronfeld K, Boewing G *et al*. (2006). Efficacy of acupuncture for the prophylaxis of migraine: a multicentre randomised controlled clinical trial. *Lancet Neurology*, **5**, 310–16.

Diener H, Krupp P, Schmitt T *et al*. (2001). Cyclandelate in the prophylaxis of migraine: a placebo-controlled study. *Cephalalgia*, **21**, 66–70.

Ferrari MD, Roon KI, Lipton RB and Goadsby PJ (2001). Oral triptans (serotonin 5-HT1B/1D agonists) in acute migraine treatment: a meta-analysis of 53 trials. *Lancet*, **358**, 1668–75.

Fratello F, Curcio G, Ferrara M *et al*. (2005). Can an inert sleeping pill affect sleep? Effects on polysomnographic, behavioral and subjective measures. *Psychopharmacology*, **181**, 761–70.

Frisaldi E, Carlino E, Lanotte M, Lopiano L and Benedetti F (2013). Characterization of the thalamic–subthalamic circuit involved in the placebo response through single-neuron recording in Parkinson patients. *Cortex*, 24 December. [Epub ahead of print]

Fulda S and Wetter TC (2008). Where dopamine meets opioids: a meta-analysis of the placebo effect in RLS treatment studies. *Brain*, **131**(Pt 4), 902–17.

Ghika J, Vingerhoets F, Albanese A and Villmeure JG (1999). Bipolar swings in mood in a patient with bilateral subthalamic deep brain stimulation (DBS) free of antiparkinsonian medication. *Parkinsonism & Related Disorders*, **5** (Suppl. 1), 104.

Goetz CG, Laska E, Hicking C *et al*. (2008a). Placebo influences on dyskinesia in Parkinson's disease. *Movement Disorders*, **23**, 700–7.

Goetz CG, Leurgans S and Raman R (2002). Placebo-associated improvements in motor function: comparison of subjective and objective sections of the UPDRS in early Parkinson's disease. *Movement Disorders*, **17**, 283–8.

Goetz CG, Leurgans S, Raman R and Stebbins GT (2000). Objective changes in motor function during placebo treatment in PD. *Neurology*, **54**, 710–14.

Goetz CG, Wuu J, McDermott MP, *et al*. (2008b). Placebo response in Parkinson's disease: comparisons among 11 trials covering medical and surgical interventions. *Movement Disorders*, **23**, 690–9.

Gospic K, Gunnarsson T, Fransson P, Ingvar M, Lindefors N and Petrovic P (2008). Emotional perception modulated by an opioid and a cholecystokinin agonist. *Psychopharmacology*, **197**, 295–307.

Haber SN (2003). The primate basal ganglia: parallel and integrative networks. *Journal of Chemical Neuroanatomy*, **26**, 317–30.

Halgren E (1982). Mental phenomena induced by stimulation in the limbic system. *Human Neurobiology*, **1**, 251–60.

Hauser RA, Freeman TB, Snow BJ *et al*. (1999). Long-term evaluation of bilateral fetal nigral transplantation in Parkinson disease. *Archives of Neurology*, **56**, 179–87.

Henry P, Hiesseprovost O, Dillenschneider A, Ganry H and Insuaty J (1995). Efficacy and tolerance of effervescent aspirin metoclopramide association in the treatment of migraine attack. Randomized double-blind study using a placebo. *Le Presses Médicale*, **24**, 254–8.

Holroyd KA, Penzien DB and Cordingley GE (1991). Propranolol in the management of recurrent migraine: a meta-analytic review. *Headache*, **31**, 333–40.

Hrobjartsson A and Gøtzsche PC (2001). Is the placebo effect powerless? An analysis of clinical trials comparing placebo with no-treatment. *New England Journal of Medicine*, **344**, 1594–602.

Hutchinson WD, Allan RJ, Opitz H *et al.* (1998). Neurophysiological identification of the subthalamic nucleus in surgery for Parkinson's disease. *Annals of Neurology*, 44, 622–8.

Ikemoto S and Panksepp J (1999). The role of nucleus accumbens dopamine in motivated behavior: a unifying interpretation with special reference to reward-seeking. *Brain Research Reviews*, 31, 6–41.

Kaufmann H, Bhattacharya KFm, Voustianiouk A and Gracies JM (2002). Stimulation of the subthalamic nucleus increases heart rate in patients with Parkinson disease. *Neurology*, 59, 1657–8.

Kaur D and Andersen J (2002). Ironing out Parkinson's disease: is therapeutic treatment with iron chelators a real possibility? *Aging Cell*, 1, 17–21.

Keitel A, Ferrea S, Südmeyer M, Schnitzler A and Wojtecki L (2013a). Expectation modulates the effect of deep brain stimulation on motor and cognitive function in tremor-dominant Parkinson's disease. *PLoS One*, 8, e81878.

Keitel A, Wojtecki L, Hirschmann J, *et al.* (2013b). Motor and cognitive placebo-/nocebo-responses in Parkinson's disease patients with deep brain stimulation. *Behavioral Brain Research*, 250C, 199–205.

Klapper J (1997). Divalproex sodium in migraine prophylaxis: a dose-controlled study. *Cephalalgia*, 17, 103–8.

Knutson B and Cooper JC (2005). Functional magnetic resonance imaging of reward prediction. *Current Opinion in Neurology*, 18, 411–17.

Krack P, Kumar R, Ardouin C *et al.* (2001). Laughter induced by subthalamic nucleus stimulation. *Movement Disorders*, 16, 867–75.

Kumar R, Krack P and Pollak P (1999). Transient acute depression-induced by high-frequency deep-brain stimulation. *New England Journal of Medicine*, 341, 1003–4.

Lanotte M, Lopiano L, Torre E, Bergamasco B, Colloca L and Benedetti F (2005). Expectation enhances autonomic responses to stimulation of the human subthalamic limbic region. *Brain Behavior Immunity*, 19, 500–9.

Laverdure-Dupont D, Rainville P, Montplaisir J and Lavigne G (2009). Changes in rapid eye movement sleep associated with placebo-induced expectations and analgesia. *Journal of Neuroscience*, 29, 11745–52.

Levy R, Dostrovsky JO, Lang AE, Sime E, Hutchison WD and Lozano AM (2001). Effects of apomorphine on subthalamic nucleus and globus pallidus internus neurons in patients with Parkinson's disease. *Journal of Neurophysiology*, 86, 249–60.

Lidstone SC, Schulzer M, Dinelle K *et al.* (2010). Effects of expectation on placebo-induced dopamine release in Parkinson disease. *Archives of General Psychiatry*, 67, 857–65.

Limousin P, Greene J, Pollak P, Rothwell J, Benabid AL and Frackowiak R (1997). Changes in cerebral activity pattern due to subthalamic nucleus or internal pallidum stimulation in Parkinson's disease. *Annals of Neurology*, 42, 283–91.

Limousin P, Krack P, Pollak P *et al.* (1998). Electrical stimulation of the subthalamic nucleus in advanced Parkinson's disease. *New England Journal of Medicine*, 339, 1105–11.

Linde K, Streng A, Jurgens S *et al.* (2005). Acupuncture for patients with migraine: a randomized controlled trial. *Journal of American Medical Association*, 293, 2118–25.

Linde K, Witt CM, Streng A *et al.* (2007). The impact of patient expectations on outcomes in four randomised controlled trials of acupuncture in patients with chronic pain. *Pain*, 128, 264–71.

Lou JS, Dimitrova DM, Hammerschlag R, *et al.* (2013). Effect of expectancy and personality on cortical excitability in Parkinson's disease. *Movement Disorders*, 28, 1257–62.

Lozano AM, Lang AE, Levy R, Hutchison W and Dostrovsky J (2000). Neuronal recordings in Parkinson's disease patients with dyskinesias induced by apomorphine. *Annals of Neurology*, **47**, S141–6.

Macedo A, Farre M and Banos JE (2006). A meta-analysis of the placebo response in acute migraine and how this response may be influenced by some of the characteristics of clinical trials. *European Journal of Clinical Pharmacology*, **62**, 161–72.

Mathew NT, Saper JR, Silberstein SD et al. (1995). Migraine prophylaxis with divalproex. *Archives of Neurology*, **52**, 281–6.

McCall WV, D'Agostino R Jr and Dunn A (2003). A meta-analysis of sleep changes associated with placebo in hypnotic clinical trials. *Sleep Medicine*, **4**, 57–62.

McRae C, Cherin E, Yamazaki G et al. (2004). Effects of perceived treatment on quality of life and medical outcomes in a double-blind placebo surgery trial. *Archives of General Psychiatry*, **61**, 412–20.

Mercado R, Constantoyannis C, Mandat T et al. (2006). Expectation and the placebo effect in Parkinson's disease patients with subthalamic nucleus deep brain stimulation. *Movement Disorders*, **21**, 1457–61.

Middleton FA and Strick PL (1996). The temporal lobe is a target of output from the basal ganglia. *Proceedings of the National Academy of Sciences of the United States of America*, **93**, 8683–7.

Mitsikostas DD (2012). Nocebo in headaches: implications for clinical practice and trial design. *Current Neurology and Neuroscience Reports*, **12**, 132–7.

Mitsikostas DD, Mantonakis LI and Chalarakis NG (2011). Nocebo is the enemy, not placebo. A meta-analysis of reported side effects after placebo treatment in headaches. *Cephalalgia*, **31**, 550–61.

Olanow CW, Goetz CG, Kordower JH et al. (2003). A double-blind controlled trial of bilateral fetal nigral transplantation in Parkinson's disease. *Annals of Neurology*, **54**, 403–14.

Papadopoulos D and Mitsikostas DD (2010). Nocebo effects in multiple sclerosis trials: a meta-analysis. *Multiple Sclerosis*, **16**, 816–28.

Parent A and Hazrati LN F (1995). Functional anatomy of the basal ganglia. II. The place of subthalamic nucleus and external pallidum in basal ganglia circuitry. *Brain Research Reviews*, **20**, 128–54.

Peikert A, Wilimzig C and Köhne-Volland R (1996). Prophylaxis of migraine with oral magnesium: results from a prospective, multi-center, placebo-controlled and double-blind randomized study. *Cephalalgia*, **16**, 257–63.

Pollo A, Torre E, Lopiano L et al. (2002). Expectation modulates the response to subthalamic nucleus stimulation in Parkinsonian patients. *NeuroReport*, **13**, 1383–6.

Priori A, Cinnante C, Genitrini S et al. (2001). Non-motor effects of deep brain stimulation of the subthalamic nucleus in Parkinson's disease: preliminary physiological results. *Neurological Sciences*, **22**, 85–6.

Schmidt D, Beyenburg S, D'Souza J and Stavem K (2013). Clinical features associated with placebo response in refractory focal epilepsy. *Epilepsy Behavior*, **27**, 393–8.

Schultz W (2002). Getting formal with dopamine and reward. *Neuron*, **36**, 241–63.

Schultz W, Tremblay L and Hollerman JR (2000). Reward processing in primate orbitofrontal cortex and basal ganglia. *Cerebral Cortex*, **10**, 272–8.

Scott DJ, Stohler CS, Egnatuk CM, Wang H, Koeppe RA and Zubieta JK (2007). Individual differences in reward responding explain placebo-induced expectations and effects. *Neuron*, **55**, 325–36.

Shetty N, Friedman JH, Kieburtz K, Marshall FJ and Oakes D (1999). The placebo response in Parkinson's disease. Parkinson Study Group. *Clinical Neuropharmacology*, **22**, 207–12.

Spencer SE, Sawyer WB and Loewy AD (1988). L-glutamate stimulation of the zona incerta in the rat decreases heart rate and blood pressure. *Brain Research*, **458**, 72–81.

Stefani A, Bassi A, Mazzone P *et al.* (2002). Subdyskinetic apomorphine responses in globus pallidus and subthalamus of parkinsonian patients: lack of clear evidence for the "indirect pathway." *Clinical Neurophysiology*, **113**, 91–100.

Stepnowsky CJ, Mao WC, Bardwell WA, Loredo JS and Dimsdale JE (2012). Mood predicts response to placebo CPAP. *Sleep Disorders*, **2012**, 404196.

Stovner LJ, Oftedal G, Straume A and Johnsson A (2008). Nocebo as headache trigger: evidence from a sham-controlled provocation study with RF fields. *Acta Neurologica Scandinavica Supplementum*, **188**, 67–71.

Strafella AP, Ko JH and Monchi O (2006). Therapeutic application of transcranial magnetic stimulation in Parkinson's disease: the contribution of expectation. *NeuroImage*, **31**, 1666–72.

Tachibana Y and Narukawa M (2013). Investigation of influencing factors on higher placebo response in East Asian versus Western clinical trials for partial epilepsy: a meta-analysis. *Clinical Drug Investigation*, **33**, 315–24.

Tfelt-Hansen P, Henry P, Mulder LJ, Schaeldewaert RG, Schoenen J and Chazot G (1995). The effectiveness of combined oral lysine acetylsalicylate and metoclopramide compared with oral sumatriptan for migraine. *Lancet*, **346**, 923–6.

Thornton JM, Aziz T, Schlugman D and Paterson DJ (2002). Electrical stimulation of the midbrain increases heart rate and arterial blood pressure in awake humans. *Journal of Physiology*, **539**, 615–21.

Turner MS, Lavin A, Grace AA and Napier TC (2001). Regulation of limbic information outflow by the subthalamic nucleus: excitatory amino acid projections to the ventral pallidum. *Journal of Neuroscience*, **21**, 2820–32.

Van del Plas J, Wiersinga-Post JE, Maes FW and Bohus B (1995). Cardiovascular effects and changes in midbrain periaqueductal gray neuronal activity induced by electrical stimulation of the hypothalamus in the rat. *Brain Research Bulletin*, **37**, 645–56.

van de Ven LLM, Franke CL and Koehler PJ (1997). Prophylactic treatment of migraine with bisoprolol: a placebo-controlled study. *Cephalalgia*, **17**, 596–9.

Voon V, Mehta AR and Hallett M (2011). Impulse control disorders in Parkinson's disease: recent advances. *Current Opinion in Neurology*, **24**, 324–30.

Walsh JK, Roth T, Randazzo A *et al.* (2000). Eight weeks of non-nightly use of zolpidem for primary insomnia. *Sleep*, **23**, 1087–96.

Watts RL, Freeman TB, Hauser RA *et al.* (2001). A double-blind, randomised, controlled, multicenter clinical trial of the safety and efficacy of stereotaxic intrastriatal implantation of fetal porcine ventral mesencephalic tissue (Neurocelli-PD) vs. imitation surgery in patients with Parkinson's disease (PD). *Parkinsonism & Related Disorders*, **7**, 87.

Chapter 6

Mental and behavioral disorders

Summary points

♦ In depression, fluoxetine treatment and a placebo treatment affect similar brain regions.

♦ Covert (unexpected) administration of antianxiety drugs is less effective than overt (expected) administration, which indicates the key role of expectation in antianxiety therapy.

♦ The disruption of prefrontal executive control in Alzheimer's disease may decrease the magnitude of placebo responses.

♦ Expectations appear to be particularly important when associated with the effects of drugs of abuse.

♦ Placebo effects appear to be powerful in psychotherapy, and the brain areas involved in the psychotherapeutic outcome are different from those involved in the placebo effect.

6.1 Depression

6.1.1 The rate of improvement in placebo groups is high and has increased over the past years

Depression, with its many variants, is a mood disorder, characterized by a persistent lowering of mood, loss of interest in usual activities, and diminished ability to experience pleasure (see Box 6.1 for a definition of negative emotions). The causes of depression involve neurotransmitters, like serotonin and norepinephrine, and neurogenesis in the hippocampus has been found to play a role (Santarelli et al., 2003). The treatment of depression may be pharmacological and psychotherapeutic, but in certain circumstances electroconvulsive therapy is also used. One of the most frequently used classes of antidepressant drugs is represented by the selective serotonin reuptake inhibitors (SSRIs) which increase the availability of serotonin in the extracellular compartment. Interestingly, it was shown that these antidepressants increase hippocampal neurogenesis in animal models, thus suggesting a relationship between depression and neuronal formation in the hippocampus (Santarelli et al., 2003).

The response rate in the placebo groups in antidepressant clinical trials is very high. In 1998, a meta-analysis was conducted by Kirsch and Sapirstein (1998) in 19 double-blind clinical trials which included 2318 patients. These investigators found that 75%

of the response to the active drug is attributable to a placebo effect, thus the specific pharmacodynamic effect of the drug would account for only 25%. In addition, a high correlation was found between the placebo effect and the drug effect, which indicates that virtually all the variation in drug effect size was due to the placebo component. In the same study, Kirsch and Sapirstein (1998) also assessed natural history effects, in order to evaluate how much of the 75% was attributable to real placebo responses and how much to other factors. To do this, another 19 trials of psychotherapy, where the use of no-treatment groups is more common, were analyzed. Natural history accounted for 23.87%, drug effects for 25.16%, and placebo effect for 50.97%. Therefore, in clinical trials for major depression, one-quarter is due to the specific action of the active medication, one-quarter is due to other factors, like spontaneous remission, and one-half is due to a placebo effect.

Evidence of significant and increasing rates of placebo responses in antidepressant trials has been documented in several studies (Khan et al., 2000; Andrews, 2001; Walsh et al., 2002), although little is known on the cause of such an increase. For example, Walsh et al. (2002) identified 75 clinical trials of antidepressants between 1981 and 2000 and found that the mean percentage of patients who showed symptom reduction in the placebo group was 29.7% 8.3 SD (range 12.5–51.8%), whereas in the active medication group with the greatest response, the mean percentage of patients responding was 50.1% 9.0 SD (range 31.6–70.4%). The proportion of patients responding to tricyclic antidepressants was 46.9% 10.6 SD (range 27.5–65.6%) and to SSRIs was 48.9% 10.3 SD (range 25.0–70.4%). Therefore, the response in the placebo groups was really high in these trials, although there is no way of knowing whether the symptom reduction was due to real placebo responses, spontaneous remissions, regression to the mean, or other factors.

Box 6.1 Some definitions of positive and negative emotions

Positive and negative emotions can be described from different perspectives. For example, they can be conceptualized in terms of opposite subjective experiences, like pleasure on the one hand and discomfort on the other, or otherwise they can be viewed as opposite action tendencies, whereby approaching behavior characterizes positive emotions whereas avoidance behavior represents negative emotions. The level of arousal can be considered as well, with calmness and relaxation as the main components of positive emotional states and alertness and excitation as the main characteristics of negative emotional states. While excitement involves urges to move, depression is associated with lack of desire to move, and whereas satisfaction is associated with calmness and warmth, anxiety is associated with inner tension in the viscera. Many overlaps do exist though, for example, high arousal levels are often shared by both negative and positive emotions, such as fear and happiness, respectively. Indeed, rather than two opposite emotional states only, positive and negative, several discrete emotional states have been recognized and described over

> **Box 6.1 Some definitions of positive and negative emotions (continued)**
>
> the last centuries. Several discrete emotions have been recognized such as happiness, surprise, sadness, anger, disgust, and fear. These are better described as representing subsets of positive and negative emotional states, and both positive and negative emotions can be further subdivided into subgroups of basic, general, and specific emotions. For example, basic emotions are deprivation of food and water or satisfaction by sex; general emotions are sadness, fear or happiness and enthusiasm; specific emotions are bad/nice sound or disgusting/good taste.

Interestingly, in Walsh's study (Walsh et al., 2002) both the proportion of patients who responded in the placebo groups and the proportion who responded to medication were significantly positively correlated with the year of publication, with a more statistically robust correlation for placebo than medication. From this study it appears that, in the last two decades, the proportion of patients who show symptom reduction in the placebo group has increased at a rate of approximately 7% per decade, and a similar increase has occurred in the fraction of patients responding to the active drug. There is little reason to think that a shift in diagnostic systems with time is responsible for such changes in response rate, as the specific criteria for the nature and duration of symptoms required for diagnosis of major depressive disorder have not changed very much over the past two decades. Although the age of patients has increased, the study by Walsh et al. (2002) showed the relationship between age and positive responses in the placebo groups was not significant. It is noteworthy that, although the length of the trials has increased over the past years and it has long been known that positive responses in the placebo group increase with trial length, in a multiple regression model that included year of publication and length of trial, only the year of publication was a significant predictor of positive response in the placebo group (Walsh et al., 2002). Hence there is not a clear explanation for the increase in symptom reduction in placebo groups of antidepressant clinical trials, and many factors may contribute, such as the natural course of depressive symptoms and real psychobiological placebo responses. Whatever the case, some factor or factors must have changed significantly in placebo groups during the period 1981–2000, but a satisfactory explanation has not yet been provided.

It is also interesting to note that expectations about the therapeutic benefit also affect antidepressant clinical trials. For example, in a 9-week, single-blind, experimental antidepressant treatment study with reboxetine, subjects were asked to self-rate their expectations of the effectiveness of the study medication by using forced-choice responses: (1) "Not at all effective," (2) "Somewhat effective," or (3) "Very effective" (Krell et al., 2004). The patients with a higher pretreatment expectation of medication effectiveness had a greater likelihood of response. In fact, 90% of patients who reported an expectation that the medication would be very effective responded to treatment, whereas only 33.3% of those who reported expecting medication to be "somewhat effective" responded to treatment. Therefore, individuals with high expectations of clinical improvement showed significantly more powerful responses to reboxetine than those with low expectations. This is yet another example of how expectations may affect the outcome of clinical trials (as described previously for trials on pain and Parkinson's disease).

Many clinical trials of antidepressants, several meta-analyses, and many reviews have been performed in more recent years, but unfortunately they do not help understand the mechanisms underlying the placebo responses in depression (e.g., Kirsch, 2008; Bridge et al., 2009; Brunoni et al., 2009; Rief et al., 2009; Gueorguieva et al., 2011; Hughes et al., 2012; Iovieno and Papakostas, 2012; Rihmer et al., 2012; Rutherford et al., 2012; Rutherford and Roose, 2013). Certainly, the placebo response is substantial. For example, in the meta-analysis by Rief et al. (2009) the placebo effect accounted for 68% of the effect in the drug groups, but in all these studies it is often difficult to separate spontaneous remissions, regression to the mean and placebo responses. The reason why it is so difficult to identify the biological underpinnings of the placebo response in depression is explained in the next section.

6.1.2 Placebos and antidepressants affect similar areas of the brain

Unlike single-dose trials of an intervention, such as oral or intravenous analgesia or anti-Parkinson acute therapy studies, antidepressants do not work acutely, requiring on average a minimum of 2–3 weeks to see any clinical effect. Therefore, investigating placebo effects in depression is more problematic from both an ethical and methodological point of view. In fact, if one wants to see what happens in the patient's brain by means of neuroimaging techniques, it is necessary to follow the patient for a long period of time or, otherwise, to devise pre- and post-treatment assessment with adequate control groups. Of course, if one wants to compare a placebo group with a no-treatment group to rule out spontaneous remission, this requires that some patients are not treated for a long period of time, with the inherent ethical problems and limitations. This is one of the main reasons why depression, albeit an interesting and exciting model for studying placebo effects, has not been investigated in detail so far.

The first attempt to uncover some neural correlates of the placebo antidepressant response was performed by Leuchter et al. (2002). They used quantitative electroencephalography and "cordance," a new tool of analysis developed by the authors themselves. This study involved a 9-week, double-blind, placebo-controlled trial in which either fluoxetine (24 patients) or venlafaxine (27 patients) were the active medication. After 9 weeks of placebo or fluoxetine or venlafaxine treatment, the investigators found that patients who showed symptom reduction in the placebo group were characterized by an increase in prefrontal cordance, particularly in the right hemisphere, starting early in treatment. In contrast, patients who responded to medication showed decreased cordance in prefrontal areas, thus suggesting that placebo treatment induces prefrontal changes that are distinct from those associated with antidepressant medication.

In a subsequent study, Leuchter et al. (2004) analyzed the neurophysiological, symptomatic, and cognitive characteristics of subjects who were likely to respond to placebo in clinical trials for major depressive disorder. It was found that placebo responders had lower pretreatment frontocentral electroencephalographic cordance in the theta-frequency band than all other subjects, particularly the medication responders. Placebo responders also showed faster cognitive processing time and lower reporting of late insomnia. A logistic regression analysis showed that these three pretreatment measures (cordance, cognitive processing time, and late insomnia) accurately identified 97.6% of eventual placebo responders.

In 2002, another brain imaging study was carried out (Mayberg et al., 2002). Changes in brain glucose metabolism were measured by means of positron emission tomography in male patients with unipolar depression who were treated with either placebo or fluoxetine for 6 weeks. Common and unique responses were described. In fact, both placebo and fluoxetine treatment induced regional metabolic increases in the prefrontal, anterior cingulate, premotor, parietal, posterior insula, and posterior cingulate, and metabolic decreases in the subgenual, parahippocampus and thalamus. The magnitude of regional fluoxetine changes was generally greater than placebo. However, fluoxetine responses were associated with additional subcortical and limbic changes in the brainstem, striatum, anterior insula, and hippocampus (Fig. 6.1). There were no regional changes unique to placebo at 6 weeks. Although no natural history group was run in these studies, psychotherapy induced brain changes that were different from both fluoxetine and placebo treatment (Mayberg et al., 2002; Benedetti et al., 2005) (Fig. 6.1). These differences rule out the hypothesis that placebo responses are mediated by changes in a common antidepressant response pathway. Moreover, they suggest that the placebo antidepressant effect is not the result of uncontrolled, nonspecific psychological treatment effects, as brain changes associated with placebo therapy match those of the active drug.

Interestingly, there were unique ventral striatal and orbital frontal changes in both placebo and drug responders at 1 week of treatment, that is, well before clinical benefit was seen (Fig. 6.2). Thus these changes are not associated with the clinical response, but rather to expectation and anticipation of the clinical benefit. Such changes were seen neither in the eventual drug nonresponders nor at 6 weeks when the antidepressant response was well established, consistent with an expectation pattern of response (Mayberg et al., 2002; Benedetti et al., 2005). This is in keeping with other brain imaging studies in which an involvement of the ventral striatum (nucleus accumbens) was found after placebo administration in Parkinson's disease (de la Fuente-Fernandez et al., 2001) and in pain (Scott et al., 2007). This pattern of activation of the ventral striatum is in agreement with an involvement of reward mechanisms in some types of placebo responses, because the nucleus accumbens is one of the most important brain regions involved in reward (Ikemoto and Panksepp, 1999; Schultz et al., 2000; Schultz, 2002; Knutson and Cooper, 2005).

As fluoxetine is an inhibitor of serotonin reuptake (Box 6.2), the anatomically concordant responses to both placebo and fluoxetine lead to the hypothesis that serotonin mechanisms might be involved in the placebo antidepressant effect. However, at least two mechanisms can be envisaged. First, serotonin reuptake inhibition could be a common mechanism shared by both fluoxetine and placebo-induced expectation of clinical improvement. Second, serotonin reuptake could be involved only in the metabolic responses to fluoxetine, the placebo response being mediated by completely different mechanisms (Benedetti, 2008).

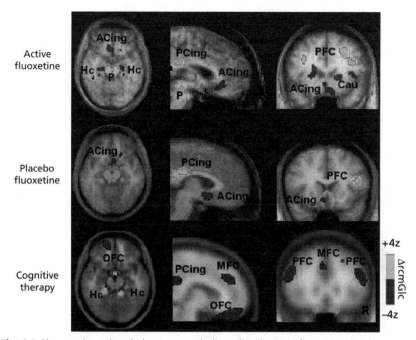

Fig. 6.1 Changes in regional glucose metabolism. (FDG) PET in fluoxetine (top), placebo (middle), and cognitive (bottom) therapy responders measured before and after a standard course of each respective treatment. Axial (left), sagittal (middle), and coronal (right) views show increases in red and decreases in blue. The fluoxetine and placebo group were studied as part of the same double-blind controlled experiment. A common pattern of cortical increases and limbic–paralimbic decreases is seen in both groups, with the active fluoxetine group showing additional changes in the brainstem, hippocampus, insula and caudate nucleus. In contrast, responses to cognitive therapy are associated with a distinctly different pattern—dorsolateral and medial frontal decreases and hippocampal increases. ACing, subgenual anterior cingulate; Cau, caudate nucleus; Hc, hippocampus; MFC, medial frontal cortex; OFC, orbital frontal cortex; P, pons; PCing, posterior cingulate; PFC, prefrontal cortex. Reproduced from Fabrizio Benedetti, Helen S. Mayberg, Tor D. Wager, Christian S. Stohler, and Jon-Kar Zubieta, Neurobiological mechanisms of the placebo effect, *Journal of Neuroscience*, 25 (45), pp. 10390–402 Copyright 2005, The Society for Neuroscience. doi: 10.1523/ JNEUROSCI.3458–05.2005 and from Helen S. Mayberg, J. Arturo Silva, Steven K. Brannan, Janet L. Tekell, Roderick K. Mahurin, Scott McGinnis, and Paul A. Jerabek, The Functional Neuroanatomy of the Placebo Effect, *The American Journal of Psychiatry*, 159 (5), pp. 728–737 Copyright 2002, American Psychiatric Association. doi: 10.1176/ appi.ajp.159.5.728 (See plate 7.)

6.1.3 Some genetic polymorphisms are involved in the antidepressant placebo response

In one study, patients with major depression were classified for 5-HTT (serotonin) promoter region polymorphism and platelet 5-HTT kinetics before treatment with

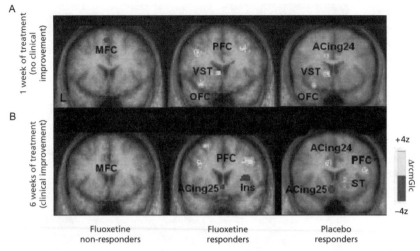

Fig. 6.2 Time course of regional metabolic changes in fluoxetine nonresponders (left), fluoxetine responders (middle), and placebo responders (right). The top panel (A) represents 1 week of treatment (no clinical improvement) and the lower panel (B) represents 6 weeks of treatment (clinical improvement). Ventral striatal and orbital frontal increases are seen uniquely at 1 week in (A) (middle and right) of both active and sham treatment in patients that go on to show clinical response at 6 weeks (B). Such changes are not seen in patients who failed to respond and are no longer present in either group of responders once clinical remission has been achieved (6-week time-point in B). In contrast, response-specific changes in the prefrontal cortex and subgenual cingulate are seen only at 6 weeks (B) and not at the 1-week (A) time-point. ACing24, anterior cingulate Brodmann area 24; ACing25, subgenual anterior cingulate Brodmann area 25; Ins, anterior insula; MFC, medial frontal cortex; OFC, orbital frontal cortex; PFC, prefrontal cortex; VST, ventral striatum. Reproduced from Fabrizio Benedetti, Helen S. Mayberg, Tor D. Wager, Christian S. Stohler, and Jon-Kar Zubieta, Neurobiological mechanisms of the placebo effect, *Journal of Neuroscience*, 25 (45), pp. 10390–402 Copyright 2005, The Society for Neuroscience doi: 10.1523/JNEUROSCI.3458–05.2005 and from Helen S. Mayberg, J. Arturo Silva, Steven K. Brannan, Janet L. Tekell, Roderick K. Mahurin, Scott McGinnis, and Paul A. Jerabek, The Functional Neuroanatomy of the Placebo Effect, *The American Journal of Psychiatry*, 159 (5), pp. 728–737 Copyright 2002, American Psychiatric Association. doi: 10.1176/appi.ajp.159.5.728 (See plate 8.)

fluoxetine, and then examined for treatment outcome (Rausch et al., 2002). It was found that genotype had a significant effect on outcome not only after fluoxetine treatment but also after placebo. The long allele group was more responsive to placebo, as well as more responsive to drug dose than was the short allele group. The influence of genotype on placebo responsiveness was supported by a subsequent study. As already described in section 2.3.5, Leuchter et al. (2009) examined polymorphisms in genes encoding the catabolic enzymes catechol-O-methyltransferase (COMT) and monoamine oxidase A in patients with major depressive disorder. Small placebo responses were found in those patients with monoamine oxidase A G/T polymorphisms (rs6323)

Box 6.2 Selective serotonin reuptake inhibitors

Selective serotonin reuptake inhibitors or serotonin-specific reuptake inhibitors (SSRIs), such as fluoxetine, are the most widely prescribed antidepressants in many countries, although their efficacy in mild or moderate cases of depression has been disputed many times. They represent a class of drugs whose mechanism of action is the increase of the extracellular level of the neurotransmitter serotonin by inhibiting its reuptake into the presynaptic cell. As a consequence, more serotonin in the synaptic cleft is available to bind to the postsynaptic receptors. It is interesting to note that SSRIs are the first class of psychotropic drugs discovered using the process called rational drug design, a process that starts with a specific biological target and then creates a molecule designed to affect it. On the basis of their effect on extracellular serotonin increased availability and the supposed pathophysiological mechanism of serotonin decrease in many neuropsychiatric conditions, SSRIs are widely used to treat not only depression, but also other conditions such as generalized anxiety disorder, obsessive–compulsive disorder, and eating disorders. There are many reasons why the efficacy of SSRIs has been disputed, particularly in depression. One has to do with the high placebo response rates (discussed in section 6.1.1). Another important reason is represented by a drug that works entirely opposite to SSRIs—tianeptine—a selective serotonin reuptake enhancer (SSRE) that also exhibits antidepressant activity, especially in patients resistant to SSRI therapy (Fig. 6.3). Therefore, these two drugs have an opposite action but the same antidepressant effect. Thus the current model for the antidepressant activity of SSRIs is not satisfactory and further research is needed to better clarify the nature of serotonin signaling in the areas of the brain related to mood and cognition.

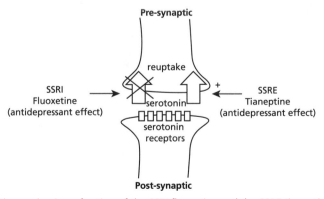

Fig. 6.3 The mechanism of action of the SSRI fluoxetine and the SSRE tianeptine. Whereas the former blocks serotonin reuptake, the latter enhances it.

coding for the highest activity form of the enzyme (G or G/G). Likewise, lower placebo responses were found in those patients with ValMet catechol-O-methyltransferase polymorphisms coding for a lower-activity form of the enzyme (2 Met alleles).

6.2 **Anxiety**

6.2.1 **Antianxiety drugs are much less effective when given covertly**

Anxiety is a mood disorder and it can be present in different circumstances. For example, whereas trait anxiety is a characteristic of the subject, and is present throughout life, state anxiety is situational, presenting only in a given circumstance. Anxiety is the main symptom of many disorders, such as social phobia, and it undergoes substantial improvement after placebo administration. For example, in the series of meta-analyses performed by Hrobjartsson and Goetzsche (2004), significant effects of placebos were found on both pain and phobia, whereby placebo interventions were compared with no-treatment groups.

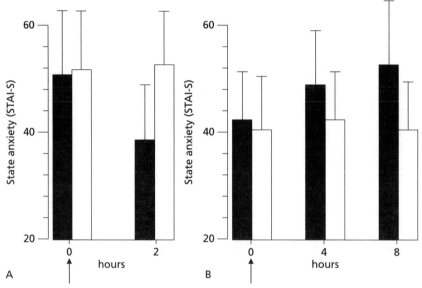

Fig. 6.4 Comparison between open (black bars) and hidden (white bars) administration (A) and interruption (B) of diazepam in postoperative state anxiety. Note that hidden diazepam administration is completely ineffective, indicating that anxiety reduction following open diazepam is only a psychological effect. Similarly, the open interruption of diazepam induces a relapse of anxiety that is psychologically mediated, since the hidden interruption does not produce any effect. The arrows represent the point of open/hidden administration or interruption of diazepam. Data from Benedetti, Fabrizio; Maggi, Giuliano; Lopiano, Leonardo; Lanotte, Michele; Rainero, Innocenzo; Vighetti, Sergio; and Pollo, Antonella, Open versus hidden medical treatments: The patient's knowledge about a therapy affects the therapy outcome. *Prevention & Treatment*, 6 (1), article 1a. doi: 10.1037/1522–3736.6.1.61a.

Compelling evidence that placebo-induced expectation plays an important role in anxiety is shown by the hidden administration of antianxiety drugs. By using the open–hidden approach (see section 2.2.4) the effectiveness of diazepam, one of the most frequently used benzodiazepines for treating anxiety, was assessed after overt and covert administration in postoperative patients with high anxiety scores (Benedetti et al., 2003; Colloca et al., 2004; Benedetti et al., 2011).

In the open group there was a clear-cut decrease of anxiety, but in the hidden group diazepam was totally ineffective, which indicates that anxiety reduction after the open diazepam was a placebo effect (Fig. 6.4A). Open–hidden interruption of a diazepam treatment has also been investigated (Benedetti et al., 2003; Colloca et al., 2004; Benedetti et al., 2011). In the open condition anxiety increased significantly after 4 and 8 hours; in the hidden condition it did not change (Fig. 6.4B). Therefore, the anxiety relapse after the expected (open) interruption of diazepam could be attributed to the negative expectation of anxiety relapse (nocebo-like effect).

6.2.2 Imaging anxiety reduction after placebo administration

Little is known about the mechanisms underlying the placebo effect in anxiety. In one brain imaging study it was found that placebo treatments can modulate emotional perception in the same way as pain perception (Petrovic et al., 2005). On the first day of the experiment, subjects were treated with either the benzodiazepine midazolam or the benzodiazepine receptor antagonist flumazenil before being shown pictures that induced unpleasantness. As expected, midazolam reduced the unpleasantness factor and flumazenil reversed the effect. Therefore, on the first day strong expectations of the treatment effect were induced. On the second day, the subjects were told that they would be treated either with the same antianxiety drug or the anxiolytic blocker, as done on the previous day. However, instead of receiving the real medication, they received a placebo. A significant and robust placebo response (reduced unpleasantness) was found when the subjects thought they had been treated with the anxiolytic drug, but no response occurred if they thought they had received the anxiolytic blocker. Functional magnetic resonance imaging showed that regional blood flow changed in both the anterior cingulate cortex and lateral orbitofrontal cortex (Fig. 6.5), which are the very same areas involved in placebo analgesia (Petrovic et al., 2002; Wager et al., 2004). This suggests that similar mechanisms might be at work in the placebo response of emotional stimuli and in placebo analgesia.

Furmark et al. (2008) used functional neuroimaging to examine patients with social anxiety disorder. Brain activity was assessed during a stressful public speaking task by means of positron emission tomography before and after an 8-week treatment period. In addition, patients were also genotyped with respect to the serotonin transporter-linked polymorphic region (5-HTTLPR) and the G-703T polymorphism in the tryptophan hydroxylase-2 (TPH2) gene promoter. The researchers found that placebo response was accompanied by reduced stress-related activity in the amygdala. However, attenuated amygdala activity occurred only in subjects who were homozygous for the long allele of the 5-HTTLPR or the G variant of the TPH2 G-703T polymorphism, and not in carriers of short or T alleles. The TPH2 polymorphism was a significant predictor of clinical placebo response, homozygosity for the G allele being associated

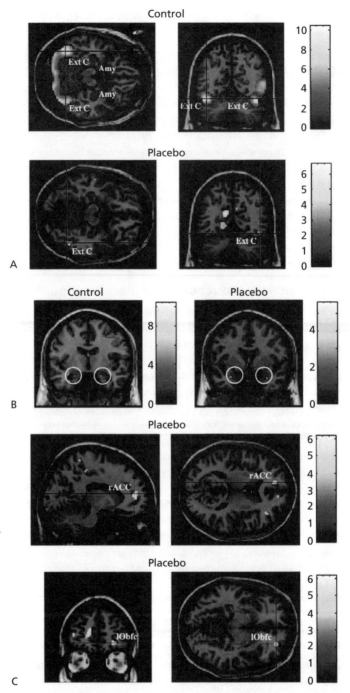

Fig. 6.5 (A) Emotional network and placebo-dependent attenuation of the same network. In the upper panel, the emotional network in the extrastriatal cortex (ExtC) activated by unpleasant pictures can be seen. In the lower panel, some regions in the ExtC show attenuated activation after placebo administration (Amy, amygdala). The t values of the

with greater improvement in anxiety symptoms. The genetic effect on symptomatic improvement with placebo was mediated by its effect on amygdala activity.

In a different study, the same group (Faria et al., 2012) examined similarities and differences in the neural response to SSRIs and placebo in patients with social anxiety disorder. Positron emission tomography was used to assess regional cerebral blood flow during an anxiogenic public speaking task, before and after 6–8 weeks of treatment under double-blind conditions. Conjunction analysis revealed a common attenuation of regional cerebral blood flow from pre- to post-treatment in responders to SSRIs and placebo in the left basomedial/basolateral and right ventrolateral amygdala. This pattern correlated with behavioral measures of reduced anxiety and differentiated responders from nonresponders. Both responders and nonresponders showed deactivation of the left lateral part of the amygdala, and no differences were found between SSRI responders and placebo responders. Therefore, drugs and placebos act on common amygdala targets.

The anxiolytic effects of placebo can be transferred to other conditions such as pain, and vice versa (Zhang and Luo, 2009). Indeed, the activity in the amygdala and insula was found to be reduced in both placebo conditions, and a greater activity in the subgenual anterior cingulate cortex under placebo conditions were found (Zhang et al., 2011). Therefore, placebo-induced expectations can use common mechanisms across different conditions.

6.3 Dementia

6.3.1 Intensive follow-up can improve cognition in demented patients

The main characteristic of dementia is the impairment of cognitive function. However, dementia is not a single entity, and its pathophysiology is complex, varying across the different types of dementia. Alzheimer's disease is by far the most common type (more than 50%), followed by vascular dementia (25–30%). The remaining 20% is distributed among frontotemporal dementia, dementia with Lewy bodies, dementia in

---

Fig. 6.5 (continued) activations are given by the color bars. (B) The amygdala is activated bilaterally by unpleasant emotions (left), and the placebo attenuates the activation of the amygdala/para-amygdaloid complex bilaterally (right). (C) The rostral anterior cingulate cortex (rACC) (upper) and the right lateral orbitofrontal cortex (lObfc) (lower) are activated by the placebo, as occurs in pain (see sections 4.1.6 and 4.1.9). Reprinted from *Neuron*, 46 (6), Predrag Petrovic, Thomas Dietrich, Peter Fransson, Jesper Andersson, Katrina Carlsson, and Martin Ingvar, Placebo in Emotional Processing—Induced Expectations of Anxiety Relief Activate a Generalized Modulatory Network, pp. 957–969, Copyright (2005), with permission from Elsevier. (See Plate 9.)

Parkinson's disease, and others (Ritchie and Lovestone, 2002; Roman et al., 2002; Emre, 2003; O'Brien et al., 2003) (see also Box 6.3). This heterogeneity plays an important role because cognitive impairment depends on the type of lesion. For example, the vascular lesions that affect mainly the frontal lobes induce a disruption of cognitive functioning that is different from that induced by parietal–temporal lesions. Likewise, the distribution of neuronal degeneration in Alzheimer's disease has a typical pattern, with sparing of the sensorimotor areas (Thompson et al., 2003), that differs from the distribution of lesions in vascular dementia. Sections 4.1.10 and 6.3.2 describe how the type of disconnection (frontal, temporal, parietal, or occipital) is important for placebo responsiveness.

There are a few studies on the role of expectation in demented patients, because most of the studies cannot identify a real placebo psychological effect (e.g., Ito et al., 2013). Although the role of expectation is not conclusive, some of these studies are worthy of mention. As explained in section 2.3.2, the Hawthorne effect refers to the patient's awareness of being under observation. This knowledge may affect the therapeutic outcomes in different ways, such as increased expectations about the therapeutic outcome. A Hawthorne effect has been suggested, and found, in several dementia trials (Rogers et al., 1998; Rosler et al., 1999; McCarney et al., 2007). For example, in a placebo-controlled trial of *Ginkgo biloba* for treating mild-to-moderate dementia, 176 participants were randomized to intensive follow-up, whereby assessment visits were performed before treatment and at 2, 4, and 6 months, or minimal follow-up, in which an abbreviated assessment was performed before treatment and a full assessment at 6 months (McCarney et al., 2007). By using cognitive functioning and participant and carer-rated quality of life as primary outcomes, these investigators found that the more intensive follow-up resulted in a better outcome than minimal follow-up for cognitive functioning.

6.3.2 Loss of prefrontal executive control affects placebo responsiveness

As already described in section 4.1.10, if there is no prefrontal control there is no placebo analgesia. Here, some more details are provided, for they are relevant to better understand the placebo response in dementia.

Box 6.3 Prevalence of dementia worldwide

According to the study by Prince et al. (2013), in 2010 there were 35.6 million people over 60 years old worldwide living with dementia. Western Europe is the region with the largest prevalence, closely followed by Southern Latin America and North America (Table 6.1).

At the country level and considering the number of people, the nine countries with the largest number of people with dementia in 2010 were: China (5.4 million), USA (3.9 million), India (3.7 million), Japan (2.5 million), Germany (1.5 million), Russia (1.2 million), France (1.1 million), Italy (1.1 million), and Brazil (1.0 million).

Box 6.3 Prevalence of dementia worldwide (continued)

Table 6.1 Prevalence of dementia worldwide in 2010

Country or global region	Prevalence (%)
Western Europe	7.2
Southern Latin America	7.0
North America	6.9
Caribbean	6.5
The Americas	6.5
Australasia	6.4
Europe	6.2
Asia Pacific	6.1
Central Latin America	6.1
Andean Latin America	5.6
Tropical Latin America	5.5
South East Asia	4.8
Eastern Europe	4.8
Central Europe	4.7
World	4.7
Central Asia	4.6
Oceania	4.0
Asia	3.9
North Africa/Middle East	3.7
South Asia	3.6
East Asia	3.2
Africa	2.6
East Sub-Saharan Africa	2.3
Southern Sub-Saharan Africa	2.1
Central Sub-Saharan Africa	1.8
West Sub-Saharan Africa	1.2

The hidden administration of a medical treatment reduces or completely abolishes the efficacy of the treatment itself (see section 2.2.4). This is due to the lack of patient expectations about the outcome when a therapy is given covertly (unexpectedly). A natural situation whereby expectations are absent exists in clinical conditions characterized by cognitive impairment. For example, in dementia of the Alzheimer's type, there is an impairment of prefrontal executive functions. This executive control by the prefrontal regions has been found to be correlated with specific areas, for example, abstract reasoning with dorsolateral frontal regions and inhibitory control with orbital and medial frontal areas (Berman et al., 1995; Nagahama et al., 1996; Rolls et al., 1996; Konishi et al., 1998, 1999a, 1999b). Interestingly, similar regions have been found to be activated by placebos (Petrovic et al., 2002, 2005; Wager et al., 2004; Zubieta et al., 2005). In addition, Alzheimer's disease is known to severely affect the frontal lobes (Thompson et al., 2003) with neuronal degeneration in those areas involved in the placebo analgesic effect, for example, the dorsolateral prefrontal cortex, the orbitofrontal cortex, and the anterior cingulate cortex.

By taking all these aspects into account, Benedetti et al. (2006) studied Alzheimer patients at the initial stage of the disease and after 1 year. They were treated with either open (expected) or hidden (unexpected) local lidocaine to reduce pain following venipuncture, in order to see whether the placebo component of the therapy, which is represented by the difference between the overt and covert application, was affected by the disease. In this study, the placebo component of the analgesic therapy was correlated with both cognitive status, as assessed by means of the Frontal Assessment Battery (FAB) test, and functional connectivity among different brain regions, as assessed by means of electroencephalographic connectivity analysis. It was found that Alzheimer's patients with reduced FAB scores showed a reduced placebo component of the analgesic treatment. In addition, the disruption of the placebo component occurred when reduced connectivity of the prefrontal lobes with the rest of the brain was present (Fig. 6.6). The loss of these placebo-related mechanisms reduced the treatment's effectiveness, and indeed an increase in dose was necessary to produce adequate analgesia.

This was the first study showing that a disruption of the placebo–psychological component of a treatment may occur in a clinical condition that affects the brain, specifically the prefrontal lobes, and that the loss of these prefrontal expectation-related mechanisms makes an analgesic treatment less effective. According to this view, the impairment of prefrontal connectivity would reduce the communication between the prefrontal lobes and the rest of the brain, so that no placebo and expectation mechanisms would be triggered.

At least two important clinical implications emerge from the disruption of placebo mechanisms in Alzheimer's disease (see also section 11.2.3). First, the reduced efficacy of the open analgesic treatment with lidocaine underscores the need for considering a possible revision of some therapies in Alzheimer patients in order to compensate for the loss of placebo-related and expectation-related mechanisms. It has been shown that the affective–emotional component of pain is impaired in Alzheimer's disease, while the sensory–discriminative component is maintained, indicating that Alzheimer patients can distinguish a painful from a tactile stimulus (Benedetti et al., 1999, 2004). Although people with Alzheimer's disease can perceive pain, there is a lower consumption of analgesics among them compared to controls, which can be due to their inability to communicate their suffering (Scherder, 2000; Scherder et al., 2005). By considering that many of these patients are likely to show severe impairment of the prefrontal lobes, and thus a loss of placebo- and expectation-related mechanisms, low doses of analgesics can be totally inadequate to relieve any kind of pain. Therefore, the analgesic treatments should be increased in order to compensate for the loss of these mechanisms.

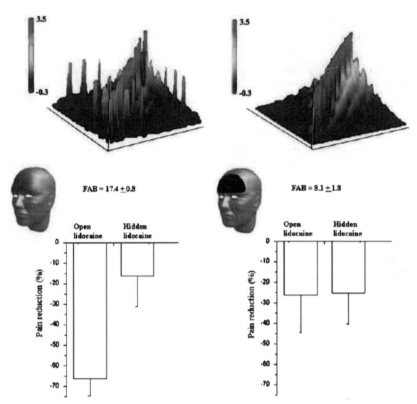

Fig. 6.6 Correlation between electroencephalographic connectivity analysis (assessed by means of mutual information: top panel), cognitive status (assessed by means of Frontal Assessment Battery or FAB) and the placebo component of open and hidden application of local analgesic lidocaine. Note the differences between normal subjects (on the left) and Alzheimer patients (on the right). Alzheimer patients show reduced electroencephalographic connectivity, as shown by the disappearance of the orange peaks (top panel), reduced FAB scores, and reduced effects of open lidocaine. Reproduced from Fabrizio Benedetti, Claudia Arduino, Sara Costa, Sergio Vighetti, Luisella Tarenzi, Innocenzo Rainero, and Giovanni Asteggiano, Loss of expectation-related mechanisms in Alzheimer's disease makes analgesic therapies less effective, *Pain*, 121 (1), pp 133–44 Copyright 2006, The International Association for the Study of Pain, with permission and from *European Journal of Applied Physiology*, 102 (4) pp. 371–380, Experimental designs and brain mapping approaches for studying the placebo analgesic effect, Luana Colloca, Fabrizio Benedetti, Carlo Adolfo Porro, Copyright 2008, Springer Science and Business Media. With kind permission from Springer Science and Business Media. (See also Plate 10.)

Second, as the prefrontal cortex can be severely affected in other neurodegenerative conditions, like frontotemporal dementia and vascular dementia (Scherder et al., 2003, 2005), the neuroanatomical localization of placebo- and expectation-related mechanisms should alert us to the potential disruption of placebo mechanisms in all those conditions whereby the prefrontal lobes are involved.

Alzheimer patients who receive placebo treatment have also been found to report a high frequency of adverse events. Amanzio et al. (2012) analyzed the rates of adverse events in patients with mild cognitive impairment and Alzheimer's disease in the placebo arms of donepezil trials. An overall comparison of 81 categories of adverse events in the placebo arm of mild cognitive impairment versus Alzheimer's disease trials showed that Alzheimer patients experienced a significantly higher number of adverse events than mildly impaired patients. The fact that Alzheimer patients are at a greater risk of developing adverse events than mild cognitive impairment patients may be related to a greater presence of somatic comorbidity predisposing them to express emotional distress as physical symptoms and/or to Alzheimer patients being frailer and therefore more susceptible to adverse events.

6.4 **Addiction**

6.4.1 **Expecting a drug of abuse makes it more pleasurable**

Reward mechanisms play a crucial role in addiction. Therefore it is not surprising to find placebo effects that are related to reward mechanisms in different types of addiction. For example, the reinforcing effects of drugs of abuse, such as cocaine, result from a complex interaction between pharmacological effects, psychological factors, and conditioned responses (Robinson and Berridge, 1993). Kirk et al. (1998) found that the response to a drug by drug abusers is more pleasurable when subjects expect to receive the drug than when they do not. In animals, the ability of drugs to activate the reward circuits (e.g., the nucleus accumbens) is larger when they are given cocaine in a context where they had previously received it than in a context where they had not (Duvauchelle et al., 2000). Today we know some mechanisms, both psychological and biological, underlying placebo and placebo-like effects in addiction.

The effect of methylphenidate on brain glucose metabolism has been analyzed in different conditions in cocaine abusers by adopting a balanced placebo design (Volkow et al., 2003) (Fig. 6.7). In one condition, cocaine abusers expected to receive the drug, and indeed received the drug. In a second condition, they expected to receive a placebo but actually received the drug. This paradigm is rather similar to the open–hidden design, as in the first case methylphenidate is expected, while in the second case its administration is unexpected. The increases in metabolism were about 50% larger, particularly in the cerebellum and the thalamus, when methylphenidate was expected than when it was not. By contrast, methylphenidate induced larger increases in left lateral orbitofrontal cortex when it was unexpected compared with when it was expected. In addition, the self-reports of "high" were also 50% greater when methylphenidate was expected than when it was not. Volkow et al. (2003) also found a correlation between the subjectively reported "high" and the metabolic activity in the thalamus but not in the cerebellum. This study strongly suggests that expectations enhance the drug effects and that the thalamus may mediate this drug enhancement by expectation, whereas the orbitofrontal cortex mediates the unexpected response to the drug.

The same research group, using the same balanced placebo design, repeated a similar experiment in nondrug abusing subjects who had minimal prior experience with

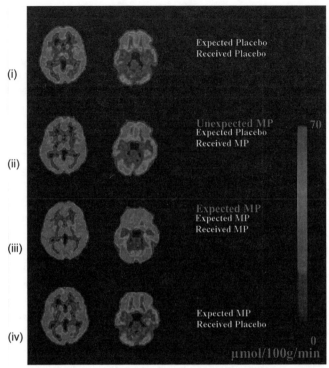

Fig. 6.7 Brain metabolic images at the thalamic and cerebellar levels in cocaine abusers in four conditions: (i) expected placebo, received placebo; (ii) expected placebo, received methylphenidate (MP); (iii) expected methylphenidate, received methylphenidate; and (iv) expected methylphenidate, received placebo. Note the larger increases in metabolism when methylphenidate was expected (iii) than when it was not (ii). Reproduced from Nora D. Volkow, Gene-Jack Wang, Yemin Ma, Joanna S. Fowler, Wei Zhu, Laurence Maynard, Frank Telang, Paul Vaska, Yu-Shin Ding, Christopher Wong, and James M. Swanson Expectation Enhances the Regional Brain Metabolic and the Reinforcing Effects of Stimulants in Cocaine Abusers, *The Journal of Neuroscience*, 23 (36), pp. 11461–11468 Copyright 2003, The Society for Neuroscience, with permission. (See Plate 11.)

stimulant drugs (Volkow et al., 2006). It was found that methylphenidate induced decreases in the striatum that were larger when the subjects expected it than when they did not. In addition, when the subjects expected to receive methylphenidate but actually received a placebo, the researchers found increases in the ventral cingulate gyrus and in the nucleus accumbens. The involvement of the nucleus accumbens following placebo administration, along with expectation to receive methylphenidate, is in agreement with the other studies in pain (Scott et al., 2007), Parkinson's disease (de la Fuente-Fernandez et al., 2001), and depression (Mayberg et al., 2002), in which the reward circuitry in the ventral striatum (nucleus accumbens) was found to be involved following placebo administration. The work by Volkow and colleagues (Volkow et al., 2003, 2006) is very informative in that it shows that expectation is an important variable to be considered whenever the reinforcing and therapeutic effects of drugs are tested both in subjects who assume drugs of abuse and in subjects who have no previous experience of drugs.

Expectation to receive methylphenidate has been found to enhance subjective arousal rather than cognitive performance. Subjects orally ingested what they believed to be methylphenidate, though actually placebo, on one visit and received no medication on the other visit. The control group received no medication on either visit. During the administration visit, experimental participants reported feeling significantly more high and stimulated compared with the non-administration visit and to the control subjects. However, there were no differences in cognitive enhancement between visits or groups which indicates that in this condition placebos affect mood but not cognition (Looby and Earleywine, 2011). Expectations of receiving marijuana may produce similar effects. For example, in a study that used the balanced placebo design, expectation of having smoked 9-tetrahydrocannabinol, regardless of active drug, decreased impulsive decision-making on a delay discounting task among participants reporting no deception and increased perception of sexual risk among women. Expectation of smoking 9-tetrahydrocannabinol in combination with active 9-tetrahydrocannabinol increased negative perceptions from risky alcohol use. Active drug and expectation independently increased subjective intoxication (Metrik et al., 2012). This study highlights the importance of marijuana expectation effects when users believe they are smoking marijuana.

6.4.2 There is no definitive role of placebo and placebo-like effects in alcohol abuse

Contrary to what should be expected, there is no clear-cut evidence of placebo and placebo-related effects in alcohol abuse (Testa et al., 2006). Placebo effects are most consistently found in studies on alcohol-induced sexual arousal (George and Stoner, 2000) but there is only modest evidence to support powerful placebo effects across different domains of social behavior (Chermack and Taylor, 1995; Fromme et al., 1999; Maisto et al., 2004). Results of a meta-analysis on 34 studies with the balanced placebo design conducted by Hull and Bond (1986) indicated that expectation of alcohol effects had significant, but heterogeneous, effects on behavior. This heterogeneity was due to the fact that alcohol expectation had powerful effects on relatively deviant social behaviors and minimal effects on nonsocial behaviors. The main effects associated with alcohol expectation involved increased sexual arousal in response to erotic stimuli. Alcohol consumption showed the opposite pattern of effects, with significant impairment of information processing and motor performance, general improvement of mood, and increased aggression. Across all the studies of this meta-analysis, alcohol consumption and expectancy interacted no more frequently than would be expected by chance.

There may be several explanations for this. One of these has to do with the credibility of the verbal instructions given by the experimenter. For example, subjects who received placebo usually report that they consumed alcohol but do not typically report feeling as intoxicated, as do subjects who received alcohol (Fromme et al.,

1999; Maisto et al., 2002). Therefore, the alcohol and the placebo conditions may not be as equivalent as researchers would like to believe. In other words, it is often difficult to manipulate verbal instructions and to deceive subjects in the setting of alcohol consumption. Within the context of the balanced placebo design, it has been proposed to replace the drug/no drug instructions with the high/low dose instructions, in order to make the instructions more credible (Ross and Pihl, 1989; Martin and Sayette, 1993).

Supporting the weak role of placebo effects and expectations is a study on the effects of alcohol and expectancies on event-related brain potentials (Marinkovic et al., 2004). By using the balanced placebo design, whereby expectancies were manipulated by verbal instructions, these investigators found no effects of expectations either on behavioral performance or on brain potentials. Conversely, although alcohol ingestion had no effect on behavioral performance, at least at the dose used in this study, it attenuated the temporoparietal N180 wave and significantly increased the amplitude of N450 and the latency of P580.

Nonetheless, some studies indicate that expectations play a role in the response to alcohol. Even when subjects receive the same dose of alcohol and attain the same blood alcohol concentration, some people show a high degree of impairment whereas others show little or no impairment. This interindividual variability may in part be due to different drinkers' expectations about the alcohol effect. Studies of alcohol effects on motor and cognitive performance have shown that those drinkers who expect the least impairment are least impaired while those who expect the most impairment are most impaired after alcohol consumption (Fillmore and Vogel-Sprott, 1995). Importantly, this same relationship is found in response to placebos.

The more recent study of the US National Institute on Alcohol Abuse and Alcoholism COMBINE (Combining Medications and Behavioral Interventions) examined 1383 alcohol-dependent patients. There appeared to be a significant "placebo effect" in this COMBINE Study, consisting of pill taking and seeing a healthcare professional. Contributing factors to the placebo response were pill taking itself, the benefits of meeting with a medical professional, repeated advice to attend Alcoholics Anonymous, and optimism about a medication effect (Weiss et al., 2008). Similarly, the meta-analysis by Schlauch et al. (2010) examined the impact of specific alcohol placebo procedures on two manipulation checks (participant reports of number of alcohol drinks consumed and subjective intoxication) to determine which procedures produced the smallest effect sizes in comparisons between alcohol and placebo conditions. Alcohol versus placebo condition comparisons generally produced large effect sizes for both interventions, but they were moderated by double-blind procedures and by peak breath-alcohol concentration attained in the alcohol condition.

Gilbertson et al. (2010) designed a double-blind, placebo-controlled alcohol administration paradigm, in which they investigated the peak breath alcohol concentration levels consistent with an episode of social drinking (about 40 mg/100 mL), and both cognitive performance and perceived levels of intoxication and impairment were assessed. A total of 63% of the participants who received placebo reported that they received alcohol, and they showed slower reaction times on an attentional task, similar to those receiving alcohol. However, accuracy was not impaired and there was no effect on self-reported measures of intoxication and impairment. As expected, participants who received alcohol had less accuracy on the attentional task and more self-reported impairment and intoxication than those who received placebo. These results indicate that belief of having received a moderate dose of alcohol has only a partial effect on some functions, such as reaction times, but not on other functions, such as accuracy and perceived intoxication.

6.4.3 Tobacco smoking and nicotine intake show large placebo effects

Smoking is a good example of how both pharmacological and nonpharmacological factors are at work in tobacco dependence. Although nicotine is necessary for maintaining tobacco dependence (Jaffe, 1990; Benowitz and Henningfield, 1994; Stolerman and Jarvis, 1995) it is generally not sufficient. In fact, despite the fact that nicotine replacement therapy is capable of delivering as much nicotine as a cigarette (and almost as rapidly), many smokers relapse to smoking (Perkins et al., 2003).

Surprisingly little research has been performed in this field, although placebo and expectation effects seem to play a crucial role. For example, a few studies have used the balanced placebo design to investigate smoking placebo effects. In one study, briefly abstinent smokers were given a stressor (embarrassing speech) while receiving a nicotine or denicotinized cigarette, along with verbal instructions about its content ("told nicotine" or "told no nicotine") (Juliano and Brandon, 2002). The researchers found an interaction of instructions and nicotine on craving. In fact, those smokers who received denicotinized cigarettes and were told there was nicotine inside reported a decrease in smoking urge. Conversely, those smokers who received nicotine cigarettes reported a decrease in urge, regardless of what they were told. Therefore, according to this study, expectations of getting nicotine induced placebo responses when placebo cigarettes were smoked, but expectations of receiving denicotinized cigarettes did not reduce the pharmacological effect of nicotine.

In a subsequent study with the balanced placebo design by Perkins et al. (2004), in which low/high dose nicotine instructions were used, expectations were found to affect both denicotinized and nicotine cigarettes. In other words, expecting high-dose nicotine but getting a denicotinized cigarette induced placebo effects, whereas expecting a denicotinized cigarette but receiving a high dose reduced the effects of nicotine. Interestingly, according to Perkins' study (Perkins et al., 2004) verbal instructions did not affect craving and withdrawal but only the number of puffs earned for those smokers who were given low nicotine, thus indicating that verbally induced expectations may affect only some responses to smoking.

While the studies just described have to do with tobacco smoking, there are some other studies that investigated the placebo effect in the context of nicotine replacement therapy. The obvious difference between these studies is that in the first case nicotine intake is through tobacco smoking whereas in the second case it is not (Perkins et al., 2003). Clinical studies with nicotine gum show placebo effects on withdrawal (Gottlieb et al., 1987; Tate et al., 1994) and gum self-administration (Hughes et al., 1989). For example, Tate et al. (1994) gave placebo gum along with the suggestion it was nicotine to different groups of subjects trying to quit smoking. One group, which was told to expect no withdrawal symptoms, showed only half as many symptoms as a second group which was given no instructions. A third group, which was given instructions to expect somatic symptoms such as headache, reported a greater increase in somatic symptoms. By contrast, a fourth group was told to expect psychological symptoms like anxiety, but they did not report any symptom worsening.

Sensory cues including the sight and smell of smoke and handling of a cigarette have also been found to relate to placebo and placebo-like effects (Perkins et al., 2003). For example, reduction in liking, satisfaction, and self-administration has been described after local anesthesia of the respiratory pathways (Rose et al., 1985) and blockade of olfactory and visual cues (Baldinger et al., 1995; Perkins et al., 2001), which suggests that salient sensory cues alone during the consumption of a denicotinized cigarette can produce substantial craving and withdrawal relief.

It is also worth mentioning the importance of placebo and expectation effects in the context of classical clinical trials. In a trial of nicotine replacement treatment for smoking reduction, smokers were randomly assigned to receive nicotine, matching placebo products, or no intervention. After 6 months, participants were asked to guess which group they believed to belong to (either nicotine or placebo). Regardless of the actual treatment received, smokers who believed they had received nicotine had significantly better outcomes than those who believed they had received the placebo (Dar et al., 2005).

6.4.4 Placebo response rates from cessation trials may inform on strength of addictions

People have long known that addictions to different substances vary in strength from weak to strong. In the first case, drug intake is easier to stop than in the second case. Although this seems to be quite obvious, explicit and rigorous scientific definitions are lacking. Indeed, comparing different forms of addiction in order to categorize the strength of addiction is not easy for reasons concerning the characteristics of the addicted subjects, the setting, and the details of study design. Now it has been shown that placebos can help categorize the strength of addiction. In fact, Moore and Aubin (2012) assessed the strength of addictions by measuring cessation rates with placebo or no treatment controls, and found that a weaker addiction has a higher cessation rate than a stronger addiction. Moore and Aubin analyzed several systematic reviews and meta-analyses of cessation trials, using randomized or quasi-randomized trials and reporting objectively measured abstinence. The outcome for comparison was the percentage of participants abstinent according to an objective test of abstinence at 6 months or longer (quit rates). A total of 28 cessation reviews, with 139,000 participants were analyzed. Most of these (127,000) came from trials of smoking cessation. Cessation rates with placebo in randomized trials using objective measures of abstinence and typically over 6 months' duration were 8% for nicotine, 18% for alcohol, 47% for cocaine, and 44% for opioids. Therefore, evidence from placebo cessation rates indicates that nicotine is more difficult to give up than alcohol, cocaine, and opioids. Although this study needs further confirmation, it represents an excellent application of placebos in a specific clinical condition, in which placebo quit rates are a useful proxy marker for the strength of different addictions.

6.5 **Psychotherapy**

6.5.1 **Does psychotherapy work through a benign human relationship?**

Psychotherapy is included in this chapter because it is mainly used to treat mental and behavioral disorders, although many other medical conditions, such as pain, are common targets of the psychotherapeutic approach. Psychotherapy is quite interesting in the context of placebo and placebo-related effects because both psychotherapy and a placebo procedure use verbal suggestions. The old debate about whether or not psychotherapy and placebos have similar mechanisms consists of ascertaining whether psychotherapy is nothing but a placebo effect, and thus whether a placebo procedure is a very simple form of psychotherapy.

Overall, there are more than 400 types of psychotherapy, each with its own theory and working hypothesis. Surprisingly, all of them seem to be effective (Parloff, 1986; Moerman, 2002). In a widely known and influential review of about 40 studies that used different psychotherapeutic approaches, Luborsky et al. (1975) found that all of them were effective, even those in which minimal treatment was carried out. In a different analysis of 375 studies of different kinds of psychotherapy by Smith and Glass (1977), negligible differences were found in the effects produced by various types of therapy. In 1982, Landman and Dawes (1982) went through these 375 studies and found that many of them did not randomly allocate patients to the different groups. Therefore, they re-analyzed the 375 studies plus a further 60 that they added, and were able to extract 42 studies that used true random assignment. Surprisingly, they found that the results were similar to those of the 375 studies analyzed by Smith and Glass (1977), which indicates that it did not matter whether the studies had a true random assignment: psychotherapy was effective regardless of its theories. Many other subsequent studies have found that, in general, psychotherapies are effective, as compared with placebo and no-treatment groups (Lipsey and Wilson, 1993; Grissom, 1996).

The conclusion appears to be that all psychotherapies work more or less fairly well and that there are little differences across the different therapeutic approaches. However, the explanation might be that psychotherapy is nothing more than a good human interaction between patient and therapist, so that trust, belief, expectation, motivation, and hope—common elements in all types of psychotherapy—are the factors responsible for the successful therapeutic outcomes (Moerman, 2002).

In this context another study is very instructive. In 1979, Strupp and Hadley (1979) conducted an interesting experiment whereby "disturbed" college students were allocated to either psychotherapy carried out by practicing psychotherapists with experience of more than 20 years each on average, or interaction with professors of English, philosophy, history, or mathematics with a renowned reputation for warmth and trustworthiness but with no previous experience as therapists. Both groups improved. Furthermore, there was no significant difference between the improvement of those who interacted with psychotherapists or with the professors. In addition, two control groups, one receiving minimal treatment and one only receiving diagnostic testing, also showed improvement, although significantly smaller than the experimental groups. Strupp and Hadley (1979) concluded that the positive changes experienced by the patients of both experimental groups was attributable to the healing effects of a benign human relationship.

The fact that all sorts of psychotherapy show negligible differences between each other (Luborsky et al., 1975; Smith and Glass, 1977) and that successful outcomes can be obtained by inexperienced therapists (Strupp and Hadley, 1979) suggests that factors other than specific elements of each psychotherapy are at work. This concept was expressed in the 1960s by Frank (1961) who proposed that all forms of psychotherapy work because they contain similar elements, such as a ritual to reinforce the therapist–patient relationship and the presence of a thoughtful listener. All these considerations lead to the question of what placebo and placebo-related effects have to do with psychotherapy.

6.5.2 It is difficult to disentangle placebo effects from psychotherapy

The main problem in studying placebo effects in psychotherapy is that it is difficult, maybe impossible, to separate the placebo component from the specific effects of a psychotherapy. There are several problems, both practical and conceptual (Borkovec and Sibrava, 2005; Herbert and Gaudiano, 2005; Kirsch, 2005). The practical problem is that placebo controls in psychotherapy are not the same as those in pharmacotherapy. In fact, in the latter, all that is needed is to omit the active ingredient from a pill or a solution and to make the pill or solution similar in all respects to the real medication, so as to disentangle the psychological component from the overall pharmacological effect. With a psychological treatment, this is not possible, as all of its ingredients are psychological. Several placebo psychotherapies have been used, such as listening to audiotapes and watching videocassettes in order to eliminate the interaction with the therapist, sitting quietly with a silent therapist, or discussing current events that have nothing to do with the psychological treatment (Prioleau et al., 1983). An additional problem is the fact that it is really difficult to devise double-blind studies in psychotherapy, as the psychotherapist by definition knows what treatment is being delivered.

The second problem is a conceptual one (Borkovec and Sibrava, 2005; Herbert and Gaudiano, 2005; Kirsch, 2005). Psychotherapy is rich in psychological ingredients, such as the supposed specific elements, the good relationship between therapist and patient, and trust, hope, and expectation, and such like. Any placebo condition that tries to eliminate these factors is per se different from the overall psychotherapeutic context, thus it is not a good placebo. This complex set of elements led Moerman (2002) to talk about a meaning effect, or response, in that the real active ingredient of a psychotherapy is the meaning of the treatment itself. Therefore, the identification of the placebo component of a psychotherapy is not as easy as it is in pharmacotherapy, from both the methodological and conceptual viewpoints. For example, if expectation is the most important ingredient in an effective psychotherapy, should we consider it nothing but a placebo effect?

In order to answer this question, a useful definition was formulated by Paul (1966, 1969). He defined the placebo condition as a treatment in which the subjects have equal faith, but which would not be expected to lead to a change in behavior on any other grounds. Of course, according to this definition, the answer to the earlier question is positive. In other words, if the most important ingredient of a psychotherapy is faith and expectation, we should consider it a placebo effect, because a really effective psychotherapy should work through mechanisms other than faith, belief, and expectation.

It is worth noting that in psychotherapy expectations do not necessarily go always in the positive direction. Bootzin and Bailey (2005) emphasized how negative iatrogenic (literally "therapist-caused") effects may also occur during psychotherapy. These nocebo and nocebo-related effects have been described in different types of psychotherapy, like critical incident stress debriefing for the treatment of post-traumatic stress disorders, group therapy for adolescents with conduct disorder, and psychotherapy for dissociative identity disorder (Bootzin and Bailey, 2005). For example, in group therapy for conduct-disorder adolescents, the interaction between juvenile delinquents during group treatments may strengthen antisocial behavior through the lack of positive expectancies (Bootzin and Bailey, 2005).

Because it is difficult both to identify and to define placebo effects in the context of psychotherapy, the debate about the role of placebo and placebo-like effects in different psychotherapies is still open, and thus the scientific evidence of their efficacy is not definitive.

6.5.3 The neural mechanisms of some psychotherapies differ from those of the placebo effect

Recent studies of clinical response in major depression to either cognitive behavioral therapy (Goldapple et al., 2004) or interpersonal psychotherapy (Brody et al., 2001; Martin et al., 2001) demonstrate very different regional brain change patterns from those seen with placebo (Mayberg et al., 2002). Both cognitive behavioral therapy and interpersonal psychotherapy are associated with substantial prefrontal decreases with other regional effects specific to each psychotherapy strategy. With clinical response to cognitive behavioral therapy, Mayberg and colleagues described additional changes in regions not affected by antidepressant drugs, like fluoxetine, including the orbital frontal and medial frontal cortex and dorsal anterior cingulate cortex (Benedetti et al., 2005). A comparison between placebo treatment and cognitive behavioral therapy is shown in Fig. 6.1. The change patterns seen with these specific psychotherapies provide evidence that refutes the hypothesis that placebo antidepressant effect is mediated by changes in a common antidepressant response pathway. These findings also suggest that the placebo antidepressant response is not the result of nonspecific psychological treatment effects. In fact, brain changes associated with placebo response most closely match the active drug-response pattern to which it was experimentally yoked (conditioned). These findings are certainly interesting, but are not definitive, as a no-treatment control group was not run in these studies, so a spontaneous remission with either treatment cannot be ruled out.

6.6 **Premenstrual dysphoric disorder**

6.6.1 **Placebos may reduce symptomatology through endogenous opioids**

In a study performed by Van Ree et al. (2005) a possible involvement of endogenous opioids, similar to that in placebo analgesia (see Chapter 4), was described. By assessing the severity of premenstrual dysphoric disorder in 22 women by means of the menstrual distress questionnaire, these researchers treated the patients with either a placebo or the opioid antagonist nalmefene. Whereas the placebo treatment significantly reduced scores on the menstrual distress questionnaire, nalmefene prevented any reduction. Although plasma levels of beta-endorphins were found to be increased, no definitive conclusion can be drawn about their role in the observed placebo effect, as the endorphin changes might represent merely an epiphenomenon. In this study there was also a general trend for the placebo treatment to attenuate plasma levels of several hormones—luteinizing hormone, follicle-stimulating hormone, estradiol, and progesterone. Although this is the only study available to date, it is quite interesting, as the blockade of the placebo response by an opioid antagonist resembles the results obtained in placebo analgesia (see Chapter 4).

6.7 **Attention-deficit hyperactivity disorder**

6.7.1 **Reducing drug intake through conditioned placebo responses**

Attention-deficit hyperactivity disorder (ADHD) is another interesting neuropsychiatric disorder, in which the placebo effect has been studied in the clinical trial setting, thus no specific factor or mechanism has been identified (Buitelaar et al., 2012). However, it is worth noting that a conditioning procedure has been found to be applicable and useful to reduce drug intake. In fact, Sandler et al. (2010) studied 99 children with ADHD who were randomized to one of three treatments of 8 weeks duration: (1) conditioned placebo dose reduction condition (50% reduced dose + placebo), or (2) a dose reduction only, or (3) a no reduction condition. The conditioned placebo dose reduction procedure involved daily pairing of mixed amphetamine salts dose with a visually distinctive placebo capsule administered in open label, with full disclosure of placebo use to subjects and parents. Seventy children completed the study. Most subjects in the reduced dose + placebo group remained stable during the treatment phase, whereas most in the reduced dose group deteriorated. There was no difference in ADHD symptoms between the reduced dose + placebo group and the full dose group, and both groups showed better ADHD control than the reduced dose group. Side effects were lowest in the reduced dose + placebo group. This is a nice clinical application of placebo conditioning mechanisms, whereby pairing placebos with stimulant medication elicits a placebo response that allows children with ADHD to be effectively treated on 50% of their optimal stimulant dose.

6.8 **Mental disorders with no available data**

A rough estimate of the improvement in placebo groups of psychopharmacology trials ranges from 20–70% (Laporte and Figueras, 1994). Although this figure seems to be large, it should be noted that many factors are involved here, including the natural history of the disease and selection bias (regression to the mean) as well as real placebo responses. Unfortunately, none of these clinical studies address the underlying mechanisms, as most of them were carried out with the purpose of validating the efficacy of psychopharmacological agents. For example, in a meta-regression analysis aimed at identifying the moderators of the improvements in placebo groups of antipsychotic trials in schizophrenia, trial duration was found to account for a substantial proportion of the between-trial variation in response (27%), with greater improvement in placebo groups observed in shorter trials with a duration of less than 6–8 weeks (Welge and Keck, 2003). Although these authors suggest that a possible explanation might be the stabilizing effect of hospitalization, clearly no conclusion can be drawn as far as the underlying mechanisms are concerned, and indeed many factors are involved in the placebo response in schizophrenia, with no clear prevalence of one relative to the others (Kinon et al., 2011; Potkin et al., 2011; Alphs et al., 2012).

6.9 **Points for further discussion**

1 Better designed trials are needed for studying the placebo effect in depression. Although this is not easy because of ethical constraints, the lack of adequate control groups in depression studies limits our understanding of the brain imaging data.

2 The action of SSRIs in depression needs to be further explored, to yield more information on the possible role of serotonin in placebo antidepressant responses.

3 The neural and biochemical pathways of different types of anxiety (e.g., state and trait anxiety) need to be elucidated. This would be very important in placebo research. For example, understanding of anticipatory anxiety is crucial to nocebo phenomena.

4 Further investigation into the effects of different types of dementia on placebo responsiveness would extend our present knowledge about reduced placebo responses in Alzheimer's disease. In particular it would be important to clarify which clinical conditions are associated with disruption of placebo and expectation mechanisms.

5 Reward mechanisms and expectations of benefit are important in drug addiction. The study of the placebo effect in this field may contribute to the development of interesting therapeutic strategies.

6 A comparison between neuroimaging studies in different psychotherapies is needed in order to better clarify whether different psychotherapeutic interventions produce a common pattern of brain responses that is attributable to a placebo effect. This issue is particularly important as it gives us insights into the mechanisms of psychotherapy.

7 Unfortunately we do not know anything about placebo mechanisms in important mental and behavioral disorders, such as schizophrenia, obsessive–compulsive disorder, phobias, and many others. Thus it would be important to devise controlled studies aimed at investigating placebo and placebo-related effects in these disorders.

References

Alphs L, Benedetti F, Fleischhacker WW and Kane JM (2012). Placebo-related effects in clinical trials in schizophrenia: what is driving this phenomenon and what can be done to minimize it? *International Journal of Neuropsychopharmacology*, **15**, 1003–14.

Amanzio M, Benedetti F and Vase L (2012). A systematic review of adverse events in the placebo arm of donepezil trials: the role of cognitive impairment. *International Psychogeriatrics*, **24**, 698–707.

Andrews G (2001). Placebo response in depression: bane of research, boon to therapy. *British Journal of Psychiatry*, **178**, 192–4.

Baldinger B, Hasenfratz M and Battig K (1995). Switching to ultralow nicotine cigarettes: effects of different tar yields and blocking of olfactory cues. *Pharmacology, Biochemistry, and Behavior*, **50**, 233–9.

Benedetti F (2008). Mechanisms of placebo and placebo-related effects across diseases and treatments. *Annual Reviews of Pharmacology and Toxicology*, **48**, 33–60.

Benedetti F, Arduino C, Costa S et al. (2006) Loss of expectation-related mechanisms in Alzheimer's disease makes analgesic therapies less effective. *Pain*, **121**, 133–44.

Benedetti F, Arduino C, Vighetti S, Asteggiano G, Tarenzi L and Rainero I (2004). Pain reactivity in Alzheimer patients with different degrees of cognitive impairment and brain electrical activity deterioration. *Pain*, **111**, 22–9.

Benedetti F, Carlino E and Pollo A (2011). Hidden administration of drugs. *Clinical Pharmacology and Therapeutics*, **90**, 651–61.

Benedetti F, Maggi G, Lopiano L et al. (2003). Open versus hidden medical treatments: the patient's knowledge about a therapy affects the therapy outcome. *Prevention & Treatment*, **6**(1).

Benedetti F, Mayberg HS, Wager TD, Stohler CS and Zubieta JK (2005). Neurobiological mechanisms of the placebo effect. *Journal of Neuroscience*, **25**, 10390–402.

Benedetti F, Vighetti S, Ricco C et al. (1999). Pain threshold and tolerance in Alzheimer's disease. *Pain*, **80**, 377–82.

Benowitz NL and Henningfield JE (1994). Establishing a nicotine threshold for addiction. *New England Journal of Medicine*, **331**, 123–5.

Berman KF, Ostrem JL, Randolph C et al. (1995). Physiological activation of a cortical network during performance of the Wisconsin Card Sorting Test: a positron emission tomography study. *Neuropsychologia*, **33**, 1027–46.

Bootzin RR and Bailey E (2005). Understanding placebo, nocebo, and iatrogenic treatment effects. *Journal of Clinical Psychology*, **61**, 871–80.

Borkovec TD and Sibrava NJ (2005). Problems with the use of placebo conditions in psychotherapy research, suggested alternatives, and some strategies for the pursuit of the placebo phenomenon. *Journal of Clinical Psychology*, **61**, 805–18.

Bridge JA, Birmaher B, Iyengar S, Barbe RP and Brent DA (2009). Placebo response in randomized controlled trials of antidepressants for pediatric major depressive disorder. *American Journal of Psychiatry*, **166**, 42–9.

Brody AL, Saxena S, Stoessel P, Gillies LA, Fairbanks LA and Alborzian S (2001). Regional brain metabolic changes in patients with major depression treated with either paroxetine or interpersonal therapy. *Archives of General Psychiatry*, **58**, 631–40.

Brunoni AR, Lopes M, Kaptchuk TJ and Fregni F (2009). Placebo response of non-pharmacological and pharmacological trials in major depression: a systematic review and meta-analysis. *PLoS One*, **4**, e4824.

Buitelaar JK, Sobanski E, Stieglitz RD, Dejonckheere J, Waechter S and Schäuble B (2012). Predictors of placebo response in adults with attention-deficit/hyperactivity disorder: data from 2 randomized trials of osmotic-release oral system methylphenidate. *Journal of Clinical Psychiatry*, **73**, 1097–102.

Chermack ST and Taylor SP (1995). Alcohol and human physical aggression: pharmacological vs expectancy effects. *Journal of Studies on Alcohol*, **56**, 449–56.

Colloca L, Benedetti F and Porro CA (2008). Experimental designs and brain mapping approaches for studying the placebo analgesic effect. *European Journal of Applied Physiology*, **102**, 371–80.

Colloca L, Lopiano L, Lanotte M and Benedetti F (2004). Overt versus covert treatment for pain, anxiety and Parkinson's disease. *Lancet Neurology*, **3**, 679–84.

Dar R, Stronguin F and Etter JF (2005). Assigned versus perceived placebo effects in nicotine replacement therapy for smoking reduction in Swiss smokers. *Journal of Consulting and Clinical Psychology*, **73**, 350–3.

de la Fuente-Fernandez R, Ruth TJ, Sossi V, Schulzer M, Calne DB and Stoessl AJ (2001). Expectation and dopamine release: mechanism of the placebo effect in Parkinson's disease. *Science*, **293**, 1164–6.

Duvauchelle CL, Ikegami A, Asami S, Robens J, Kressin K and Castaneda E (2000). Effects of cocaina context on NAcc dopamine and behavioral activity after repeated intravenous cocaina administration. *Brain Research*, **862**, 49–58.

Emre M (2003). Dementia associated with Parkinson's disease. *Lancet Neurology*, **2**, 229–37.

Faria V, Appel L, Åhs F *et al.* (2012). Amygdala subregions tied to SSRI and placebo response in patients with social anxiety disorder. *Neuropsychopharmacology*, **37**, 2222–32.

Fillmore MT and Vogel-Sprott M (1995). Expectancies about alcohol-induced motor impairment predict individual differences in responses to alcohol and placebo. *Journal of Studies on Alcohol*, **56**, 90–8.

Frank JD (1961). *Persuasion and healing*. Johns Hopkins University Press, Baltimore, MD.

Fromme K, D'Amico EJ and Katz EC. (1999). Intoxicated sexual risk taking: an expectancy or cognitive impairment explanation. *Journal of Studies on Alcohol*, **60**, 54–63.

Furmark T, Appel L, Henningsson S *et al.* (2008). A link between serotonin-related gene polymorphisms, amygdala activity, and placebo-induced relief from social anxiety. *Journal of Neuroscience*, **28**, 13066–74.

George WH and Stoner SA (2000). Understanding acute alcohol effects on sexual behavior. *Annual Review of Sexual Research*, **11**, 92–124.

Gilbertson R, Prather R and Nixon SJ (2010). Acute alcohol administration and placebo effectiveness in older moderate drinkers: influences on cognitive performance. *Journal of Studies on Alcohol and Drugs*, **71**, 345–50.

Goldapple K, Segal Z, Garson C *et al.* (2004). Modulation of cortical-limbic pathways in major depression: treatment specific effects of cognitive behavior therapy compared to paroxetine. *Archives of General Psychiatry*, **61**, 34–41.

Gottlieb AM, Killen JD, Marlatt GA and Taylor CB (1987). Psychological and pharmacological influences in cigarette smoking withdrawal: effects of nicotine gum and expectancy on smoking withdrawal symptoms and relapse. *Journal of Consulting and Clinical Psychology*, **55**, 606–8.

Grissom RJ (1996). The magical number 0.7 + 2; meta-meta-analysis of the probability of superior outcome in comparisons involving therapy, placebo, and control. *Journal of Consulting & Clinical Psychology*, **64**, 973–82.

Gueorguieva R, Mallinckrodt C and Krystal JH (2011). Trajectories of depression severity in clinical trials of duloxetine: insights into antidepressant and placebo responses. *Archives of General Psychiatry*, **68**, 1227–37.

Herbert JD and Gaudiano BA (2005). Moving from empirically supported treatment lists to practice guidelines in psychotherapy: the role of the placebo concept. *Journal of Clinical Psychology*, **61**, 893–908.

Hrobjartsson A and Goetzsche PC (2004). Is the placebo powerless? Update of a systematic review with 52 new randomized trials comparing placebo with no treatment. *Journal of Internal Medicine*, **256**, 91–100.

Hughes J, Gabbay M, Funnell E and Dowrick C (2012). Exploratory review of placebo characteristics reported in randomised placebo controlled antidepressant drug trials. *Pharmacopsychiatry*, **45**, 20–7.

Hughes JR, Strickler G, King D et al. (1989). Smoking history, instructions, and the effects of nicotine: two pilot studies. *Pharmacology, Biochemistry, and Behavior*, **34**, 149–55.

Hull JG and Bond CF (1986). Social and behavioral consequences of alcohol consumption and expectancy: a meta-analysis. *Psychological Bulletin*, **99**, 347–60.

Ikemoto S and Panksepp J (1999). The role of nucleus accumbens dopamine in motivated behavior: a unifying interpretation with special reference to reward-seeking. *Brain Research Reviews*, **31**, 6–41.

Iovieno N and Papakostas GI (2012). Correlation between different levels of placebo response rate and clinical trial outcome in major depressive disorder: a meta-analysis. *Journal of Clinical Psychiatry*, **73**, 1300–6.

Ito K, Corrigan B, Romero K, et al. (2013). Understanding placebo responses in Alzheimer's disease clinical trials from the literature meta-data and CAMD database. *Journal of Alzheimer's Disease*, **37**, 173–83.

Jaffe JH (1990). Tobacco smoking and nicotine dependence. In S Wonnacott, MAH Russell, and IP Stolerman, eds. *Nicotine psychopharmacology: molecular, cellular, and behavioral aspects*, pp. 1–37. Oxford University Press, New York.

Juliano LM and Brandon TH (2002). Effects of nicotine dose, instructional set, and outcome expectancies on the subjective effects of smoking in the presence of a stressor. *Journal of Abnormal Psychology*, **111**, 88–97.

Khan A, Warner HA and Brown WA (2000). Symptom reduction and suicide risk in patients treated with placebo in antidepressant clinical trials: an analysis of the FDA database. *Archives of General Psychiatry*, **57**, 311–17

Kinon BJ, Potts AJ and Watson SB (2011). Placebo response in clinical trials with schizophrenia patients. *Current Opinion in Psychiatry*, **24**, 107–13.

Kirk JM, Doty P and De Wit H (1998). Effects of expectancies on subjective responses to oral delta9-tetrahydrocannabinol. *Pharmacology, Biochemistry and Behavior*, **59**, 287–93.

Kirsch I (2005). Placebo psychotherapy: synonym or oxymoron? *Journal of Clinical Psychology*, **61**, 791–803.

Kirsch I (2008). Challenging received wisdom: antidepressants and the placebo effect. *McGill Journal of Medicine*, **11**, 219–22.

Kirsch I and Sapirstein G (1998). Listening to prozac but hearing placebo: a meta-analysis of antidepressant medication. *Prevention & Treatment*, **1**(2).

Knutson B and Cooper JC (2005). Functional magnetic resonance imaging of reward prediction. *Current Opinion in Neurology*, **18**, 411–17.

Konishi S, Kawazu M, Uchida I, Kikyo H, Asakura I and Miyashita Y (1999a). Contribution of working memory to transient activation in human inferior prefrontal cortex during performance of the Wisconsin Card Sorting Test. *Cerebral Cortex*, **9**, 745–53.

Konishi S, Nakajima K, Uchida I et al. (1998). Transient activation of inferior prefrontal cortex during cognitive set shifting. *Nature Neuroscience*, **1**, 80–4.

Konishi S, Nakajima K, Uchida I, Kikyo H, Kameyama M and Miyashita Y (1999b). Common inhibitory mechanism in human inferior prefrontal cortex revealed by event-related functional MRI. *Brain*, **122**, 981–91.

Krell HV, Leuchter AF, Morgan M, Cook IA and Abrams M (2004). Subject expectations of treatment effectiveness and outcome of treatment with an experimental antidepressant. *Journal of Clinical Psychiatry*, **65**, 1174–9.

Landman JT and Dawes RM (1982). Psychotherapy outcome. Smith and Glass' conclusions stand up under scrutiny. *American Psychologist*, **37**, 504–16.

Laporte J-R and Figueras A (1994). Placebo effects in psychiatry. *Lancet*, **344**, 1206–9.

Leuchter AF, Cook IA, Witte EA, Morgan M and Abrams M (2002). Changes in brain function of depressed subjects during treatment with placebo. *American Journal of Psychiatry*, **159**, 122–9.

Leuchter AF, McCracken JT, Hunter AM, Cook IA and Alpert JE (2009). Monoamine oxidase a and catechol-o-methyltransferase functional polymorphisms and the placebo response in major depressive disorder. *Journal of Clinical Psychopharmacology*, **29**, 372–7.

Leuchter AF, Morgan M, Cook IA, Dunkin J, Abrams M and Witte E (2004). Pretreatment neurophysiological and clinical characteristics of placebo responders in treatment trials for major depression. *Psychopharmacology*, **177**, 15–22.

Lipsey MW and Wilson DB (1993). The efficacy of psychological, educational, and behavioral treatment: confirmation from meta-analysis. *American Psychologist*, **48**, 1181–209.

Looby A and Earleywine M (2011). Expectation to receive methylphenidate enhances subjective arousal but not cognitive performance. *Experimental and Clinical Psychopharmacology*, **19**, 433–44.

Luborsky L, Singer B and Luborsky L (1975). Comparative studies of psychotherapies. Is it true that "everyone has won and all must have prizes"? *Archives of General Psychiatry*, **32**, 995–1008.

Maisto SA, Carey MP, Carey KB and Gordon CM (2002). The effects of alcohol and expectancies on risk perception and behavior skills relevant to safer sex among heterosexual young adult women. *Journal of Studies on Alcohol*, **63**, 476–85.

Maisto SA, Carey MP, Carey KB, Gordon CM, Schum JL and Lynch KG (2004). The relationship between alcohol and individual difference variables on attitudes and behavioral skills relevant to sexual health among heterosexual young adult men. *Archives of Sexual Behavior*, **33**, 571–84.

Marinkovic K, Halgren E and Maltzman I (2004). Effects of alcohol on verbal processing: an event-related potential study. *Alcoholism, Clinical and Experimental Research*, **28**, 415–23.

Martin SD, Martin E, Rai SS, Richardson MA and Royall R (2001). Brain blood flow changes in depressed patients treated with interpersonal psychotherapy or venlafaxine hydrochloride. *Archives of General Psychiatry,* **58**, 641–64.

Martin CS and Sayette MA (1993). Experimental design in alcohol administration research: limitations and alternatives in the manipulation of dosage-set. *Journal of Studies on Alcohol,* **54**, 750–61.

Mayberg HS, Silva JA, Brannan SK *et al.* (2002). The functional neuroanatomy of the placebo effect. *American Journal of Psychiatry,* **159**, 728–37.

McCarney R, Warner J, Iliffe S, van Haselen R, Griffin M and Fisher P (2007). The Hawthorne Effect: a randomised, controlled trial. *BMC Medical Research Methodology,* **7**, 30.

Metrik J, Kahler CW, Reynolds B, *et al.* (2012). Balanced placebo design with marijuana: pharmacological and expectancy effects on impulsivity and risk taking. *Psychopharmacology (Berlin),* **223**, 489–99.

Moerman DE (2002). *Meaning, medicine and the placebo effect.* Cambridge University Press, Cambridge, MA.

Moore RA and Aubin HJ (2012). Do placebo response rates from cessation trials inform on strength of addictions? *International Journal of Environmental Research and Public Health,* **9**, 192–211.

Nagahama Y, Fukuyama H, and Yamauchi H (1996). Cerebral activation during performance of a card sorting test. *Brain,* **119**, 1667–75.

O'Brien JT, Erkinjuntti T, Reisberg B *et al.* (2003). Vascular cognitive impairment. *Lancet Neurology,* **2**, 89–98.

Parloff MB (1986). Frank's "common elements" in psychotherapy: non-specific factors and placebos. *American Journal of Orthopsychiatry,* **56**, 521–30.

Paul GL (1966). *Insight vs desensitization in psychotherapy.* Stanford University Press, Stanford, CA.

Paul GL (1969). Behavior modification research: design and tactics. In CM Franks, ed. *Behavior therapy: appraisal and status,* pp. 29–62. McGraw-Hill, New York.

Perkins KA, Gerlach D, Vender J, Grobe JE, Meeker J and Hutchinson S (2001). Sex differences in the subjective and reinforcing effects of visual and olfactory cigarette smoke stimuli. *Nicotine & Tobacco Research,* **3**, 141–50.

Perkins KA, Jacobs L, Ciccocioppo M, Conklin C, Sayette M and Caggiula A (2004). The influence of instructions and nicotine dose on the subjective and reinforcing effects of smoking. *Experimental and Clinical Psychopharmacology,* **12**, 91–101.

Perkins KA, Sayette M, Conklin C and Caggiula A (2003). Placebo effects of tobacco smoking and other nicotine intake. *Nicotine & Tobacco Research,* **5**, 695–709.

Petrovic P, Dietrich T, Fransson P, Andersson J, Carlsson K and Ingvar M (2005). Placebo in emotional processing-induced expectations of anxiety relief activate a generalized modulatory network. *Neuron,* **46**, 957–69.

Petrovic P, Kalso E, Petersson KM and Ingvar M (2002). Placebo and opioid analgesia-imaging a shared neuronal network. *Science,* **295**, 1737–40.

Potkin S, Agid O, Siu C, Watsky E, Vanderburg D and Remington G (2011). Placebo response trajectories in short-term and long-term antipsychotic trials in schizophrenia. *Schizophrenia Research,* **132**, 108–13.

Prince M, Bryce R, Albanese E, Wimo A, Ribeiro W and Ferri CP (2013). The global prevalence of dementia: a systematic review and metaanalysis. *Alzheimer's & Dementia,* **9**, 63–75.

Prioleau L, Murdock M and Brody N (1983). An analysis of psychotherapy versus placebo studies. *Behavioral and Brain Sciences*, **6**, 275–310.

Rausch JL, Johnson ME, Fei YJ *et al.* (2002). Initial conditions of serotonin transporter kinetics and genotype: influence on SSRI treatment trial outcome. *Biological Psychiatry*, **51**, 723–32.

Rief W, Nestoriuc Y, Weiss S, Welzel E, Barsky AJ and Hofmann SG (2009). Meta-analysis of the placebo response in antidepressant trials. *Journal of Affective Disorders*, **118**, 1–8.

Rihmer Z, Dome P, Baldwin DS and Gonda X (2012). Psychiatry should not become hostage to placebo: an alternative interpretation of antidepressant-placebo differences in the treatment response in depression. *European Neuropsychopharmacology*, **22**, 782–6.

Ritchie K and Lovestone S (2002). The dementias. *Lancet*, **360**, 1759–66.

Robinson TE and Berridge KC (1993). The neural basis of drug craving: an incentive-sensitization theory of addiction. *Brain Research Reviews*, **18**, 247–91.

Rogers SL, Farlow MR, Doody RS, Mohs R and Friedhoff LT (1998). A 24-week, double-blind, placebo-controlled trial of donepezil in patients with Alzheimer's disease. *Neurology*, **50**, 136–45.

Rolls ET, Critchley HD, Mason R and Wakeman EA (1996). Orbitofrontal cortex neurons: role in olfactory and visual association learning. *Journal of Neurophysiology*, **75**, 1970–81.

Roman GC, Erkinjuntti T, Wallin A, Pantoni L and Chui HC (2002). Subcortical ischaemic vascular dementia. *Lancet Neurology*, **1**, 426–36.

Rose JE, Tashkin DP, Ertle A, Zinser MC and Lafer R (1985). Sensory blockade of smoking satisfaction. *Pharmacology, Biochemistry, and Behavior*, **23**, 289–93.

Rosler M, Anand R, Cicin-Sain A *et al.* (1999). Efficacy and safety of rivastigmine in patients with Alzheimer's disease: International randomised controlled trial. *British Medical Journal*, **318**, 633–8.

Ross DF and Pihl RO (1989). Modification of the balanced-placebo design for use at high blood alcohol levels. *Addictive Behaviors*, **14**, 91–7.

Rutherford BR, Mori S, Sneed JR, Pimontel MA and Roose SP (2012). Contribution of spontaneous improvement to placebo response in depression: a meta-analytic review. *Journal of Psychiatric Research*, **46**, 697–702.

Rutherford BR and Roose SP (2013). A model of placebo response in antidepressant clinical trials. *American Journal of Psychiatry*, **170**(7), 723–33.

Sandler AD, Glesne CE and Bodfish JW (2010). Conditioned placebo dose reduction: a new treatment in attention-deficit hyperactivity disorder? *Journal of Developmental and Behavioral Pediatrics*, **31**, 369–75.

Santarelli L, Saxe M, Gross C *et al.* (2003). Requirement of hippocampal neurogenesis for the behavioral effects of antidepressants. *Science*, **301**, 805–9.

Scherder EJ (2000). Low use of analgesics in Alzheimer's disease: possible mechanisms. *Psychiatry*, **63**, 1–12.

Scherder EJ, Oosterman J, Swaab D *et al.* (2005). Recent developments in pain in dementia. *British Medical Journal*, **330**, 461–4.

Scherder EJA, Sergeant JA and Swaab DF (2003). Pain processing in dementia and its relation to neuropathology. *Lancet Neurology*, **2**, 677–86.

Schlauch RC, Waesche MC, Riccardi CJ *et al.* (2010). A meta-analysis of the effectiveness of placebo manipulations in alcohol-challenge studies. *Psychology of Addictive Behaviors*, **24**, 239–53.

Schultz W (2002). Getting formal with dopamine and reward. *Neuron*, **36**, 241–63.

Schultz W, Tremblay L and Hollerman JR (2000). Reward processing in primate orbitofrontal cortex and basal ganglia. *Cerebral Cortex*, **10**, 272–8.

Scott DJ, Stohler CS, Egnatuk CM, Wang H, Koeppe RA and Zubieta JK (2007). Individual differences in reward responding explain placebo-induced expectations and effects. *Neuron*, **55**, 325–36.

Smith ML and Glass GV (1977). Meta-analysis of psychotherapy outcome studies. *American Psychologist*, **32**, 752–60.

Stolerman IP and Jarvis MJ (1995). The scientific case that nicotine is addictive. *Psychopharmacology*, **117**, 2–10.

Strupp HH and Hadley SW (1979). Specific vs non-specific factors in psychotherapy. A controlled study of outcome. *Archives of General Psychiatry*, **36**, 1125–36.

Tate JC, Stanton AL, Green SB, Schmitz JM, Le T and Marshall B (1994). Experimental analysis of the role of expectancy in nicotine withdrawal. *Psychology of Addictive Behaviors*, **8**, 169–78.

Testa M, Fillmore MT, Norris J et al. (2006). Understanding alcohol expectancy effects: revisiting the placebo condition. *Alcohol Clinical and Experimental Research*, **30**, 339–48.

Thompson PM, Hayashi KM, de Zubicaray G et al. (2003). Dynamics of gray matter loss in Alzheimer's disease. *Journal of Neuroscience*, **23**, 994–1005.

Van Ree JM, Schagen Van Leeuwen JH, Koppeschaar HP and Te Velde ER (2005). Unexpected placebo response in premenstrual dysphoric disorder: implication of endogenous opioids. *Psychopharmacology*, **182**, 318–19.

Volkow ND, Wang GJ, Ma Y et al. (2003). Expectation enhances the regional brain metabolic and the reinforcing effects of stimulants in cocaine abusers. *Journal of Neuroscience*, **23**, 11461–8.

Volkow ND, Wang GJ, Ma Y et al. (2006). Effects of expectation on the brain metabolic responses to methylphenidate and to its placebo in non-drug abusing subjects. *NeuroImage*, **32**, 1782–92.

Wager TD, Rilling JK, Smith EE et al. (2004). Placebo-induced changes in fMRI in the anticipation and experience of pain. *Science*, **303**, 1162–6.

Walsh BT, Seidman SN, Sysko R and Gould M (2002). Placebo response in studies of major depression: variable, substantial, and growing. *Journal of the American Medical Association*, **287**, 1840–7.

Weiss RD, O'Malley SS, Hosking JD, Locastro JS, Swift R and COMBINEStudy Research Group (2008). Do patients with alcohol dependence respond to placebo? Results from the COMBINE Study. *Journal of Studies on Alcohol and Drugs*, **69**, 878–84.

Welge JA and Keck Jr PE (2003). Moderators of placebo response to antipsychotic treatment in patients with schizophrenia: a meta-regression. *Psychopharmacology*, **166**, 1–10.

Zhang W and Luo J (2009). The transferable placebo effect from pain to emotion: changes in behavior and EEG activity. *Psychophysiology*, **46**, 626–34.

Zhang W, Qin S, Guo J and Luo J (2011). A follow-up fMRI study of a transferable placebo anxiolytic effect. *Psychophysiology*, **48**, 1119–28.

Zubieta JK, Bueller JA, Jackson LR et al. (2005). Placebo effects mediated by endogenous opioid activity on μ-opioid receptors. *Journal of Neuroscience*, **25**, 7754–62.

Chapter 7

Immune and endocrine systems

Summary points

- The placebo effect in the immune and endocrine system is basically a conditioned response, whereby classical conditioning plays a key role.
- Conditioned immunosuppression affects a number of immune mediators, like interleukin-2 (IL-2) and interferon-gamma (IFN-γ).
- Some negative allergic reactions may be induced by the administration of nocebos.
- The responses of some hormones, like insulin, growth hormone, and cortisol, have been successfully conditioned.
- The hypothalamus–pituitary–adrenal (HPA) axis may represent an important system in placebo and nocebo responsiveness.

7.1 Immunity and hormone secretion are subject to psychosocial influences

It has long been known that both immune mediators and hormones are influenced by the brain, and one of the most studied of these influences is the so-called stress response. Psychoneuroendocrinoimmunology is a biomedical discipline aimed at investigating how stress, and more in general a negative and/or positive psychosocial context, may affect the immune system and the secretion of hormones. Therefore, it is not surprising that the immune and endocrine systems are involved in placebo and placebo-related effects. As already described in section 4.2, nocebo hyperalgesia can be considered a stress response after all. Nocebo suggestions induce anxiety and activate the HPA axis, thus increasing adrenocorticotropic hormone (ACTH) and cortisol plasma concentrations (Benedetti et al., 2006, 2007). Indeed, many stress responses and many experimental models used in the psychoneuroendocrinoimmunological approach can be conceptualized as placebo-related, or nocebo-related, effects whereby negative psychosocial influences and negative expectations are at work. This is the reason why those working in the field of psychoneuroendocrinoimmunology became interested in placebo phenomena, and conceptualized many behaviorally conditioned effects of immunomodulation as placebo or placebo-like effects (Ader, 1985, 1997; Pacheco-Lopez et al., 2006).

There may be many neural and neuroendocrine pathways through which the psychosocial context affects immune and hormonal functions. For example, the HPA axis (whereby the hypothalamic corticotropin-releasing hormone, CRH, stimulates secretion of pituitary ACTH, which then stimulates cortisol secretion from the adrenal glands) is typically activated in stressful situations, and cortisol (one of the main glucocorticoids of the adrenal glands) is intimately related to immune functions. In fact, at physiological concentrations it causes a shift in immune responses from a type 1 proinflammatory cytokine pattern (e.g., tumor necrosis factor alpha) to a type 2 anti-inflammatory cytokine pattern (e.g., interleukin-10) (Elenkov and Chrousos, 1999). At higher concentrations, cortisol is immunosuppressive, thus the hyperactivity of the HPA axis tends to suppress immune responses and predisposes to infections (Sternberg, 1997a, 1997b).

It should also be remembered that during the stress response the CRH–ACTH–cortisol axis is not the only hyperactive neuroendocrine system—many other hormones can be affected as well. Many of these mechanisms are only partially known, some are even totally unknown, and psychoneuroendocrinoimmunology is trying to better understand the psychosocial influences on all these immune and endocrine functions.

Other pathways connecting the brain to the immune system involve the autonomic nervous system. For example, the ventromedial hypothalamus controls sympathetic innervation of the spleen, and the splenic nerve controls, at least in part, activity of natural killer cells (Katafuchi et al., 1993, 1994; Okamoto et al., 1996). Besides the sympathetic system (Elenkov et al., 2000) the vagus and parasympathetic cholinergic system has been found to affect immune functions (Tracey, 2002; Pavlov and Tracey, 2005). Therefore, opposing activation of the sympathetic and parasympathetic systems has profound effects on immune responses. Boxes 7.1 and 7.2 illustrate the very general organization of the immune system and of the hypersensitivity immune responses.

Box 7.1 A quick overview of the immune system

The main objective of the immune system is to defend the organism from invaders, such as viruses and bacteria. The organization of this system is quite complex and there are many variations across species. For example, even simple unicellular organisms such as bacteria possess an immune system; however, this is basically represented by enzyme systems that protect against viral infections. By contrast, vertebrates such as humans have a more sophisticated defense mechanism that consists of many types of proteins, cells, organs, and tissues, which interact in an elaborate and dynamic network. As part of this more complex immune response, the human immune system adapts over time to recognize specific pathogens more efficiently. This adaptation process is referred to as adaptive immunity and creates immunological memory, which is the basis of vaccines. Even plants possess a form of innate immunity but lack of adaptive immunity. Some immune responses are mediated by T lymphocytes, which turn into macrophages, and B lymphocytes, which turn into plasma cells (Fig. 7.1). Whereas macrophages destroy antigens through phagocytosis, plasma cells produce antibodies which bind to antigens and destroy them.

Box 7.1 A quick overview of the immune system (continued)

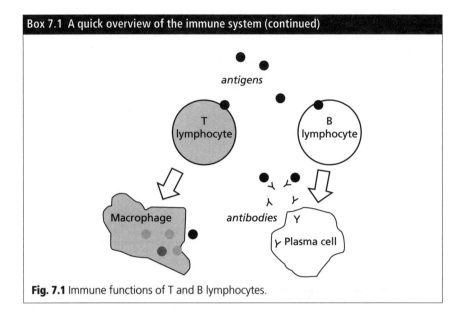

Fig. 7.1 Immune functions of T and B lymphocytes.

7.2 **The immune system**

7.2.1 **Immune responses can be conditioned**

An intriguing observation was reported in 1896 by MacKenzie (1896) who showed that some people who are allergic to flowers show an allergic reaction when presented with something that superficially looks like a flower, but contains no pollen (an artificial flower). In this case, the association between the features of the flower (color and shape, and the like) and the pollen antigen inside the flower may lead to a conditioned response, whereby the color and the shape of the flower may induce a conditioned allergic response. As described in section 2.3.3, according to this perspective a placebo response may occur on the basis of classic Pavlovian conditioning mechanisms. Indeed, the immune system provides some of the best evidence for the placebo effect as a conditioned response deriving from repeated associations between an antigen and conditioned stimulus. Most, if not all, research in this field began in animal models of behaviorally conditioned immunosuppression. Therefore, the immune system represents a very good example of placebo responses in animals via classical conditioning.

Early experimental evidence of a relationship between the brain and the immune system was obtained in the 1920s from conditioning experiments of the immune response (Metal'nikov and Chorine, 1926). However, the first compelling evidence that immunological responses can be behaviorally conditioned was obtained by a long series of experiments performed in the 1970s and 1980s. For example, Ader and Cohen (1975) employed a taste-aversion conditioning paradigm in rats. The rats were given a flavored drinking solution (saccharin) that was paired with the immunosuppressive drug, cyclophosphamide, and were subsequently immunized with sheep red blood cells. Rats that were re-exposed to saccharin at the time of antigenic stimulation were found to have low hemagglutinating antibodies 6 days after injection of the sheep red blood cells; these levels were lower than those in conditioned animals that were not re-exposed to saccharin, nonconditioned animals given saccharin, and animals given a placebo. Thus, saccharin was capable of mimicking the immunosuppressive action of cyclophosphamide. At that time, these findings were replicated at least by two studies (Rogers et al., 1976; Wayner et al., 1978).

Behavioral conditioning has also been found in a graft-versus-host response, a phenomenon that is suppressed by injections of low-dose cyclophosphamide (Whitehouse et al., 1973). In fact, three injections of low-dose cyclophosphamide are capable of reducing the weight of lymph nodes following injection of a cellular graft. By contrast, a single low dose is much less effective. However, if the single low dose of cyclophosphamide is paired to saccharin in rats that had previously been conditioned with saccharin, the single low dose is capable of inducing graft-versus-host responses like those obtained with three doses.

Over the following years, it was observed that conditioned enhancement of antibody production is possible, using an antigen as an unconditioned stimulus of the immune system. Gorczynski et al. (1982) grafted skin tissue from C57BL/6J mice to CBA mice many times. Although the recipient mice were then re-exposed to the grafting procedures, but without receiving the allogenic tissue, there was nonetheless an increase in the number of cytotoxic lymphocyte precursor cells in response to the conditioned stimulus. In another study, mice were given repeated immunizations with keyhole limpet hemocyanin paired with a gustatory conditioned stimulus (chocolate milk). A classically conditioned enhancement of antikeyhole limpet hemocyanin (anti-KLH) antibodies was observed when the mice were re-exposed to the gustatory stimulus along with a low-dose injection of keyhole limpet hemocyanin (Ader et al., 1993). Subsequently, Alvarez-Borda et al. (1995) found an increase in immunoglobulins IgG and IgM in animals re-exposed to a conditioned stimulus previously paired with an antigen (hen egg lysosome). These behaviorally conditioned immune responses have been found to undergo "extinction," thus lending support to the notion that associative processes are involved in the behavioral alteration of immune responses (Gorczynski et al., 1982; Bovbjerg et al., 1984).

Studying conditioned immune responses in humans is not as easy as in animals. In fact, some early studies produced contrasting results. Smith and McDaniels (1983) described a conditionally reduced delayed-type hypersensitivity response that was not, however, elicited by a conditioned stimulus previously paired with tuberculin. These findings were not confirmed in a subsequent study (Booth et al., 1995). Contrasting results were also obtained in human studies on conditioned increases in natural killer cell activity (Kirschbaum et al., 1992a), in allergic rhinitis patients (Gauci et al., 1994), and on recombinant IFN-γ as an unconditioned stimulus (Longo et al., 1999).

Another study provided convincing evidence that behavioral conditioning of immunosuppression is possible in humans (Goebel et al., 2002). Repeated associations between ciclosporin A and a flavored drink induced conditioned immunosuppression in healthy male volunteers, in which the flavored drink alone suppressed immune functions as assessed by means of interleukin-2 (IL-2) and IFN-γ mRNA expression, in vitro release of IL-2 and IFN-γ, as well as lymphocyte proliferation (Fig. 7.2). It is

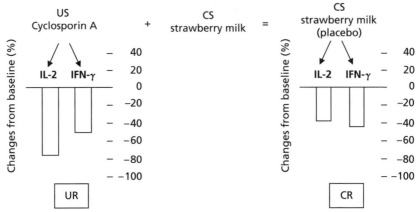

Fig. 7.2 Repeated associations between the immunosuppressive drug ciclosporin A (US, unconditioned stimulus)—which inhibits both IL-2 and IFN-γ (UR, unconditioned response)—and strawberry milk (CS, conditioned stimulus) induce conditioned responses (CR) whereby the CS alone (a placebo in all respects) is capable of inhibiting both IL-2 and IFN-γ. Data from Goebel MU, Trebst AE, Steiner J, Xie YF, Exton MS et al., Behavioral conditioning of immunosuppression is possible in humans, *FASEB Journal*, 16, pp. 1869–73, Federation of American Societies for Experimental Biology.

interesting to note that the effects of the conditioned stimulus were the same as those of the specific effects of ciclosporin A. In fact, ciclosporin A binds to cyclophilins, leading to inhibition of intracellular phosphatase calcineurin, and selectively reduces the expression of some cytokines (e.g., IL-2 and IFN-γ) which finally results in the suppression of T-cell function. A later study by the same group suggested that more than a single associative learning trial would be needed in order to produce immune conditioned effects (Goebel et al., 2005), thus emphasizing the important role of learning in placebo responsiveness.

Overall, different immune parameters have been found to be affected by behavioral conditioning paradigms. A summary of these is shown in Table 7.1 (Pacheco-Lopez et al., 2006). As described in section 2.2.3, it is worth noting that these responses can be considered placebo effects in all respects, as the conditioned (neutral) stimulus is an inert substance that acquires the capacity of producing drug-like effects.

It is important to point out that behavioral conditioning seems to be a necessary condition in order to induce immune placebo responses. In fact, cognitive factors alone do not seem to work. For example, Albring et al. (2012) investigated whether a single re-exposition to the conditioned stimulus is able to induce a behaviorally conditioned immunosuppression, and found that, in contrast to four conditioned stimulus re-expositions, a single re-exposition was not sufficient to significantly suppress IL-2 production. In addition, the mere expectation of taking an immunosuppressant did not cause an immunosuppressive response. However, it is worth mentioning that recent research provides some evidence that in some circumstances

Table 7.1 Immune parameters affected by behavioral conditioning paradigms (CTL, cytotoxic T lymphocyte; NK, natural killer). Reprinted from *Brain, Behavior, and Immunity*, 20 (5), Gustavo Pacheco-López, Harald Engler, Maj-Britt Niemi, and Manfred Schedlowski, Expectations and associations that heal: Immunomodulatory placebo effects and its neurobiology, pp. 430–446, Copyright (2006), with permission from Elsevier

Conditioned stimulus	Unconditioned stimulus	Conditioned response
Taste/odor	Immunosuppressant drugs	↓ Antibody production
		↓ Lymphocyte proliferation
		↓ Hypersensitivity
		↓ Allergic response
		↓ Allograft rejection
		↓ NK-cell activity
		↓ Cytokines
Taste/odor	Immunostimulating drugs/antigens	↑ Skin hypersensitivity
Auditory/visual Touch		↑ NK-cell activity
		↑ CTL activity
		↑ Neutrophil activity
		↑ Antibody production
		↑ Histamine release
		↑ Anaphylaxis
		↑ Complement

the immune system can be modulated by expectations. Vits et al. (2013) found that in patients with house dust mite allergy immune placebo responses do not require a learning procedure, but they can also be induced by cognitive factors such as expectations.

Interestingly, Klein et al. (2008) studied the effect of a vaccination-like procedure with a placebo on immunocompetent cells from healthy individuals. These subjects were injected subcutaneously with 1 mL physiological saline twice a week for up to 12 weeks. Lymphocytes were isolated before and during exposure and incubated with recall antigens (purified protein derivative, tetanus toxoid, bacillus Calmette–Guérin). Then, the production of T-helper type 1-, type 2-, and macrophage/monocyte-related cytokines was analyzed, and a significant increase of the recall-antigen-induced production of IFN-γ, IL-5, IL-13, TNF-α, and granulocyte-macrophage colony-stimulating factor (GM-CSF) was found. This study shows that subcutaneous injection of placebo enhances immunoreactivity, although the underlying mechanism is not clear: many factors might be involved, such as psychological aspects, activation of the autonomic nervous system, or local activation of mast cells or dendritic cells.

Box 7.2 Hypersensitivity

Undesirable reactions produced by the normal immune system are collected, as a whole, under the term hypersensitivity. These reactions may be damaging, uncomfortable, and sometimes fatal. According to the classification by Gell and Coombs (1963), there are four types of hypersensitivity:

Hypersensitivity type I. This refers to allergy, that is, reactions occurring when the immune system reacts to normally harmless substances in the environment. These substances are called allergens. Typical allergies are anaphylaxis and asthma. The antibodies that mediate this reaction are IgE and IgG4.

Hypersensitivity type II. This refers to antibody-dependent cell-mediated cytotoxicity, whereby an effector cell of the immune system attacks a target cell, whose membrane-surface antigens have been bound by specific antibodies. Typical disorders are represented by autoimmune hemolytic anemia and myasthenia gravis. This type is mediated by IgM, IgG, and complement.

Hypersensitivity type III. In this type, an immune complex is formed from the binding of an antibody to a soluble antigen. These immune complexes can be subject to a variety of responses, such as phagocytosis and processing by proteases, and may themselves cause disease when they are deposited in organs. This deposition is a typical feature of systemic lupus erythematosus and rheumatoid arthritis. IgG and complement mediate this hypersensitivity.

Hypersensitivity type IV. This is a delayed type hypersensitivity, that is, the reaction takes 2–3 days to develop and, differently from the other types, it is not mediated by antibodies but by cells, like T cells and macrophages. Typical examples are chronic transplant rejection, multiple sclerosis, and contact dermatitis.

7.2.2 Can conditioning of immune placebo responses affect the course of autoimmune diseases and allergies?

In order to see whether conditioned immune responses could be of any biological or clinical relevance, it is necessary to study immune functions and responses in pathological conditions to see whether behavioral conditioning affects immune diseases. Ader and Cohen (1982) paired a conditioned stimulus (again, a solution of saccharin) with an unconditioned stimulus (cyclophosphamide) in NZB/NZW hybrid mice. This is a standard model for systemic lupus erythematosus in humans (Steinberg et al., 1981; Theofilopoulos and Dixon, 1981). The mice developed a lethal glomerulonephritis at 8–14 months of age, and progression of this disease can be delayed by cyclophosphamide (Casey, 1968; Morris et al., 1976). Ader and Cohen (1982) continued to give one group saccharin alone and found that the mice that were conditioned by pairing saccharin and cyclophosphamide showed less severe glomerulonephritis (as assessed through proteinuria measurements) and longer survival times compared with nonconditioned mice. Similarly, the severity of adjuvant-induced arthritis in rats was found to be reduced by conditioned stimuli that had been previously associated with immunosuppressive stimuli (Klosterhalfen and Klosterhalfen, 1983; Lysle et al., 1992).

The possible clinical implications of behavioral conditioning are also evident in transplantation models of graft reject. On the basis of the fact that A/J mice reject skin grafts from BALB/c or C57BL/6 donors and that cyclophosphamide promotes survival of the allograft, Gorczynski (1990) paired saccharin with cyclophosphamide and subsequently re-exposed conditioned A/J mice to saccharin alone. Survival of the skin allograft was prolonged by saccharin. Similar findings were obtained in other studies (Grochowicz et al., 1991; Exton et al., 1998).

Besides these studies in animals, there is little experimental evidence suggesting that conditioned immune placebo responses are relevant in autoimmune diseases (Box 7.3) in humans. For example, a clinical case study of a child with lupus erythematosus has been described by Olness and Ader (1992). The child received Cytoxan® (cyclophosphamide) paired with taste and smell stimuli, according to the conditioning procedure used in animals. During the course of 12 months a clinically successful outcome was obtained by using taste and smell stimuli alone on half the monthly chemotherapy sessions. In another study, multiple sclerosis patients received four monthly intravenous treatments with cyclophosphamide paired with anise-flavored syrup (Giang et al., 1996). After 6 months of administering the placebo treatment paired with the drink, eight out of ten patients displayed decreased peripheral leukocyte counts—mimicking the effects of cyclophosphamide.

Goebel et al. (2008) investigated the conditionability of antiallergic effects in patients suffering from house-dust mite allergy and treated with a histamine-1 receptor antagonist. During the association phase, 30 patients received a novel-tasting drink once daily, followed by a standard dose of the histamine-1 receptor antagonist, desloratadine, on 5 consecutive days. After 9 days of drug washout, the evocation trial commenced: ten patients received water together with an identically looking placebo pill (water group), 11 patients were re-exposed to the novel-tasting drink and received a placebo pill (conditioned stimulus group), and nine patients received water and desloratadine (drug group). During the association phase, desloratadine treatment decreased the subjective total symptom scores, attenuated the effects of the skin prick test for histamine, and reduced basophil activation ex vivo in all groups. During the evocation trial, the water group, in which subjects were not re-exposed to the gustatory stimulus, showed a reduction in subjective total symptom scores and skin prick test results, but no inhibition of basophil activation. In contrast, re-exposure to the novel-tasting drink decreased basophil activation, the skin prick test result and the subjective symptom score in the conditioned stimulus group to a degree that was similar to the effects of desloratadine in the drug group. Therefore, behaviorally conditioned effects are not only able to relieve subjective rhinitis symptoms and allergic skin reactions, but also to induce changes in effector immune functions.

Box 7.3 Autoimmune diseases

Inappropriate immune responses of the body against substances and tissues normally present in the body give rise to autoimmune diseases. This may be restricted to certain organs or may involve a particular tissue in different places, for example, the basement membrane both in the lung and in the kidney (Goodpasture's disease). Whereas the autoimmune origin of many diseases is widely accepted, the autoimmune pathophysiology for other diseases is only suspected. This distinction makes a big difference, because the treatment of an autoimmune disorder is typically based on the use of immunosuppressant agents. Table 7.2 gives some examples.

Table 7.2 Diseases with an accepted or suspected autoimmune origin

Accepted autoimmune origin	Suspected autoimmune origin
Autoimmune hemolytic anemia	Ankylosing spondylitis
Autoimmune hepatitis	Chronic obstructive pulmonary disease
Autoimmune pancreatitis	Endometriosis
Celiac disease	Interstitial cystitis
Crohn's disease	Multiple sclerosis
Diabetes mellitus type 1	Narcolepsy
Guillain–Barré syndrome	Progressive inflammatory neuropathy
Hashimoto's thyroiditis	Raynaud phenomenon
Lupus erythematosus	Restless leg syndrome
Myasthenia gravis	Sarcoidosis
Pernicious anemia	Schizophrenia
Psoriasis	Scleroderma
Rheumatoid arthritis	Vitiligo

7.2.3 Specific and discrete neural networks are responsible for immune placebo effects

Conditioning of immune placebo responses represents an example of the intimate relationship between the brain and the immune system. The mechanisms underlying the brain–immune interaction and the pathways responsible for behavioral conditioning of immune responses have been partially elucidated (Fig. 7.3). Some experimental evidence of neural networks involved in immune placebo effects comes from lesion studies. Lesions of the insular cortex in rats have been found to disrupt the acquisition of conditioned immunosuppression by taste aversion (Ramirez-Amaya et al., 1996). Likewise, the lesion of the amygdala interferes with the acquisition of conditioned immunosuppressive responses, but has no effect on the performance of pre-existing conditioned responses when the experimental model is the pairing of saccharin taste with cyclophosphamide administration (Ramirez-Amaya et al., 1998). In addition, the insular cortex and the amygdala (but not the hippocampus) have been found to be involved in conditioned enhancement of antibody production when taste or smell stimuli are paired with antigenic stimuli (Ramirez-Amaya and Bermudez-Rattoni, 1999; Chen et al., 2004).

By using the association between saccharin as conditioned stimulus and ciclosporin A as unconditioned stimulus, it has been demonstrated that lesions of specific and discrete brain regions affect the conditioned reduction of splenocyte responsiveness and the conditioned decrease of cytokine (IL-2 and IFN-γ) production (Pacheco-Lopez et al., 2005). The insular cortex is essential for acquiring and evoking these conditioned placebo responses, whereas the amygdala is likely to mediate the input of visceral information necessary at the time of acquisition. By contrast, the ventromedial hypothalamic nucleus seems to participate in the output pathway to the immune system, which is necessary to evoke the behaviorally conditioned immune response (Pacheco-Lopez et al., 2005, 2006).

7.2.4 Several neurotransmitters are implicated in conditioned immune placebo effects

From a neurochemical perspective, several neurotransmitters have been found to be implicated in conditioned immune effects. For example, the recall stage of the conditioned increase of natural killer cell activity in rodents has been found to require catecholamines (Hsueh et al., 1999) and glutamate (Kuo et al., 2001). By employing a behaviorally conditioned immunosuppression paradigm in healthy men to analyze predictors of learned placebo responses, Ober et al. (2012) showed that plasma norepinephrine and state anxiety levels predict placebo response in learned immunosuppression. During acquisition, the subjects received either the immunosuppressant ciclosporin A (unconditioned stimulus) or a placebo together with a novel-tasting drink (conditioned stimulus). During evocation, the subjects were re-exposed to the conditioned stimulus alone. In responders, the conditioned stimulus alone caused a significant inhibition of IL-2 production by anti-CD3-stimulated peripheral blood T cells, closely mimicking the drug effect. Conversely, nonresponders did not show responses different from those of the controls. Baseline IL-2, plasma norepinephrine, and state anxiety predicted nearly 60% of the variance in the conditioned IL-2 response. Other systems, such as the cholinergic and serotoninergic, have been found to play a role in the conditioned natural killer cell response, at both the association and recall stages (Hsueh et al., 2002).

Opioids seem to play a role as well. Morphine decreases natural killer cell activity (Mellon and Bayer, 1998, 1999; Gomez-Flores and Weber, 1999) and opioids in general suppress many immune responses, like antibody production, and delayed-type hypersensitivity. This occurs in part through desensitization of chemokine receptors on neutrophils, monocytes, and lymphocytes (Grimm et al., 1998; Rogers et al., 2000). Pavlovian conditioning of morphine-induced immunomodulating effects has been described (Coussons-Reed et al., 1994a). The opioid antagonist, naltrexone, when injected before conditioning, has been found to prevent acquisition of the conditioned

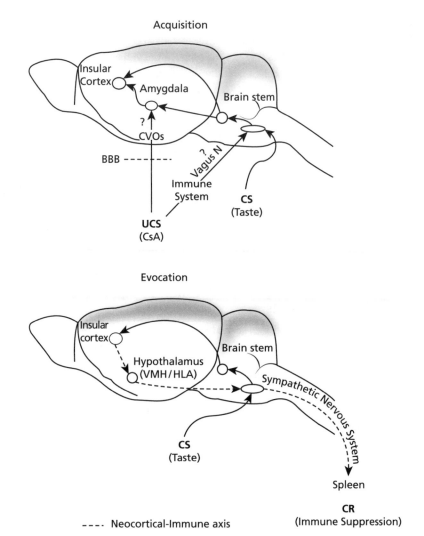

Fig. 7.3 Conditioned immunosuppression model in the rat. The insular cortex may play an associative role, being necessary to acquire and evoke the behavioral conditioned immune response. The amygdala seems to mediate the input of visceral information that is required at the acquisition time (A), whereas lesions of the ventromedial nucleus of the hypothalamus (VMH) disrupt the brain–immune communication necessary to evoke the immunological conditioned response. At the acquisition time, two main afferent routes are possible for the unconditioned stimulus (UCS), which is represented by intraperitoneal ciclosporin A (CsA)—in the indirect afferent route, CsA may disrupt peripheral cytokine homeostasis, which could be detected by the brain's immune-sensing capacities (e.g., vagus nerve); in the direct afferent route, CsA might reach the brain through brain areas with a weak blood–brain barrier (BBB), like the circumventricular organs (CVOs), subsequently signaling to forebrain structures. At the evocation time (B), the

suppression of splenic proliferation of lymphocytes, of natural killer cell activity, and of IL-2 production (Coussons-Reed et al., 1994a). When opioid antagonists were injected before testing (after conditioning) they were found to block the expression of conditioned lymphoproliferative responses, to reduce the suppression of natural killer cell activity, and to have no effect on IL-2 production (Coussons-Reed et al., 1994a). Therefore, opioid receptor activity is involved in the acquisition of conditioned morphine-induced immune responses, as well as in the expression of a subset of these conditioned responses (splenic lymphoproliferation and suppression of natural killer cell activity). Conditioning of morphine-induced immunomodulation has also been found to involve peripheral beta-adrenergic receptors (Coussons-Reed et al., 1994b).

In light of the many neural pathways connecting the brain to the immune system, the involvement of all these neurotransmitters in conditioned immune responses is not surprising. Both the noradrenergic sympathetic system and the cholinergic parasympathetic system are connected to immune functions. For example, the sympathetic system innervates immune organs such as the thymus, spleen, and lymph nodes (Felten, 2000); adrenergic receptors are expressed on lymphocytes and different lymphocyte populations have been found to be differentially sensitive to beta-adrenergic stimulation (Coussons-Reed et al., 1994b). Systemic administration of norepinephrine and epinephrine has also been shown to inhibit the production of type 1 proinflammatory cytokines like IL-12, TNF-α, and IFN-γ, and to stimulate the production of type 2 anti-inflammatory cytokines, such as IL-10 and transforming growth factor TGF-β (Elenkov et al., 2000).

It is also worth remembering that an important pathway that connects the brain to the immune system is the HPA axis, whereby the CRH–ACTH–cortisol axis plays a fundamental role in modulation of many immune functions, with a shift from a proinflammatory pattern of cytokines to an anti-inflammatory pattern (Elenkov and Chrousos, 1999).

7.2.5 Inducing nocebo allergic reactions and adverse events

Untoward effects of drugs and other substances, like food, that are due to allergic reactions are frequent in clinical practice. However, some studies have shown that some of these adverse reactions are nocebo effects. Although few studies have been carried out in this field, some trials show that allergic reactions to inert substances may indeed occur. For example, Jewett et al. (1990) tested adverse effects following placebo administration in double-blind trials of symptom provocation to determine food sensitivity.

Fig. 7.3 (continued) neocortical–immune axis (dotted pathway), with hypothalamic relays and sympathetic peripheral mechanisms, seems to be the efferent pathway through which the brain is able to modify peripheral immune functions. CR: conditioned response; CS: conditioned stimulus; HLA: lateral hypothalamic area. Reproduced from Gustavo Pacheco-López, Maj-Britt Niemi, Wei Kou, Margarete Härting, Joachim Fandrey, and Manfred Schedlowski, Neural Substrates for Behaviorally Conditioned Immunosuppression in the Rat, *The Journal of Neuroscience*, 25 (9), pp. 2330–2337, figure 5 Copyright 2005, The Society for Neuroscience, with permission.

They found that nasal stuffiness, dry mouth, nausea, fatigue, headache, and depression occurred in 27% of the subjects who received the active substance, and in 24% of the patients who received the inert substance. In a similar trial, it was found that 70% of subjects experienced symptoms after saline injections and 15% experienced a skin reaction (Fox et al., 1999).

Passalacqua et al. (2002) performed a study in 452 patients with well-documented reactions, such as urticaria, respiratory symptoms, laryngeal edema, and anaphylaxis. Each oral challenge of a drug was preceded by a placebo: if a reaction occurred, a second placebo was administered. It was found that about 22% of the patients (most of them were women) had untoward reactions after the first placebo and about 35% of these reacted to the second placebo as well. In a subsequent study, Liccardi et al. (2004) evaluated the occurrence and clinical characteristics of nocebo responses in 600 patients with a history of reactions to drugs. They underwent a blind oral challenge with an inert substance, and observed untoward reactions in 27% of patients. Most of these were subjective symptoms, such as itching and headache, and were perceived as troublesome by all patients. Occurrence was significantly higher in women than in men. Another study (Lombardi et al., 2008) obtained similar results.

Although additional studies with adequate control groups need to be performed, these findings are interesting for at least two reasons. First, they show the frequent occurrence of nocebo reactions in the clinical setting of allergic drug and food reactions. Second, they raise the issue of whether all untoward reactions described in the literature are real drug reactions. From a clinical and practical perspective, this leads to the conclusion that oral challenge of an inert substance would be useful to distinguish real allergic reactions from nocebo responses.

Disease-specific adverse events following nonlive vaccines have been described. Nonlive vaccine, because they are inactivated and they do not replicate in vaccinees, do not cause disease-specific adverse reactions. However, Okaïs et al. (2011) found that vaccinees and healthcare professionals tend to report preferentially the symptoms of the disease against which the nonlive vaccine is administered. They found that this is true particularly for the following pairs: gynecological symptoms and the quadrivalent human papillomavirus vaccine, trismus and tetanus vaccines, hepatobiliary disorders and hepatitis B vaccines. Therefore, the adverse reactions following vaccination for these conditions can be attributable to nocebo effects.

7.3 The endocrine system

7.3.1 Insulin conditioning can induce both hypoglycemic and hyperglycemic placebo responses

The first studies on insulin conditioning showed that the hypoglycemic effects of insulin could be conditioned by pairing insulin with a conditioned stimulus in animals (Lichko, 1959; Alvarez-Buyalla and Carrasco-Zanini, 1960; Alvarez-Buyalla et al., 1961). This conditioned hypoglycemia was analyzed in detail by Woods and collaborators in a long series of animal experiments. In a typical experiment, a conditioned stimulus was paired with insulin in rats; in the control group the conditioned stimulus was paired with saline solution. After repeated pairings, the experimental group showed a significant decrease of blood glucose compared to the control group (Woods et al., 1968); this was a conditioned effect that underwent extinction (Woods et al., 1969). Conditioned hypoglycemia was found to be mediated by the vagus nerve, as both vagotomy and pharmacological blockade with atropine abolished it (Woods, 1972). By performing a conditioning procedure with tolbutamide, a drug that stimulates insulin release, Woods et al. (1972) also showed a conditioned insulin secretion that was mediated by the vagus nerve. Interestingly, conditioned insulin secretion was also found by using food as an unconditioned stimulus (Morrell et al., 1988).

In contrast to the studies on conditioned hypoglycemia, Siegel (1972, 1975) found that repeated pairings between a conditioned stimulus and insulin induced an increase in blood glucose. In other words, if hypoglycemia was induced several times by injecting insulin, its replacement with a placebo induced a conditioned response in the opposite direction (see also section 2.3.3). At least two hypotheses have been put forward to explain the discrepancy between the hypo- and hyperglycemic findings. The first comes from a series of experiments performed by Flaherty and Becker (1984) and Flaherty et al. (1987). These investigators found that the conditioned stimulus context (type of cage, smell, etc.) and novelty influenced the direction of the glycemic conditioned response. A novel conditioned stimulus produced conditioned hyperglycemia, while a familiar conditioned stimulus produced conditioned hypoglycemia.

A second explanation for the discrepancy between hypo- versus hyperglycemic conditioned responses resides in the very nature of the unconditioned response (Siegel, 2002). In other words, whenever the conditioned response is opposite to the unconditioned response, the unconditioned response must be defined correctly. For example, the administration of insulin will reduce glucose concentration in the blood. This hypoglycemia, however, is not the unconditioned response, but rather the unconditioned stimulus that is detected by receptors in the central nervous system (see also section 2.3.3). The real unconditioned response should be considered to be the compensatory hyperglycemic response that the central nervous system adopts once the hypoglycemic status has been detected. Therefore, it is clear that by defining the unconditioned response correctly the conditioned response does not go in the opposite direction.

Hypoglycemia can also be conditioned in humans, as shown in Fig. 7.4 (Stockhorst et al., 1999, 2000). The first human observations were performed in schizophrenic patients who underwent insulin shock therapy, whereby high doses of insulin were administered. When insulin was replaced with a placebo, symptoms of hypoglycemia occurred, like sweating, tiredness, and changes in heart rate and blood pressure (Lichko, 1959). Subsequent studies gave contrasting results (Fehm-Wolfsdorf et al., 1993a, 1993b) and the number of acquisition trials was found to be a possible explanation for these discrepant findings (Fehm-Wolfsdorf et al., 1999). In fact, a substantial change in blood glucose was found in nine of 16 subjects after four acquisition trials, whereas only two of 16 subjects showed substantial changes after two acquisition trials. This difference emphasizes once again the important role of learning in the placebo effect, and the reason why sometimes the interindividual variability in placebo responsiveness may be high.

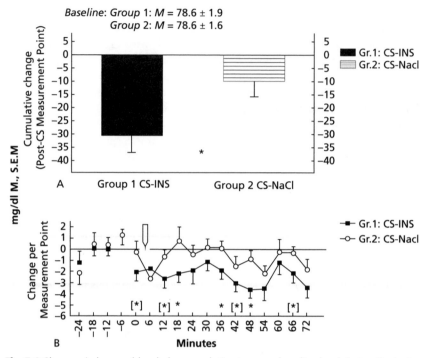

Fig. 7.4 Changes in human blood glucose relative to mean baseline level during the test phase under conditioned stimulus (CS) saline (NaCl) in group 1 (conditioned with insulin, INS; black bar) and group 2 (conditioned with saline; white bar). (A) Cumulative change over the post-CS measurement points (mean SEM). Baseline level is also shown. Note that the decrease in mean cumulative blood glucose was significantly larger in group 1. (B) Change per measurement point. Pre-CS measurements (minutes −24 to −6) are interconnected by dotted lines; post-CS measurements are interconnected by solid lines. Group 1 (black squares) reached lower values than group 2 (white circles). **p < 0.10; *p < 0.05. Reproduced from Ursula Stockhorst, Eva Gritzmann, Kerstin Klopp, Yolanda Schottenfeld-Naor, Achim Hübinger, Hans-Walter Berresheim, Hans-Joachim Steingrüber, and Friedrich Arnold Gries, Classical Conditioning of Insulin Effects in Healthy Humans, *Psychosomatic Medicine*, 61, (4), pp. 424–435, fig 3 Copyright 1999, American Psychosomatic Society, with permission.

Another study that used a placebo control group provided evidence that conditioned hypoglycemia can be obtained in humans (Stockhorst et al., 1999, 2000). Although in this study the conditioned placebo response was not large, the response pattern was consistent. In this study, a trend for a conditioned insulin increase was also found. In addition, there was a first hint that cortisol increased as part of a counter-regulatory response.

7.3.2 **Inducing placebo insulin secretion**

Stimuli that signal food, such as the sight and smell of food (Sjostrom et al., 1980; Johnson and Wildman, 1983; Simon et al., 1986) and imagination or thinking about food

(Goldfine et al., 1970) are all capable of inducing insulin secretion in the beta cells of the pancreas. This is called the cephalic phase of insulin release (see Stockhorst et al., 2000 for a review). Although cephalic-phase insulin secretion, like many other functions described in this book, has never been conceptualized in terms of a placebo effect, it is a good example of how contextual cues can trigger the activation of an endogenous system. Cephalic-phase insulin secretion is mediated by the vagus nerve, as it is abolished by vagotomy (Louis-Sylvestre, 1976; Woods and Bernstein, 1980). In addition, the blockade of vagal activity with atropine in obese humans abolishes the cephalic-phase insulin response (Sjostrom et al., 1980).

Cephalic-phase insulin release is highly variable, both in animals and humans. For example, a different pattern of response has been described, ranging from insulin increase, but not hypoglycemia, to decrease of glucose, but not insulin increase, and to a decrease of both insulin and glucose (Stockhorst et al., 2000). As pointed out by Stockhorst et al. (2000) these different responses may be explained by the involvement of other hormonal responses, like glucagon and catecholamines, in the cephalic phase of insulin secretion. It should also be stressed that while animals show quite consistent responses, human studies show very high variability. Stockhorst et al. (2000) say that high interindividual variability can be explained, at least in part, by responder characteristics. They list a number of factors that could explain such a variability, such as obesity, degree of cognitive control of food intake, gender, and eating disorders, as well as other variables like palatability of food, degree of deprivation, and number and type of stimuli.

Although cephalic-phase insulin release can be conceptualized as a conditioned response whereby conditioned stimuli (like the sight, smell, and taste of food) had previously been associated with food, the demonstration that the cephalic-phase insulin response is a true conditioned response requires the association of a neutral stimulus with an unconditioned stimulus that induces insulin secretion (Stockhorst et al., 2000). To do this, several studies have been aimed at pairing a conditioned stimulus with glucose, which represents the most physiological and natural stimulus for insulin secretion.

Animal studies have shown that the pairing of a conditioned stimulus, such as flavor (Deutsch, 1974), smell (Morrell et al., 1988), and contextual cues of the conditioning cage (Roozendaal et al., 1990) with oral glucose administration induces either conditioned hyperinsulinemia or hypoglycemia. Atropine was found to prevent the response, thus indicating the involvement of the vagus nerve (Woods et al., 1977), and lesions of the amygdala abolished the conditioned response (Roozendaal et al., 1990). Moreover, Holmes et al. (1989) found an increase in serotonin and its metabolite 5-hydroxyindoleacetic acid in both the lateral and ventromedial hypothalamus. Similar results were obtained by pairing a conditioned stimulus with intravenous administration of glucose (Mityushov, 1954; Russek and Pina, 1962; Matysiak and Green, 1984).

There are only a few studies of conditioned hyperinsulinemia in humans. Overduin and Jansen (1997) paired peppermint flavor as a conditioned stimulus with oral administration of glucose in the experimental group, and peppermint with aspartame, which does not induce insulin secretion, in the control group. Although a small increase in insulin secretion was found, no effects on glycemia occurred. In another placebo-controlled experiment in humans, conditioned hyperinsulinemia after glucose conditioning was found to be less pronounced than conditioned hypoglycemia after insulin conditioning (Stockhorst et al., 1999, 2000). Therefore, in contrast to the consistency of the results in animals, to date only a few data are available in humans.

7.3.3 Hypothalamic–pituitary–adrenal activity can be conditioned

The hyperactivity of the HPA axis (Box 7.4) is related to stress, and is typical of the stress response. It can be assessed through measurement of plasma concentrations of hypothalamic CRH and/or pituitary ACTH and/or the adrenal glucocorticoids

---

Box 7.4 The hypothalamus–pituitary system

The hypothalamus–pituitary system controls many endocrine functions in the body. The hormones of the anterior pituitary gland are controlled by hypothalamic hormones. For example, the thyroid-stimulating hormone (TSH) is controlled by the hypothalamic TSH-releasing hormone (TRH); the adrenocorticotropic hormone (ACTH) is controlled by the hypothalamic corticotropin-releasing hormone (CRH); and the two gonadotropins, follicle-stimulating hormone (FSH) and luteinizing hormone (LH), are controlled by the hypothalamic gonadotropin-releasing hormone (GnRH). The hypothalamus also controls the growth hormone (GH) through a GH-releasing hormone (GHRH) and a GH-inhibiting hormone (GHIH), and prolactin (PRL) through a PRL-releasing hormone (PRH) and a PRL-inhibiting hormone (PIH) (Fig. 7.5). ACTH is secreted, together with the melanocyte-stimulating hormone (MSH) and β-endorphin, by the pro-opiomelanocortin (POMC) cells. The CRH–ACTH–cortisol system is better known as the hypothalamus–pituitary–adrenal (HPA) system.

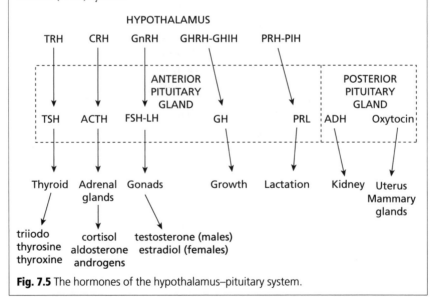

Fig. 7.5 The hormones of the hypothalamus–pituitary system.

Box 7.4 The hypothalamus–pituitary system (continued)

The hormones of the posterior pituitary gland, antidiuretic (ADH or vasopressin) and oxytocin, are synthetized in the hypothalamus, transported to the posterior pituitary gland through the pituitary peduncle, and then released into the bloodstream.

There are other endocrine glands in the body that are not under the hypothalamus–pituitary control. These include the parathyroid glands, which release the parathyroid hormone (regulating calcium metabolism), and the endocrine pancreas, which secretes insulin (regulating glucose metabolism).

(e.g., cortisol). Some animal studies show that the activity of the HPA axis can be conditioned by pairing a conditioned stimulus, such as a contextual cue or flavor, with an unconditioned aversive stimulus that triggers a stress response, such as an electric shock or injection of cytotoxic drug (Ader, 1976; Stanton and Levine, 1988). Similarly, a conditioned decrease in activity of the HPA axis, as assessed by plasma glucocorticoid concentration, has been shown in rats by pairing a conditioned stimulus with daily feeding (Coover et al., 1977).

Only limited information exists in humans. In one randomized, double-blind, placebo-controlled study, a flavored beverage was paired with oral administration of dexamethasone (Sabbioni et al., 1997). After three pairings (separated by 1 week from each other) researchers found that the flavored beverage alone induced an increase in plasma cortisol. This is a typical example of a compensatory conditioned response, whereby the conditioned response goes in the opposite direction of the unconditioned response, as already discussed for hypo- and hyperglycemia. In fact, the administration of dexamethasone induces a decrease in plasma cortisol levels, whereas the conditioned response in the study by Sabbioni et al. (1997) was an increase in cortisol. As discussed previously (sections 2.3.3 and 7.3.1) for insulin conditioning, the unconditioned response is not so much the direct effect of the drug, but rather the response of the central nervous system to the effects of the drug. In the study by Sabbioni et al. (1997) the unconditioned response is not the dexamethasone-induced decrease of cortisol, but rather the response of the central nervous system to the decrease of cortisol; that is, a compensatory increase in hypothalamic CRH, pituitary ACTH, and adrenal cortisol. By this reasoning, the conditioned increase in cortisol does not go in the opposite direction of the unconditioned response.

It is worth noting that in the human study by Sabbioni et al. (1997) the conditioned cortisol changes are quite small (about 15%) compared to the effects of dexamethasone (more than 50%), or the treadmill exercise (more than 100%) (Luger et al., 1987), or the psychological stress of public speaking (up to 250%) (Kirschbaum et al., 1992b). Nonetheless, this study in humans is in keeping with the data obtained in animals.

7.3.4 Conditioning but not expectation induces growth hormone and cortisol placebo responses

In order to assess whether conditioning on the one hand and expectation on the other affect hormone secretion, it would be necessary to devise experiments in which the

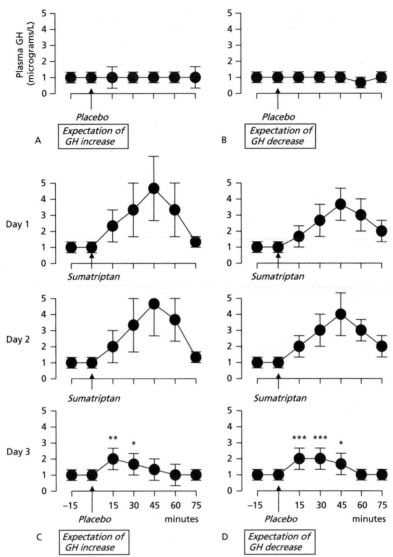

Fig. 7.6 Verbal suggestions of growth hormone (GH) increase (A) and decrease (B) have no effect on GH plasma concentrations. (C) After 2 days of sumatriptan preconditioning, suggestion of GH increase (placebo) mimics the effects of sumatriptan. (D) This effect is not caused by the suggestion itself, however, because the same sumatriptan-like effect is present after the opposite verbal instruction. *p < 0.05; ***p < 0.01. Reproduced from Fabrizio Benedetti, Antonella Pollo, Leonardo Lopiano, Michele Lanotte, Sergio Vighetti, and Innocenzo Rainero, Conscious Expectation and Unconscious Conditioning in Analgesic, Motor, and Hormonal Placebo/Nocebo Responses, *The Journal of Neuroscience*, 23 (10), pp. 4315–4323, fig 5 Copyright 2003, The Society for Neuroscience, with permission.

same hormones are tested by means of conditioning procedures or manipulation of expectation. In one study aimed at differentiating the effects of conditioning and expectation, plasma levels of both growth hormone and cortisol were measured in different conditions (Benedetti et al., 2003).

First, verbal suggestions of growth hormone increase and cortisol decrease were delivered to healthy volunteers, so as to make them expect hormonal changes. These verbal instructions did not have any effect on either hormone and, in fact, no change in plasma concentration was detected. Second, sumatriptan (an agonist of serotonin type 1B/1D receptors that stimulates growth hormone and inhibits cortisol secretion; Rainero et al., 2001) was administered for 2 days in a row and then replaced with a placebo on the third day. After placebo administration there was a significant increase in growth hormone and a decrease in cortisol concentration (Figs. 7.6 and 7.7). These conditioned effects occurred regardless of the verbal suggestions the subjects received. In other words, the placebo mimicked the sumatriptan-induced increase in growth hormone, even though the subjects expected a decrease in growth hormone. Likewise, the placebo mimicked the sumatriptan-induced decrease in cortisol, even though subjects expected an increase. It can be assumed in this case that the conditioned stimulus was represented by the act of injecting the pharmacological agent (the context around the treatment).

7.4 **Points for further discussion**

1 Behavioral conditioning of the immune system is a robust phenomenon that is worthy of further scientific inquiry. What we need to know is which immune functions are affected as well as the role of placebo responsiveness within the context of psychoneuroendocrinoimmunology.

2 One crucial point is the applicability of behavioral immunosuppression in the real clinical setting, for example, to reduce the intake of immunosuppressive drugs. In this sense, we need to explore several medical conditions, such as lupus, and to perform trials in humans.

3 Unwanted allergic reactions are a fruitful field of research for nocebo phenomena and may have important clinical implications. For example, is a first trial with nocebo indicated to see whether the allergic reaction has a psychological origin?

4 As for the immune system, we need to investigate the conditioned responses of different hormones, ranging from pituitary to pancreatic hormones and from thyroid to sex hormones. This would give a clearer picture of the applicability of the hormonal conditioned responses in the clinic.

5 A critical point is the differentiation between conditioning and expectation mechanisms. Although classical conditioning seems to play a key role in hormone and immune secretion, is there any role for expectation? Are there immune mediators and/or hormones that are affected by expectation and anticipatory mechanisms?

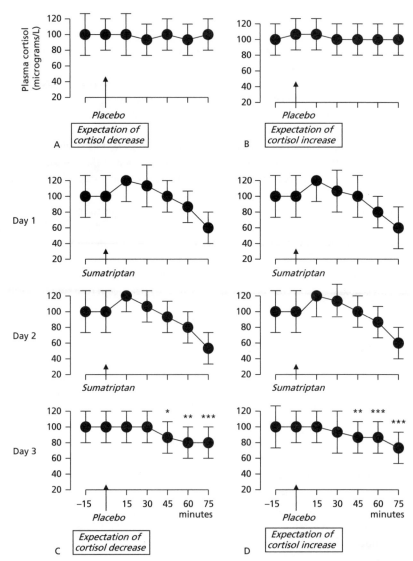

Fig. 7.7 Verbal suggestions of cortisol decrease (A) and increase (B) have no effect on cortisol plasma concentrations. (C) After 2 days of sumatriptan preconditioning, suggestion of cortisol decrease (placebo) mimics the effects of sumatriptan. (D) This effect is not caused by the suggestion itself, however, because the same sumatriptan-like effect is present after the opposite instruction. *$p < 0.04$; **$p < 0.02$; ***$p < 0.01$. Reproduced from Fabrizio Benedetti, Antonella Pollo, Leonardo Lopiano, Michele Lanotte, Sergio Vighetti, and Innocenzo Rainero, Conscious Expectation and Unconscious Conditioning in Analgesic, Motor, and Hormonal Placebo/Nocebo Responses, *The Journal of Neuroscience*, 23 (10), pp. 4315–4323, fig 6 Copyright 2003, The Society for Neuroscience, with permission.

References

Ader R (1976). Conditioned adrenocortical steroid elevations in the rat. *Journal of Comparative Physiology and Psychology*, **90**, 1156–63.

Ader R (1985). Conditioned immunopharmacological effects in animals: implications for a conditioning model of pharmacotherapy. In L White, B Tursky and GE Schwartz, eds. *Placebo: theory, research, and mechanisms*, pp. 306–23. Guilford Press, New York.

Ader R (1997). The role of conditioning in pharmacotherapy. In A Harrington, ed. *The placebo effect: an interdisciplinary exploration*, pp. 138–65. Harvard University Press, Cambridge, MA.

Ader R and Cohen N (1975). Behaviorally conditioned immunosuppression. *Psychosomatic Medicine*, **37**, 333–40.

Ader R and Cohen N (1982). Behaviorally conditioned immunosuppression and murine systemic lupus erythematosus. *Science*, **215**, 1534–6.

Ader R, Kelly K, Moynihan JA, Grota LJ and Cohen N (1993). Conditioned enhancement of antibody production using antigen as the unconditioned stimulus. *Brain, Behavior and Immunity*, **7**, 334–43.

Albring A, Wendt L, Benson S *et al.* (2012). Placebo effects on the immune response in humans: the role of learning and expectation. *PLoS One*, **7**, e49477.

Alvarez-Borda B, Ramirez-Amaya V, Pèrez-Montfort R and Bermùdez-Rattoni F (1995). Enhancement of antibody production by a learning paradigm. *Neurobiology of Learning and Memory*, **64**, 103–5.

Alvarez-Buyalla R and Carrasco-Zanini J (1960). A conditioned reflex which reproduces the hypoglycemic effect of insulin. *Acta Physiologica Latino Americana*, **10**, 153–8.

Alvarez-Buyalla R, Segura ET and Alvarez-Buyalla ER (1961). Participation of the hypophysis in the conditioned reflex which reproduces the hypoglycemic effect of insulin. *Acta Physiologica Latino Americana*, **11**, 113–19.

Benedetti F, Amanzio M, Vighetti S and Asteggiano G (2006). The biochemical and neuroendocrine bases of the hyperalgesic nocebo effect. *Journal of Neuroscience*, **26**, 12014–22.

Benedetti F, Lanotte M, Lopiano L and Colloca L (2007). When words are painful—unraveling the mechanisms of the nocebo effect. *Neuroscience*, **147**, 260–71.

Benedetti F, Pollo A, Lopiano L, Lanotte M, Vighetti S and Rainero I (2003). Conscious expectation and unconscious conditioning in analgesic, motor and hormonal placebo/nocebo responses. *Journal of Neuroscience*, **23**, 4315–23.

Booth RJ, Petrie KJ and Brook RJ (1995). Conditioning allergic skin responses in humans: a controlled study. *Psychosomatic Medicine*, **57**, 492–5.

Bovbjerg D, Ader R and Cohen N (1984). Acquisition and extinction of conditioned suppression of a graft-versus-host response in the rat. *Journal of Immunology*, **132**, 111–13.

Casey TP (1968). Immunosuppression by cyclophosphamide in NZB/NZW mice with lupus nephritis. *Blood*, **32**, 436–44.

Chen J, Lin W, Wang W *et al.* (2004). Enhancement of antibody production and expression of c-Fos in the insular cortex in response to a conditioned stimulus after a single-trial learning paradigm. *Behavioral Brain Research*, **154**, 557–65.

Coover GD, Sutton BR and Heybach JP (1977). Conditioning decreases in plasma corticosterone level in rats by pairing stimuli with daily feeding. *Journal of Comparative Physiology and Psychology*, **91**, 716–26.

Coussons-Reed ME, Dykstra LA and Lysle DT (1994a). Pavlovian conditioning of morphine-induced alterations of immune status: evidence for opioid receptor involvement. *Journal of Neuroimmunology*, **55**, 135–42.

Coussons-Reed ME, Dykstra LA and Lysle DT (1994b). Pavlovian conditioning of morphine-induced alterations of immune status: evidence for peripheral beta-adrenergic receptor involvement. *Brain, Behavior, and Immunity*, **8**, 204–17.

Deutsch R (1974). Conditioned hypoglycemia: a mechanism for saccharin-induced sensitivity to insulin in the rat. *Journal of Comparative Physiology and Psychology*, **95**, 350–8.

Elenkov IJ and Chrousos GP (1999). Stress hormones, Th1/Th2 patterns, pro/anti-inflammatory cytokines and susceptibility to disease. *Trends in Endocrinology and Metabolism*, **10**, 359–68.

Elenkov IJ, Wilder RL, Chrousos GP and Vizi ES (2000). The sympathetic nerve—an integrative interface between two supersystems: the brain and the immune system. *Pharmacological Reviews*, **52**, 595–638.

Exton MS, von Horsten SB, Schult M *et al.* (1998). Behaviorally conditioned immunosuppression using cyclosporine A: central nervous system reduces IL-2 production via splenic innervation. *Journal of Neuroimmunology*, **88**, 182–91.

Fehm-Wolfsdorf G, Beermann U, Kern W and Fehm HL (1993a). Failure to obtain classical conditioned hypoglycemia in man. In H Lehnert, R Murison, H Weiner, D Hellhammer and J Beyer Jr, eds. *Neuronal control of bodily function: basic and clinical aspects. Endocrine and nutritional control of basic biological functions*, pp. 257–61. Hogrefe & Huber Publishers, Seattle, WA.

Fehm-Wolfsdorf G, Gnadler M, Kern W, Klosterhalfen W and Kerner W (1993b). Classically conditioned changes of blood glucose level in humans. *Physiology and Behavior*, **54**, 155–60.

Fehm-Wolfsdorf G, Pohl J and Kerner W (1999). Classically conditioned changes of blood glucose level in humans. *Integrative Physiological and Behavioral Sciences*, **34**, 132.

Felten DL (2000). Neural influence on immune responses: underlying suppositions and basic principles of neural-immune signalling. *Progress in Brain Research*, **122**, 381–9.

Flaherty CF and Becker HC (1984). Influence of conditioned stimulus context on hyperglycaemic conditioned responses. *Physiology and Behavior*, **33**, 587–93.

Flaherty CF, Grigson PS and Brady A (1987). Relative novelty of conditioning context influences directionality of glycemic conditioning. *Journal of Experimental Psychology: Animal Behavior Process*, **13**, 144–9.

Fox RA, Sabo BM, Williams TP and Joffres MR (1999). Intradermal testing for food and chemical sensitivities: a double-blind controlled study. *Journal of Allergy and Clinical Immunology*, **103**, 907–11.

Gauci M, Husband AJ, Saxarra H and King MG (1994). Pavlovian conditioning of nasal tryptase release in human subjects with allergic rhinitis. *Physiology and Behavior*, **55**, 823–5.

Gell PGH and Coombs RRA, eds (1963). *Clinical aspects of immunology*. Blackwell, Oxford.

Giang DW, Goodman AD, Schiffer RB *et al.* (1996). Conditioning of cyclophosphamide-induced leukopenia in humans. *Journal of Neuropsychiatry and Clinical Neuroscience*, **8**, 194–201.

Goebel MU, Hubell D, Kou W *et al.* (2005). Behavioral conditioning with interferon beta-1a in humans. *Physiology and Behavior*, **84**, 807–14.

Goebel MU, Meykadeh N, Kou W, Schedlowski M and Hengge UR (2008). Behavioral conditioning of antihistamine effects in patients with allergic rhinitis. *Psychotherapy and Psychosomatics*, **77**, 227–34.

Goebel MU, Trebst AE, Steiner J, Xie YF, Exton MS *et al.* (2002). Behavioral conditioning of immunosuppression is possible in humans. *FASEB Journal*, **16**, 1869–73.

Goldfine ID, Abraira C, Gruenewald D and Goldstein MS (1970). Plasma insulin levels during imaginary food ingestion under hypnosis. *Proceedings of the Society of Experimental Biology and Medicine*, **133**, 274–6.

Gomez-Flores R and Weber RJ (1999). Inhibition of interleukin-2 production and downregulation of IL-2 and transferring receptors on rat splenic lymphocytes following PAG morphine administration: a role in natural killer and T-cell suppression. *Journal of Interferon and Cytokine Research*, **19**, 625–30.

Gorczynski RM (1990). Conditioned enhancement of skin allograft in mice. *Brain, Behavior, and Immunity*, **4**, 85–92.

Gorczynski RM, Macrae S and Kennedy M (1982). Conditioned immune response associated with allogeneic skin grafts in mice. *Journal of Immunology*, **129**, 704–9.

Grimm MC, Ben-Baruch A, Taub DD *et al.* (1998). Opiates transdeactivate chemokine receptors: delta and mu opiate receptor-mediated heterologous desensitization. *Journal of Experimental Medicine*, **188**, 317–25.

Grochowicz P, Schedlowski M, Husband AJ, King MG, Hibberd AD and Bowen KM (1991). Behavioral conditioning prolongs heart allograft survival in rats. *Brain, Behavior, and Immunity*, **5**, 349–56.

Holmes LJ, Smythe GA and Storlien LH (1989). Monoaminergic activity at the level of the hypothalamus and striatum: relationship to anticipated feeding and pancreatic insulin responses. *Brain Research*, **496**, 204–10.

Hsueh C, Chen S, Lin R and Chao H (2002). Cholinergic and serotonergic activities are required in triggering conditioned NK cell response. *Journal of Neuroimmunology*, **123**, 102–11.

Hsueh C, Kuo J, Chen S *et al.* (1999). Involvement of catecholamines in recall of the conditioned NK cell response. *Journal of Neuroimmunology*, **94**, 172–81.

Jewett DL, Fein G and Greenberg MH (1990). A double-blind study of symptom provocation to determine food sensitivity. *New England Journal of Medicine*, **323**, 429–33.

Johnson WG and Wildman HE (1983). Influence of external and covert food stimuli on insulin secretion in obese and normal persons. *Behavioral Neuroscience*, **97**, 1025–8.

Katafuchi T, Ichijo T, Take S and Hori T (1993). Hypothalamic modulation of splenic natural killer cell activity in rats. *Journal of Physiology*, **471**, 209–21.

Katafuchi T, Okada E, Take S and Hori T (1994). The biphasic changes in splenic natural killer cell activity following ventromedial hypothalamic lesions in rats. *Brain Research*, **652**, 164–8.

Kirschbaum C, Jabaij L, Buske-Kirschbaum A *et al.* (1992a). Conditioning of drug-induced immunomodulation in human volunteers: a European collaborative study. *British Journal of Clinical Psychology*, **31**, 459–72.

Kirschbaum C, Wit S and Hellhammer D (1992b). Consistent sex differences in cortisol responses to psychological stress. *Psychosomatic Medicine*, **54**, 648–57.

Klein R, Buck S, Classen K, Rostock M and Huber R (2008). Enhanced in vitro activation of immunocompetent cells in healthy individuals being subcutaneously "vaccinated" with placebo (physiological saline). *Clinical Immunology*, **126**, 322–31.

Klosterhalfen W and Klosterhalfen S (1983). Pavlovian conditioning of immunosuppression modifies adjuvant arthritis in rats. *Behavioral Neuroscience*, **97**, 663–6.

Kuo J, Chen S, Huang H, Yang C, Tsai P and Hsueh C (2001). The involvement of glutamate in recall of the conditioned NK cell response. *Journal of Neuroimmunology*, **118**, 245–55.

Liccardi G, Senna G, Russo M *et al.* (2004). Evaluation of the nocebo effect during oral challenge in patients with adverse drug reactions. *Journal of Investigational Allergology and Clinical Immunology*, **14**, 104–7.

Lichko AE (1959). Conditioned reflex hypoglycaemia in man. *Pavlovian Journal of High Nervous Activity*, **9**, 731–7.

Lombardi C, Gargioni S, Canonica GW and Passalacqua G (2008). The nocebo effect during oral challenge in subjects with adverse drug reactions. *European Annals of Allergy and Clinical Immunology*, **40**, 138–41.

Longo DL, Duffey PL, Kopp WC *et al.* (1999). Conditioned immune response to interferon-gamma in humans. *Clinical Immunology*, **90**, 173–81.

Louis-Sylvestre J (1976). Preabsorptive insulin release and hypoglycaemia in rats. *American Journal of Physiology*, **230**, 56–60.

Luger A, Deuster PA, Kyle SB *et al.* (1987). Acute-hypothalamic-pituitary-adrenal responses to the stress of treadmill exercise. Physiologic adaptations to physical training. *New England Journal of Medicine*, **316**, 1309–15.

Lysle DT, Luecken LJ and Maslonek KA (1992). Suppression of the development of adjuvant arthritis by a conditioned aversive stimulus. *Brain, Behavior, and Immunity*, **6**, 64–73.

Matysiak J and Green L (1984). On the directionality of classically-conditioned glycemic responses. *Physiology and Behavior*, **32**, 5–9.

McKenzie JN (1896). The production of the so-called "rose-cold" by means of an artificial rose. *American Journal of the Medical Sciences*, **91**, 45.

Mellon RD and Bayer BM (1998). Role of central opioid receptor subtypes in morphine-induced alterations in peripheral lymphocyte activity. *Brain Research*, **789**, 56–67.

Mellon RD and Bayer BM (1999). The effects of morphine, nicotine and epibatidine on lymphocyte activity and hypothalamic-pituitary-adrenal axis responses. *Journal of Pharmacology and Experimental Therapeutics*, **288**, 635–42.

Metal'nikov S and Chorine V (1926). Role des reflexes conditionnels dans l'immunitè. *Annals de l'Institute Pasteur*, **40**, 893–900.

Mityushov MI (1954). Conditioned reflex secretion of insulin. *Pavlovian Journal of High Nervous Activity*, **4**, 206–12.

Morrell EM, Surwit RS, Kuhn CM, Feinglos MN and Cochrane C (1988). Classically conditioned enhancement of hyperinsulinemia in the ob/ob mouse. *Psychosomatic Medicine*, **50**, 586–90.

Morris AD, Esterly J, Chase G and Sharp GC (1976). Cyclophosphamide protection in NZB/NZW disease. *Arthritis and Rheumatism*, **19**, 49–55.

Ober K, Benson S, Vogelsang M, *et al.* (2012). Plasma noradrenaline and state anxiety levels predict placebo response in learned immunosuppression. *Clinical Pharmacology and Therapeutics*, **91**, 220–6.

Okamoto S, Ibaraki K, Hayashi S and Saito M (1996). Ventromedial hypothalamus suppresses splenic lymphocyte activity through sympathetic innervation. *Brain Research*, **739**, 308–13.

Okaïs C, Gay C, Seon F, Buchaille L, Chary E and Soubeyrand B (2011). Disease-specific adverse events following nonlive vaccines: a paradoxical placebo effect or a nocebo phenomenon? *Vaccine*, **29**, 6321–6.

Olness K and Ader R (1992). Conditioning as an adjunct in the pharmacotherapy of lupus erythematosus. *Journal of Developmental and Behavioral Pediatrics*, **13**, 124–5.

Overduin J and Jansen A (1997). Conditioned insulin and blood sugar responses in humans in relation to binge eating. *Physiology and Behavior*, **61**, 569–75.

Pacheco-Lopez G, Engler H, Niemi MB and Schedlowski M (2006). Expectations and associations that heal: immunomodulatory placebo effects and its neurobiology. *Brain, Behavior, and Immunity*, **20**, 430–46.

Pacheco-Lopez G, Niemi MB, Kou W, Harting M, Fandrey J and Schedlowski M (2005). Neural substrates for behaviorally conditioned immunosuppression in the rat. *Journal of Neuroscience*, **25**, 2330–7.

Passalacqua G, Milanese M, Mincarini M *et al.* (2002). Single-dose oral tolerance test with alternative compounds for the management of adverse reactions to drugs. *International Archives of Allergy and Immunology*, **129**, 242–7.

Pavlov V and Tracey K (2005). The cholinergic anti-inflammatory pathway. *Brain, Behavior, and Immunity*, **19**, 493–9.

Rainero I, Valfre` W, Savi L *et al.* (2001). Neuroendocrine effects of subcutaneous sumatriptan in patients with migraine. *Journal of Endocrinological investigation*, **24**, 310–15.

Ramirez-Amaya V, Alvarez-Borda B and Bermudez-Rattoni F (1998). Differential effects of NMDA-induced lesions into the insular cortex and amigdala on the acquisition and evocation of conditioned immunosuppression. *Brain, Behavior, and Immunity*, **12**, 149–60.

Ramirez-Amaya V, Alvarez-Borda B, Ormsby C, Martinez R, Pèrez-Montfort R and Bermudez-Rattoni F (1996). Insular cortex lesions impair the acquisition of conditioned immunosuppression. *Brain, Behavior, and Immunity*, **10**, 103–14.

Ramirez-Amaya V and Bermudez-Rattoni F (1999). Conditioned enhancement of antibody production is disrupted by insular cortex and amygdale but not hippocampal lesions. *Brain, Behavior, and Immunity*, **13**, 46–60.

Rogers MP, Reich P, Strom TB and Carpenter CB (1976). Behaviorally conditioned immuno-suppression: replication of a recent study. *Psychosomatic Medicine*, **38**, 447–52.

Rogers TJ, Steele AD, Howard OMZ and Oppenheim JJ (2000). Bidirectional heterologous desensitization of opioid and chemokine receptors. *Annals of the New York Academy of Sciences*, **917**, 19–28.

Roozendaal B, Oldenburger WP, Strubbe JH, Koolhaas JM and Bohus B (1990). The central amygdale is involved in the conditioned but not in the meal-induced cephalic insulin response in the rat. *Neuroscience Letters*, **116**, 210–15.

Russek M and Pina S (1962). Conditioning of adrenalin anorexia. *Nature*, **193**, 1296–7.

Sabbioni MEE, Bovbjerg DH, Mathew S, Sikes C, Lasley B and Stokes PE (1997). Classically conditioned changes in plasma cortisol levels induced by dexamethasone in healthy men. *FASEB Journal*, **11**, 1291–6.

Siegel S (1972). Conditioning of insulin-induced glycemia. *Journal of Comparative Physiology and Psychology*, **78**, 233–41.

Siegel S (1975). Conditioning insulin effects. *Journal of Comparative Physiology and Psychology*, **89**, 189–99.

Siegel S (2002). Explanatory mechanisms for placebo effects: Pavlovian conditioning. In HA Guess, A Kleinman, JW Kusek, and LW Engel, eds. *The science of the placebo: toward an interdisciplinary research agenda*, pp. 133–57. BMJ Books, London.

Simon C, Schlienger JL, Sapin R and Imler M (1986). Cephalic phase insulin secretion in relation to food presentation in normal and overweight subjects. *Physiology and Behavior*, **36**, 465–9.

Sjostrom L, Garellick G, Krotkiewski M and Luyckx A (1980). Peripheral insulin in response to the sight and smell of food. *Metabolism*, **10**, 901–9.

Smith GR and McDaniels SM (1983). Psychologically mediated effect on the delayed hypersensitivity reaction to tuberculin in humans. *Psychosomatic Medicine*, **45**, 65–70.

Stanton ME and Levine S (1988). Pavlovian conditioning of endocrine responses. In E Ader, H Weiner and A Baum, eds. *Experimental foundation of behavioral medicine: conditioning approaches*, pp. 25–46. Lawrence Erlbaum Associates, Hillsdale, NJ.

Steinberg AD, Huston DP, Taurog JD, Cowdery JS and Raveche ES (1981). The cellular and genetic basis of murine lupus. *Immunology Reviews*, **55**, 121–54.

Sternberg EM (1997a). Emotions and disease: from balance of humors to balance of molecules. *Nature Medicine*, **3**, 264–7.

Sternberg EM (1997b). Neural-immune interactions in health and disease. *Journal of Clinical Investigation*, **100**, 2641–7.

Stockhorst U, Gritzmann E, Klopp K *et al.* (1999). Classical conditioning of insulin effects in healthy humans. *Psychosomatic Medicine*, **61**, 424–35.

Stockhorst U, Steingruber HJ and Scherbaum WA (2000). Classically conditioned responses following repeated insulin and glucose administration in humans. *Behavioral Brain Research*, **110**, 143–59.

Theofilopoulos AN and Dixon FJ (1981). Etiopathogenesis of murine SLE. *Immunology Reviews*, **55**, 179–216.

Tracey K (2002). The inflammatory reflex. *Nature*, **420**, 853–9.

Vits S, Cesko E, Benson S, *et al.* (2013). Cognitive factors mediate placebo responses in patients with house dust mite allergy. *PLoS One*, **8**, e79576.

Wayner EA, Flannery GR and Singer G (1978). The effects of taste aversion conditioning on the primary antibody response to sheep red blood cells and Brucella abortus in the albino rat. *Physiology and Behavior*, **21**, 995–1000.

Whitehouse MW, Levy L and Beck FJ (1973). Effect of cyclophosphamide on a local graft-versus-host reaction in the rat: influence of sex, disease and different dosage regimens. *Agents and Actions*, **3**, 53–60.

Woods SC (1972). Conditioned hypoglycemia: effect of vagotomy and pharmacological blockade. *American Journal of Physiology*, **223**, 1424–7.

Woods SC, Alexander KR and Porte D Jr (1972). Conditioned insulin secretion and hypoglycemia following repeated injections of tolbutamide in rats. *Endocrinology*, **90**, 227–31.

Woods SC and Bernstein IL (1980). Cephalic insulin response as a test for completeness of vagotomy to the pancreas. *Physiology and Behavior*, **24**, 485–8.

Woods SC, Makous W and Hutton RA (1968). A new technique for conditioned hypoglycemia. *Psychonomic Science*, **10**, 389–90.

Woods SC, Makous W and Hutton RA (1969). Temporal parameters of conditioned hypoglycemia. *Journal of Comparative Physiology and Psychology*, **69**, 301–7.

Woods SC, Vasselli JR, Kaestner E, Szakmary GA, Milburn P and Vitiello MV (1977). Conditioned insulin secretion and meal feeding in rats. *Journal of Comparative Physiology and Psychology*, **91**, 128–33.

Disease-based classification of placebo effects—less-studied conditions

Part 3 is the continuation of Part 2. However, in these medical conditions little is known about the mechanisms of the placebo effect. Although many clinical trials have been performed, little information is available about the psychological and biological placebo mechanisms in the cardiovascular system, the respiratory system, the gastrointestinal and genitourinary apparatus, as well as in special conditions such as oncology, surgery, physical therapy, and complementary and alternative medicine.

Chapter 8

Cardiovascular and respiratory systems

Summary points

- Compared to other systems, little is known about the mechanisms of placebo and placebo-related effects in both the cardiovascular and respiratory systems.

- Side effects in placebo groups of cardiovascular clinical trials are common and might represent the basis of nocebo effects, although no definitive conclusion can be drawn.

- Heart activity can be conditioned and can also be affected during a placebo analgesic response.

- Not only may placebo-activated endogenous opioids act on pain transmission, but on the heart and the respiratory centers as well.

- Asthma and cough are powerfully affected by placebos, but the underlying mechanisms are unknown.

8.1 The cardiovascular system

8.1.1 There are a few and contrasting placebo studies in cardiovascular health

The data on real placebo effects in the cardiovascular system and circulatory diseases are scanty and somehow contrasting, mainly due to the lack of systematic analysis of cardiovascular placebo responses. In addition, some studies that claim powerful placebo effects in cardiovascular diseases suffer from methodological flaws that limit the interpretation of the results. There are in fact many studies in which either short-lasting or long-lasting placebo effects are described, but actually they cannot be distinguished from spontaneous remission and regression to the mean.

For example, the first Vasovagal Pacemaker Study (VPS-I) (Connolly et al., 1999) compared implantation versus no implantation of a pacemaker device for the treatment of neurocardiogenic syncope. Although the investigators found a reduction in the rate of syncope in the group that was implanted, they considered the possibility that the implant itself had an important placebo component. This reasoning led to a second VPS (VPS-II) (Connolly et al., 2003). Here, all the patients were implanted with a pacemaker, but the devices were maintained either on or off according to a double-blind design. No significant benefit was found in the active pacing group. Although these studies are generally considered a good example of the placebo effect in the field of cardiology, neither spontaneous remission nor regression to the mean or other factors can be ruled out completely. Thus, we cannot conclude that the reduction in the rate of syncope is a true psychobiological phenomenon.

However, an interesting study comparing two placebo treatments was performed in 2001 by Ammirati et al. (2001). The comparison between two placebos is an interesting experimental approach in order to demonstrate a real placebo effect. In fact, if a placebo is inert and does not produce any psychological effect, two different placebos should not differ from each other. By contrast, if the psychological effect of a placebo treatment is superior to that of a different placebo treatment, different outcomes should be expected (see also section 4.1.3). According to this point of view, Ammirati et al. (2001) compared a placebo pill of atenolol, a beta-blocker, with a placebo pacemaker device, and showed that the device was far superior to the drug, which indicates that placebo strength varies by intervention type.

Another example of circulatory diseases and therapeutic interventions that can mistakenly be taken as an example of powerful placebo effects is highlighted by a study on therapeutic angiogenesis and laser myocardial revascularization in patients with coronary heart disease (Rana et al., 2005). In this study, fibroblast growth factor-2 and laser revascularization were compared with placebo. Long-lasting placebo effects were found, with improvements of symptoms and exercise tolerance times lasting up to 2 years. However, it is not possible to be sure that these are true placebo effects, as no information about the natural course of the disease is available.

Many other studies do not allow clear identification of the placebo effect in cardiovascular health, nor do they clearly define its magnitude (Olshansky, 2007). Moreover, several treatments that are currently in use do not have a placebo-controlled design, thus the placebo component of the therapy is unknown. For example, using catheter ablation to treat atrial fibrillation is considered an effective treatment for many supraventricular tachycardias and placebo-controlled trials are often considered unnecessary (Olshansky, 2007). Therefore, it is not known whether the successful outcomes frequently reported following this procedure (Pappone et al., 2003; Nademanee et al., 2004) are merely a placebo effect.

The occurrence of placebo effects in hypertension has been investigated in detail but unfortunately contrasting results have been obtained. In some studies, a reduction of blood pressure in hypertensive patients who received a placebo has been found (Bienenfeld et al., 1996; Preston et al., 2000; Asmar et al., 2001). However, some other studies found substantial differences between hospital and ambulatory blood pressure measurements, suggesting that many factors may be involved, including the method used for measurement (Sassano et al., 1987; Mutti et al., 1991; Prager et al., 1994; Mancia et al., 1995). Even in more recent and well controlled studies on the role of placebos in the modulation of blood pressure, contrasting results were obtained (Meissner and Ziep, 2011; Redwine et al., 2012; Weiss et al., 2013; Zimmermann et al., 2013).

8.1.2 **Some cardiac effects can be conditioned**

Although experiments in animals and humans show that cardiac effects can be conditioned, surprisingly little research has been pursued in this field within the context of placebo research. Some experimental evidence suggests that heart responses to a number of pharmacological agents can be conditioned in the same way seen for other systems, such as the immune and endocrine systems. In fact, neutral stimuli can acquire the ability to induce heart responses after several pairings with drugs. Bykov was one of the first scientists who realized that some cardiac effects can be conditioned (Bykov, 1959). He paired intravenous injections of nitroglycerin (the unconditioned stimulus) with a bicycle horn (the conditioned stimulus) several times in dogs, and found that after several pairings the bicycle horn alone was capable of mimicking the electrocardiographic changes induced by nitroglycerin; for example, increased heart rate and alterations in both the ST segment and T wave were elicited by the presentation of the conditioned stimulus.

Lang et al. (1967) obtained similar results and emphasized the important clinical implications of these phenomena in the context of the placebo effect. In addition, Lang and Rand (1969) paired sublingual nitroglycerin with peppermint flavor in healthy women about eight times. In the test session, nitroglycerin was replaced with a peppermint-flavored placebo, and a conditioned tachycardic response occurred, along with some side effects that are typically reported after nitroglycerin administration (e.g., headache).

More recently, the effects of conditioning on the heart have been studied in different fields. One of these is conditioned bradycardia in fear conditioning. In a typical experiment of this kind, a conditioned stimulus (a sound, for example) is paired with an unconditioned stimulus (e.g., an electric shock) many times. After repeated pairings, the conditioned stimulus induces a conditioned bradycardic response. This effect has been found both in animals and in humans. In animals, many brain regions seem to be involved in conditioned bradycardia, like the amygdala, hippocampus, hypothalamus, and medial prefrontal cortex (Powell, 1994; Powell et al., 1997; Sacchetti et al., 2005), but the cerebellum appears to play a crucial role (Supple and Kapp, 1993).

Lesions of the anterior cerebellar vermis severely attenuate the acquisition of conditioned bradycardia without disrupting the baseline heart rate or unconditioned heart rate responses. Furthermore, lesions of the vermis after acquisition of conditioned bradycardia eliminate evidence of prior conditioning. In contrast, lesions of the cerebellar hemispheres affect neither conditioned nor unconditioned heart rate responses, thus confirming the crucial role of the anterior cerebellar vermis in both the acquisition and retention of conditioned bradycardia (Supple and Kapp, 1993). The role of the cerebellum in fear conditioning was also confirmed by Sacchetti et al. (2004); they found a long-lasting potentiation of the synapse between the parallel fibers and Purkinje cells in vermal lobules V–VI, in which a postsynaptic mechanism is involved. In addition, these researchers found that hotfoot mice with a primary deficiency of the parallel fiber–Purkinje cell synapse (an important neuronal circuit in the cerebellum) show an impairment of fear conditioning.

Interestingly, there is some experimental evidence that the same circuit is involved in humans. By using a classical conditioning paradigm with a tone as the conditioned stimulus and an electrical shock as the unconditioned stimulus, Maschke et al. (2002) tested five patients with medial cerebellar lesions (due to surgery for astrocytoma) and five controls. Compared to the controls, the patients did not show a significant decrease of heart rate during fear conditioning, thus suggesting that the medial cerebellum is involved in fear-conditioned bradycardia in humans.

Although these studies have always been considered to be outside the placebo literature, it is clear they are relevant to the conditioned placebo response. In fact, they indicate that the heart beat can be affected by neutral stimuli (placebos) that are repeatedly paired with unconditioned stimuli.

8.1.3 Placebo-induced activation of endogenous opioids may affect heart activity

Conditioned bradycardia has been found to involve the endogenous opioid systems, as pharmacological manipulation with opioid antagonists, like naloxone, impairs learning of classically conditioned heart rate changes (Hernandez and Powell, 1983; Harris and Fitzgerald, 1989; Hernandez et al., 1990; Hernandez and Watson, 1997). Unfortunately there is no study testing placebo-activated endogenous opioids on the heart. However, there is some indication that during placebo analgesia the activation of the endogenous opioid systems may also affect the heart.

In a study by Pollo et al. (2003), a placebo was given to subjects who underwent induction of experimental pain, along with the suggestion that it was a painkiller. Besides the assessment of the analgesic effect, both heart rate and heart rate variability were measured. This was done in both the clinical and experimental settings (Pollo et al., 2003). In the clinical setting, patients who were assessed for their autonomic functions were delivered noxious stimuli and a placebo was applied to the skin along with the verbal suggestions that it was a potent local anesthetic. These subjects showed consistent placebo analgesic responses that were accompanied by reduced heart rate. Because of ethical constraints in the clinical setting, these subjects were not tested further.

In order to investigate this effect from a pharmacological viewpoint, the same placebo effect was reproduced in the laboratory setting, using experimental ischemic arm pain (Pollo et al., 2003). It was found that the opioid antagonist naloxone completely antagonized both placebo-analgesia and the concomitant reduced heart rate, whereas the beta-blocker propranolol antagonized the placebo heart-rate reduction but not placebo analgesia. By contrast, both placebo responses were present during muscarinic blockade with atropine, indicating no involvement of the parasympathetic system (Fig. 8.1A). To better understand the effects of naloxone and propranolol, a spectral analysis of heart rate variability was also carried out (Box 8.1). This allows identification of the sympathetic and parasympathetic activity of the heart. In fact, this procedure makes it possible to identify a low-frequency component (0.1–0.15 Hz) that corresponds to sympathetic activity, and a high-frequency component (0.25–0.4 Hz) that corresponds to parasympathetic activity (Malliani et al., 1991).

Pollo et al. (2003) found that the beta-adrenergic low-frequency (0.15 Hz) spectral component was reduced during placebo analgesia, which suggests a reduction of sympathetic activity during placebo analgesia. Importantly, this effect was reversed by

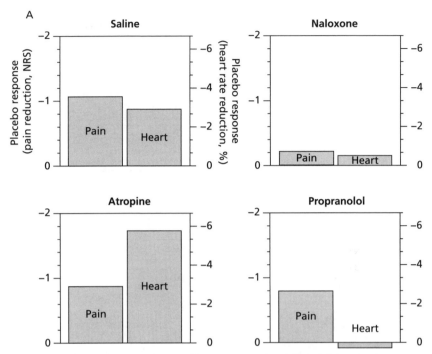

Fig. 8.1 (A) Different pharmacological effects, expressed as the size of the placebo response (difference between hidden and open injections) on placebo analgesic and placebo heart responses. Significant placebo effects occur with saline and atropine for both pain and heart rate, and with propranolol for pain only. By contrast, naloxone blocks both pain and heart placebo responses, whereas propranolol blocks placebo heart responses. (B) Spectral analysis of heart-rate variability from four representative subjects during ischemic arm pain. Note the placebo reduction (solid line = open injection; dashed line = hidden injection) of the sympathetic low-frequency peak (0.15 Hz) under the effect of both saline and atropine, whereas no placebo reduction was present with naloxone and propranolol. PSD, power spectrum density. Reproduced from Antonella Pollo, Sergio Vighetti, Innocenzo Rainero, and Fabrizio Benedetti, Placebo analgesia and the heart, *Pain*, 102 (1), pp. 125–33 Copyright 2003, The International Association for the Study of Pain, with permission.

naloxone, suggesting the possible involvement of endogenous opioids (Fig. 8.1B). It should be pointed out, however, that the underlying opioid mechanism is unknown. A possible explanation for the effects of naloxone on the heart is that the reduced sympathetic and heart responses during placebo analgesia are a consequence of the effects of endogenous opioids on the pain itself. Another possible explanation is that expectation of analgesia triggers the release of endogenous opioids which, in turn, inhibits both pain transmission and the beta-adrenergic sympathetic system. In other words, reduction of sympathetic control of the heart might be due to either a direct effect of endogenous opioids on the heart or an indirect effect through reduction of pain itself.

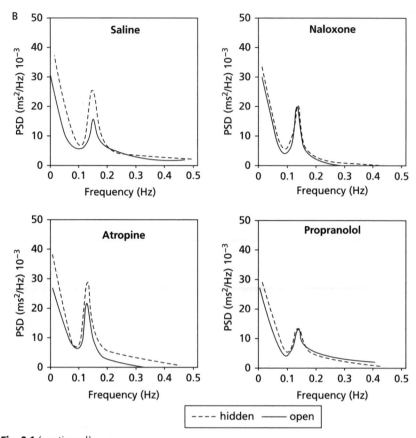

Fig. 8.1 (continued)

8.1.4 **Side effects are common in placebo groups of cardiovascular clinical trials**

As emphasized several times throughout this book, many side effects of drugs are attributable to nocebo effects. In treatments related to the circulatory system, one study on beta-blocker therapy is notable because it has important practical aspects (Ko et al., 2002). It was based on the fact that many other studies found beta-blocker therapy to be associated with several side effects, such as depression, fatigue, and sexual dysfunction (Koch-Weser and Frishman, 1981; Weiss, 1991; Lue, 2000). Indeed, the Food and Drug Administration cited these negative effects in the package inserts of beta-blockers (*Physicians' desk reference*, 2002).

In 2002, Ko et al. (2002) performed a quantitative review of 15 randomized trials of beta-blockers in a large population of 35,000 patients suffering from myocardial infarction, heart failure, and hypertension. The main finding was that beta-blockers were not associated with a greater risk of depression, leading only to a small associated risk of fatigue and sexual dysfunction. In fact, in seven trials that included 10,662 patients, the overall frequency of depressive symptoms was 20.1% in the beta-blocker groups,

Box 8.1 Extracting sympathetic and parasympathetic activity from the electrocardiogram

Efferent sympathetic and vagal (parasympathetic) activities directed to the heart are characterized by discharge largely synchronous with each cardiac cycle that can be modulated by central vasomotor and respiratory centers as well as by peripheral oscillations in arterial pressure and respiratory movements. These oscillations generate rhythmic fluctuations in efferent neural discharge that result in short- and long-term oscillations in the heart period. As a consequence, the analysis of these rhythms through the recording of the electrocardiogram (ECG) permits inferences on the state and function of the sympathetic and parasympathetic nervous system. To do this, ECG is recorded by using conventional techniques with two electrodes on the chest. Heart rate is analyzed by measuring the R–R intervals of the ECG and then transforming them into frequency (1/R–R). Therefore, the ECG is transformed into a tachocardiogram (R–R intervals over time), which represents heart rate variability. Then, spectral analysis of the tachocardiogram is carried out to identify the sympathetic and parasympathetic components of the ECG, which are expressed as power spectrum densities (PSD) (Fig. 8.2).

By using this procedure, it is possible to identify a low-frequency (LF) component (0.04–0.15 Hz), which corresponds to sympathetic activity, and a high-frequency (HF) component (0.15–0.4 Hz), which corresponds to parasympathetic activity. Whereas the HF component reflects the influence of vagal efferents on respiration, the LF component is less understood and is thought to be related to sympathetic-mediated influences on vasomotor activity and arterial pressure. Due to the interference between vagal parasympathetic activity and respiratory rate, HF responses are better detectable if breathing is kept constant, so that the subject has to synchronize his breathing with a metronome. For an example of the application of this technique, see Malliani et al. (1991), Benedetti et al. (2004) and Lanotte et al. (2005).

The balance between sympathetic and parasympathetic activity is expressed with the ratio LF/HF. A typical example is represented by a stressful versus a nonstressful condition. The former is characterized by a prominent sympathetic activity (large LF/small HF), the latter by a prominent vagal activity (small LF/large HF).

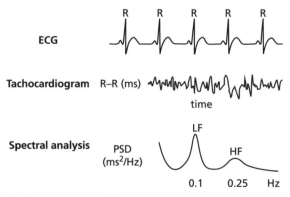

Fig. 8.2 Analysis of heart rate variability.

and as large as 20.5% in the placebo groups. In addition, withdrawal of medication due to depression was assessed in four trials, on 5803 patients; these found that 0.4% of patients were withdrawn from the beta-blocker groups and 0.5% from the placebo groups. Likewise, in 10 trials that included 17,682 patients, the overall frequency of fatigue symptoms was 33.4% in the beta-blocker groups, but as large as 30.4% in the placebo groups. Moreover, withdrawal of medication due to fatigue was assessed in ten trials on 29,454 patients; medication was withdrawn from 2.4% of patients in the beta-blocker groups and 0.5% in the placebo groups. Similar findings were found for sexual dysfunction. In six trials on a total of 14,897 patients the overall frequency of sexual dysfunction was 21.6% in the beta-blocker groups, and it was as large as 17.4% in the placebo groups. Four trials (11,260 patients) assessed withdrawal of medication due to sexual dysfunction, with 1.3% of patients withdrawn from the beta-blocker groups and 0.3% from the placebo groups.

The study by Ko et al. (2002) does not furnish information regarding possible mechanisms of the side effects and the occurrence of real nocebo effects in the placebo groups, but it is important for two reasons. First, it shows the high rate of side effects in placebo groups of cardiovascular clinical trials. Second, beta-blockers are underused as physicians are reluctant to prescribe them because of these possible side effects (Krumholz et al., 1998; Ko et al., 2002). This reluctance persists despite the fact that beta-blockers after myocardial infarction have been shown to reduce mortality by approximately 20% (Freemantle et al., 1999). Indeed, patients may be discouraged by listings of harmful effects provided in good faith by doctors, drug information sheets, and media. This holds true not only for severe side effects but also for minor adverse events. For example, Barron et al. (2013) found that 28 of the 33 classically described side effects are not significantly more common on beta-blockers than placebo. Of 100 patients developing dizziness on beta-blockers, 81 would have developed it on placebo. For diarrhea this proportion is 82/100, and for hyperglycemia 83/100.

8.2 The respiratory system

8.2.1 Placebos can mimic the depressant effects of narcotics on ventilation

Most of the studies on the placebo effect in diseases of the respiratory system are clinical trials aimed at assessing the effectiveness of a medical treatment. Thus, there is no way to understand the relative contribution of different factors, like spontaneous remission, regression to the mean, or real placebo responses. A notable exception is narcotic-induced respiratory depression.

Narcotics are widely used as analgesics. However, they may induce several side effects, such as respiratory depression, nausea, constipation, or urinary retention. Placebos have been found to induce respiratory depression (Benedetti et al., 1998, 1999). In a clinical study in the postoperative setting, buprenorphine (a narcotic used to treat postoperative pain) was given for 3 days consecutively and both analgesia and respiratory depressant effects were measured (Benedetti et al., 1999). Ventilation was assessed by means of a spirometer and expressed as minute ventilation (liters per minute). After every infusion of buprenorphine, a mild reduction in ventilation was observed. On the fourth day, buprenorphine was replaced with a placebo, and this mimicked the respiratory depressant effect of buprenorphine. These placebo respiratory-depressant responses could be prevented by the opioid antagonist naloxone, which suggests involvement of endogenous opioids at the level of the respiratory centers (Fig. 8.3). Interestingly, the patients themselves did not expect any effect and did not notice any decrease in ventilation, which suggests this effect is an unconscious conditioning mechanism whereby the act of giving the drug was the conditioned stimulus.

It is worth noting that the effects of placebos on the respiratory function may be independent of those on pain. In fact, Benedetti et al. (1998) showed that when buprenorphine is given for several days consecutively and then replaced with a placebo, the placebo analgesic response depends on the analgesic effectiveness of buprenorphine over the previous days. Likewise, the magnitude of the placebo respiratory-depressant response was larger in patients with post-buprenorphine respiratory depression of the previous days, regardless of the analgesic efficacy. This dissociation between placebo respiratory depression and placebo analgesia suggests that the mechanisms of the two effects are independent of each other. Considering the involvement of the endogenous opioids in both cases, they might involve different subpopulations of opioid receptors. For example, after systemic administration of morphine, antinociception has been found to be mediated mainly by the supraspinal μ_1 receptors (Pasternak, 1993). In fact, the μ_1 selective antagonists naloxonazine and naloxazone block the analgesia induced by morphine and other opioids in rodents (Pasternak et al., 1980a, 1980b; Zhang and Pasternak, 1981; Ling and Pasternak, 1983). Conversely, the μ_2 receptors appear to be important in the respiratory depressant effects of opioids in rodents (Pasternak, 1988; 1993). In fact, administration of the μ_1 antagonist naloxonazine antagonizes morphine analgesia without affecting respiratory depression, as assessed by the drop in oxygen pressure and the rise in carbon dioxide pressure (Ling et al., 1983, 1985). On the basis of these findings, it has been postulated that the effects of placebos on pain might be mediated by the μ_1 opioid receptors, while those affecting respiration might be brought about by μ_2 receptors (Benedetti et al., 1998).

8.2.2 Placebos reduce bronchial hyper-reactivity in asthma

Asthma has been reported to be influenced by many psychological factors (McQuaid et al., 2000; Liu et al., 2002; Sandberg et al., 2004; Chen et al., 2006). In 1968, Luparello et al. (1968) showed that administration of a placebo, along with verbal suggestions that the inhaled substance contained irritants, induced a dramatic increase in airway resistance and breathing difficulty in asthmatic patients. However, if placebo was administered again, but the patients were told it was therapeutic, airway resistance decreased and easy breathing returned.

In many placebo-controlled trials of asthma, the forced expiratory volume in one second (FEV_1; a measure of bronchoconstriction: see Box 8.2) has been found to improve in patients who had received a placebo (Creticos et al., 1996; Balon et al., 1998; Knorr et al., 1998; Milgrom et al., 1999; Robinson et al., 2001), although spontaneous

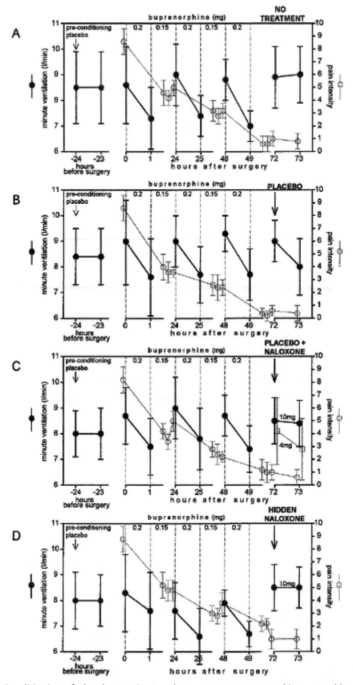

Fig. 8.3 Conditioning of placebo respiratory depressant response and its reversal by naloxone. The black circles represent the minute ventilation VE and the white circles represent the pain scores. In the preconditioning placebo test, no placebo respiratory

remissions or other factors could not be ruled out in these studies. In a meta-analysis of 33 randomized, double-blind, placebo-controlled clinical trials, on a total of 1243 patients, about 6% of those who received placebo treatment showed clinically relevant changes in pulmonary function, and the mean percentage increase in FEV_1 was about 5% (Joyce et al., 2000). Compared to other medical conditions, this percentage is quite small. However, in another study 18% were found to be placebo responders (Kemeny et al., 2007) although it should be noted that the criteria for placebo responsiveness were different in the two studies.

In the study by Kemeny et al. (2007) 55 patients with mild intermittent and persistent asthma with stable airway hyper-reactivity were subdivided into two groups. The first group received salmeterol, an antiasthma bronchodilator agent, before a methacholine challenge. In fact, methacholine induces bronchoconstriction, with a decrease in FEV_1, and salmeterol prevents this effect of methacholine. The second group received a placebo before the methacholine challenge. The investigators found that the placebo increased the dose of methacholine required to induce a 20% decrease in FEV_1, which indicates that bronchial reactivity to methacholine was reduced (Fig. 8.4). The response to salmeterol was larger than that to the placebo, and the placebo component represented 29% of the total effect attributable to salmeterol. Interestingly, the same study assessed the effects of the physician–patient interaction on placebo responsiveness, but neither the magnitude nor the frequency of the placebo response was affected by the physician's behavior.

Although the precise mechanisms of the effects of placebos on bronchial reactivity are not known, Kemeny et al. (2007) hypothesize that they can be mediated either by inhibition of efferent cholinergic pathways or by activation of noradrenergic efferent pathways, or even through regulation of inflammatory mediators like tumor necrosis factor TNF-α and arachidonic acid metabolites.

Interestingly, Leigh et al. (2003) studied both placebo and nocebo suggestions in suggestible and suggestion-resistant subjects (as assessed by means of the Creative Imagination Scale). These investigators measured the FEV_1 in patients after inhalation of saline solution which the subjects believed to be either a bronchodilator or a

---

Fig. 8.3 (continued) depressant effect was found, whereas 0.2 mg buprenorphine always produced a VE reduction at 1 h, 25 h and 49 h. (A) The no-treatment group did not receive any treatment at 72 h such that no difference of VE was observed between 72 h and 73 h. (B) The placebo group received an open injection of saline at 72 h which produced a placebo respiratory depressant effect at 73 h. (C) 10 mg naloxone blocked completely the placebo response at 73 h whereas 4 mg were ineffective (white squares). (D) A hidden injection of 10 mg naloxone did not produce any change in VE at 72–73 h, indicating that naloxone per se did not affect VE. Note that the time course of pain was similar in all groups and that pain disappeared almost completely at 72 h, such that all patients were almost pain-free when tested with open and hidden injections. Reproduced from Fabrizio Benedetti, Martina Amanzio, Sergio Baldi, Caterina Casadio, and Giuliano Maggi, Inducing placebo respiratory depressant responses in humans via opioid receptors, *European Journal of Neuroscience*, 11 (2), pp. 625–31 Copyright 1999, John Wiley and Sons.

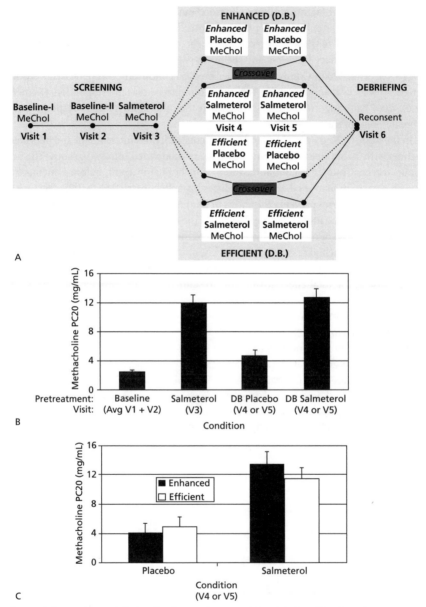

Fig. 8.4 (A) Experimental design for the assessment of the placebo effect in asthma. Eligibility was determined at three screening visits (V), after which subjects were randomized to "enhanced" or "efficient" physician interactions and to order of pre-methacholine (MeChol) challenge treatment (with a crossover between salmeterol and placebo), followed by a final visit for re-consenting the patients. (B) Bronchoprovocation response by visit. All subjects demonstrated bronchial hyper-responsiveness (PC20 ≤ 4 mg/mL) at baseline (average of visits 1 and 2), whereby PC20 is the concentration of methacholine required to induce a 20% decrease in FEV1. This was significantly reduced by pretreatment with

bronchoconstrictor. Suggestible asthmatics showed a significant fall in FEV_1 when they believed that the saline was a bronchoconstrictor whereas the suggestions of bronchodilation did not produce any decrease in FEV_1. Therefore, suggestible asthmatic patients are more likely to respond to a sham bronchoconstrictor.

In order to better understand the mechanisms of the placebo response in asthma, Wechsler et al. (2011) compared the effects of a bronchodilator with two placebo interventions and no intervention. In a double-blind crossover study, 46 patients with asthma were randomly assigned to active treatment with an albuterol inhaler, a placebo inhaler, sham acupuncture, or no intervention. Each of these four interventions was administered in random order during four sequential visits, and this procedure was repeated in two more blocks of visits, for a total of 12 visits by each patient. At each visit, FEV_1 was measured and patients' self-reported improvement was recorded. Among the 39 patients who completed the study, albuterol resulted in a 20% increase in FEV_1, as compared with approximately 7% with each of the other three interventions. However, patients' reports of improvement after the intervention did not differ significantly for the albuterol inhaler (50% improvement), placebo inhaler (45%), or sham acupuncture (46%), but the subjective improvement with all three of these interventions was significantly greater than that with the no-intervention control (21%). Therefore, although albuterol, but not the two placebo interventions, improved FEV_1, albuterol provided no incremental benefit with respect to the self-reported outcomes. This study highlights the difference, at least in asthma, between the objective measurements performed by health professionals and the subjective symptoms reported by patients in the outcome following a placebo treatment.

8.2.3 Cough is powerfully reduced by placebo treatments

Clinical trials comparing active treatments for cough with placebo treatments show that the difference between the two therapies is small, with medication a little more effective than placebo (Schroeder and Fahey, 2001, 2002; Eccles, 2002, 2006, 2009, 2010). Patients who receive the placebo show a reduction in cough up to 85% of the total effect of active medication. Therefore, only 15% of the reduction in cough is attributable to the

---

Fig. 8.4 (continued) salmeterol at visit 3, according to a single-blind design, as shown by the methacholine PC20 increase. Visits 4 and 5 included pretreatment with double-blind (DB) placebo or salmeterol (in a randomized order) before methacholine challenge. Double-blind placebo induced a significant increase in methacholine PC20 (> 4 mg/mL) compared with baseline values. (C) Bronchoprovocation response by physician interaction. Subjects were randomized to enhanced physician interaction style (black bars) or efficient physician interaction style (white bars) for visits 4 and 5, and to pre-methacholine treatment order (placebo/salmeterol or salmeterol/placebo). No physician–interaction-style effect was present. Reprinted from *Journal of Allergy and Clinical Immunology*, 119 (6), Margaret E. Kemeny, Lanny J. Rosenwasser, Reynold A. Panettieri, Robert M. Rose, Steve M. Berg-Smith, and Joel N. Kline, Placebo response in asthma: A robust and objective phenomenon, pp. 1375–81, Copyright (2007), with permission from Elsevier.

Box 8.2 Forced expiratory volume in 1 second

The forced expiratory volume 1 (FEV_1) is the volume exhaled during the first second of a forced expiratory maneuver following a maximal inspiratory act, that is, started from the level of total lung capacity. FEV_1 is the most frequently used index for assessing airway obstruction and bronchoconstriction. Therefore, it is often used to assess bronchoconstriction in asthma. In a normal adult subject, FEV_1 is about 80%. This means that we are able to exhale 80% of the air in the lung during the first second. If there is an obstruction in the airways, for example, bronchoconstriction in asthma, the air flow during expiration slows down, thus the air exhaled in the first second drops to lower values (e.g., 50–60%) (Fig. 8.5).

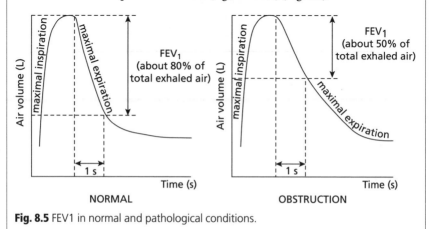

Fig. 8.5 FEV1 in normal and pathological conditions.

active pharmacological component (Pavesi et al., 2001; Eccles, 2002). Lee et al. (2000) studied patients with coughs associated with the common cold; cough frequency was measured at baseline and at 90, 135, and 180 minutes following administration of either a single dose of 30 mg dextromethorphan or a matched placebo capsule containing lactose. Both treatments produced exactly the same reduction in cough frequency at all the three time points.

Most clinical trials on cough medication did not include a no-treatment group, so they did not quantify a real placebo effect. However, Lee et al. (2005) conducted a trial on cough associated with acute upper respiratory infection with a no-treatment group and a placebo group. They found that the placebo treatment, compared with the no-treatment group, induced both a decrease in cough frequency and an increase in cough suppression time (the length of time patients can suppress their cough for). The no-treatment group had a 7% decrease in cough frequency compared to a 50% decrease in the placebo group.

Leech et al. (2012) investigated the effects of a placebo treatment on capsaicin-evoked urge to cough. Healthy participants were unknowingly conditioned to believe that an inert inhaler temporarily suppressed capsaicin-induced urge to cough by deceptively modifying the challenge concentration of capsaicin. In the test session, there was a significant decrease in mean urge-to-cough ratings to capsaicin challenge following placebo compared with a no treatment group and with a group in which participants were aware that no active medication was given. In a subsequent study by the same group (Leech et al., 2013), functional magnetic resonance imaging was used to investigate the regional changes in human brain activity related to the urge-to-cough following placebo antitussive administration. It was found that the decrease in participants' ratings of capsaicin-induced urge-to-cough following placebo administration was associated to reduced activity in the somatosensory, primary motor, insular, and cingulate cortices. This finding suggests that beliefs about treatment can modify the central processing of inputs arising from the airways.

8.3 **Points for further discussion**

1 To date, only a few studies on placebo mechanisms have been conducted on both the cardiovascular and respiratory systems. Therefore, one priority in placebo research is to investigate these functions, as has been done in other systems and apparatuses. Pathologies like arrhythmias, congestive heart failure or chronic respiratory diseases all deserve further analysis.

2 Stress plays an important role in many pathologies of the heart, so the effect of nocebos on cardiovascular health is a promising field of investigation that will contribute to our understanding of the stress–heart relationship.

3 Conditioned bradycardia in fear conditioning should be studied within the context of placebo and placebo-related effects. It would be interesting to study the effects of repeated associations between a neutral stimulus and a pharmacological agent acting on the heart. Can bradycardia and tachycardia be easily reproduced with a placebo after several conditioning sessions?

4 Do the endogenous opioid systems also affect the heart? The pharmacological and in vivo receptor binding studies performed in placebo analgesia should be extended to the cardiovascular system.

5 The possibility that placebos act on subpopulations of opioid receptors, such as the μ_2, during placebo respiratory depression should be investigated further.

6 There are a couple of respiratory diseases which have been investigated carefully— asthma and cough. They are known to undergo powerful placebo effects, thus we need to know the biological underpinnings. Asthma is a particularly good model because several biochemical pathways, like the cholinergic innervation of the bronchi, could be analyzed in detail.

References

Ammirati F, Colivicchi F and Santini M (2001). Permanent cardiac pacing versus medical treatment for the prevention of recurrent vasovagal syncope: a multicenter, randomised, controlled trial. *Circulation*, **104**, 52–7.

Asmar R, Safar M and Queneau P (2001). Evaluation of the placebo effect and reproducibility of blood pressure measurement in hypertension. *American Journal of Hypertension*, **14**, 546–52.

Balon J, Aker PD, Crowther ER *et al.* (1998). A comparison of active and simulated chiropractic manipulation as adjunctive treatment for childhood asthma. *New England Journal of Medicine*, **339**, 1013–20.

Barron AJ, Zaman N, Cole GD, Wensel R, Okonko DO and Francis DP (2013). Systematic review of genuine versus spurious side-effects of beta-blockers in heart failure using placebo control: recommendations for patient information. *International Journal of Cardiology*, **168**, 3572–9.

Benedetti F, Amanzio M, Baldi S *et al.* (1998). The specific effects of prior opioid exposure on placebo analgesia and placebo respiratory depression. *Pain*, **75**, 313–19.

Benedetti F, Amanzio M, Baldi S, Casadio C and Maggi G (1999). Inducing placebo respiratory depressant responses in humans via opioid receptors. *European Journal of Neuroscience*, **11**, 625–31.

Benedetti F, Colloca L, Lanotte M, Bergamasco B, Torre E and Lopiano L (2004). Autonomic and emotional responses to open and hidden stimulations of the human subthalamic region. *Brain Research Bulletin*, **63**, 203–11.

Bienenfeld L, Frishman W and Glasser SP (1996). The placebo effect in cardiovascular disease. *American Heart Journal*, **132**, 1207–21.

Bykov KM (1959). *The cerebral cortex and the internal organs*. Foreign Languages Publishing House, Moscow.

Chen E, Hanson MD, Paterson LQ, Griffin MJ, Walker HA and Miller GE (2006). Socioeconomic status and inflammatory processes in childhood asthma: the role of psychological stress. *Journal of Allergy and Clinical Immunology*, **117**, 1014–20.

Connolly SJ, Sheldon R, Roberts RS and Gent M (1999). The North American Vasovagal Pacemaker Study (VPS). A randomized trial of permanent cardiac pacing for the prevention of vasovagal syncope. *Journal of the American College of Cardiology*, **33**, 16–20.

Connolly SJ, Sheldon R, Thorpe KE *et al.* (2003). Pacemaker therapy for prevention of syncope in patients with recurrent severe vasovagal syncope: second Vasovagal Pacemaker Study (VPS II): a randomized trial. *Journal of the American Medical Association*, **289**, 2224–9.

Creticos PS, Reed CE, Norman PS *et al.* (1996). Ragweed immunotherapy in adult asthma. *New England Journal of Medicine*, **334**, 501–6.

Eccles R (2002). The powerful placebo in cough studies. *Pulmonary Pharmacology and Therapeutics*, **15**, 303–8.

Eccles R (2006). Mechanisms of the placebo effect of sweet cough syrups. *Respiratory Physiology & Neurobiology*, **152**, 340–8.

Eccles R (2009). Central mechanisms IV: conscious control of cough and the placebo effect. *Handbook of Experimental Pharmacology*, **187**, 241–62.

Eccles R (2010). Importance of placebo effect in cough clinical trials. *Lung*, **188**(Suppl. 1), S53–61.

Freemantle N, Cleland J, Young P, Mason J and Harrison J (1999). Beta blockade after myocardial infarction: systematic review and meta regression analysis. *British Medical Journal*, **318**, 1730–7.

Harris GC and Fitzgerald RD (1989). Impaired learning of classically conditioned bradycardia in rats following fourth ventricle administration of D-Ala2-methionine-enkephalinamide. *Behavioral Neuroscience*, **103**, 77–83.

Hernandez LL and Powell DA (1983). Naloxone induces multiple effects on aversive Pavlovian conditioning in rabbits. *Behavioral Neuroscience*, **97**, 478–91.

Hernandez LL, Powell DA and Gibbs CM (1990). Amygdaloid central nucleus neuronal activity accompanying pavlovian cardiac conditioning: effects of naloxone. *Behavioral Brain Research*, **41**, 71–9.

Hernandez LL and Watson KL (1997). Opioid modulation of attention-related responses: delta-receptors modulate habituation and conditioned bradycardia. *Psychopharmacology*, **131**, 140–7.

Joyce DP, Jackevicius C, Chapman KR, McIvor RA and Kesten S (2000). The placebo effect in asthma drug therapy trials: a meta-analysis. *Journal of Asthma*, **37**, 303–18.

Kemeny ME, Rosenwasser LJ, Panettieri RA, Rose RM, Berg-Smith SM and Kline JN (2007). Placebo response in asthma: a robust and objective phenomenon. *Journal of Allergy and Clinical Immunology*, **119**, 1375–81.

Knorr B, Matz J, Bernstein JA *et al.* (1998). Montelukast for chronic asthma in 6- to 14-year-old children: a randomized, double-blind trial. Pediatric Montelukast Study Group. *Journal of the American Medical Association*, **279**, 1181–6.

Ko DT, Hebert PR, Coffey CS, Sedrakyan A, Curtis JP and Krumholz HM (2002). Beta-blocker therapy and symptoms of depression, fatigue, and sexual dysfunction. *Journal of the American Medical Association*, **288**, 351–7.

Koch-Weser J and Frishman WH (1981). Beta-adrenoceptor antagonists: new drugs and new indications. *New England Journal of Medicine*, **305**, 500–6.

Krumholz HM, Radford MJ, Wang Y, Chen J, Heiat A and Marciniak TA (1998). National use and effectiveness of beta-blockers for the treatment of elderly patients after acute myocardial infarction: National Cooperative Cardiovascular Project. *Journal of the American Medical Association*, **280**, 623–9.

Lang W and Rand MA (1969). A placebo response as a conditional reflex to glycerol trinitrate. *Medical Journal of Australia*, **1**, 912–4.

Lang WJ, Ross P and Glover A (1967). Conditional responses induced by hypotensive drugs. *European Journal of Pharmacology*, **2**, 169–74.

Lanotte M, Lopiano L, Torre E, Bergamasco B, Colloca L and Benedetti F (2005). Expectation enhances autonomic responses to stimulation of the human subthalamic limbic region. *Brain Behavior Immunity*, **19**, 500–9.

Lee PCL, Jawad MS, Eccles R (2000). Antitussive efficacy of dextromethorphan in cough associated with acute upper respiratory tract infection. *Journal of Pharmacy and Pharmacology*, **52**, 1137–42.

Lee PCL, Jawad MSM, Hull JD, West WHL, Shaw K and Eccles R (2005). The antitussive effect of placebo treatment on cough associated with acute upper respiratory infection. *Psychosomatic Medicine*, **67**, 314–17.

Leech J, Mazzone SB and Farrell MJ (2012). The effect of placebo conditioning on capsaicin-evoked urge to cough. *Chest*, **142**, 951–7.

Leech J, Mazzone SB and Farrell MJ (2013). Brain activity associated with placebo suppression of the urge-to-cough in humans. *American Journal of Respiratory and Critical Care Medicine*, **188**, 1069–75.

Leigh R, MacQueen G, Tougas G, Hargreave FE and Bienenstock J (2003). Change in forced expiratory volume in 1 second after sham bronchoconstrictor in suggestible but not suggestion-resistant asthmatic subjects. A pilot study. *Psychosomatic Medicine*, 65, 791–5.

Ling GSF and Pasternak GW (1983). Spinal and supraspinal analgesia in the mouse: the role of subpopulations of opioid binding sites. *Brain Research*, **271**, 152–6.

Ling GSF, Spiegel K, Lockhart SH and Pasternak GW (1985). Separation of opioid analgesia from respiratory depression: evidence for different receptor mechanisms. *Journal of Pharmacology and Experimental Therapeutics*, **232**, 149–55.

Ling GSF, Spiegel K, Nishimura SL and Pasternak GW (1983). Dissociation of morphine's analgesic and respiratory depressant actions. *European Journal of Pharmacology*, **86**, 487–8.

Liu LY, Coe CL, Swenson CA, Kelly EA, Kita H and Busse WW (2002). School examinations enhance airway inflammation to antigen challenge. *American Journal of Respiratory Critical Care Medicine*, **165**, 1062–7.

Lue TF (2000). Erectile dysfunction. *New England Journal of Medicine*, **342**, 1802–13.

Luparello TJ, Lyons HA, Bleeker ER and McFadden ER (1968). Influence of suggestion on airways reactivity in asthmatic subjects. *Psychosomatic Medicine*, **30**, 819–25.

Malliani A, Pagani M, Lombardi F and Cerutti S (1991). Cardiovascular neural regulation explored in the frequency domain. *Circulation*, **84**, 482–92.

Mancia G, Omboni S, Parati G, Ravogli A, Villani A and Zanchetti A (1995). Lack of placebo effect on ambulatory blood pressure. *American Journal of Hypertension*, **8**, 311–15.

Maschke M, Schugens M, Kindsvater K *et al.* (2002). Fear conditioned changes of heart rate in patients with medial cerebellar lesions. *Journal of Neurology, Neurosurgery and Psychiatry*, **72**, 116–18.

McQuaid EL, Fritz GK, Nassau JH, Lilly MK, Mansell A and Klein RB (2000). Stress and airways resistance in children with asthma. *Journal of Psychosomatic Research*, **49**, 239–45.

Meissner K and Ziep D (2011). Organ-specificity of placebo effects on blood pressure. *Autonomic Neuroscience*, **164**, 62–6.

Milgrom H, Fick RB Jr, Su JQ *et al.* (1999). Treatment of allergic asthma with monoclonal anti-IgE antibody. rhuMAb-E25 Study Group. *New England Journal of Medicine*, **341**, 1966–73.

Mutti E, Trazzi S, Omboni S, Parati G and Mancia G (1991). Effect of placebo on 24-h noninvasive ambulatory blood pressure. *Journal of Hypertension*, **9**, 361–4.

Nademanee K, McKenzie J, Kosar E *et al.* (2004). A new approach for catheter ablation of atrial fibrillation: mapping of the electrophysiologic substrate. *Journal of the American College of Cardiology*, **43**, 2044–53.

Olshansky B (2007). Placebo and nocebo in cardiovascular health. Implications for healthcare, research, and the doctor-patient relationship. *Journal of the American College of Cardiology*, **49**, 415–21.

Pappone C, Rosanio S, Augello G *et al.* (2003). Mortality, morbidity, and quality of life after circumferential pulmonary vein ablation for atrial fibrillation: outcomes from a controlled nonrandomized long-term study. *Journal of the American College of Cardiology*, **42**, 185–97.

Pasternak GW (1988). Multiple morphine and enkephalin receptors and the relief of pain. *Journal of the American Medical Association*, **259**, 1362–7.

Pasternak GW (1993). Pharmacological mechanisms of opioid analgesics. *Clinical Neuropharmacology*, **16**, 1–18.

Pasternak GW, Childer SR and Snyder SH (1980a). Naloxazone, a long-acting opiate antagonist: effects in intact animals and on opiate receptors binding in vitro. *Journal of Pharmacology and Experimental Therapeutics*, **214**, 455–62.

Pasternak GW, Childer SR and Snyder SH (1980b). Opiate analgesia: evidence for mediation by a subpopulation of opiate receptors. *Science*, **208**, 514–16.

Pavesi L, Subburaj S and Porter-Shaw K (2001). Application and validation of a computerized cough acquisition system for objective monitoring of acute cough—a meta-analysis. *Chest*, **120**, 1121–8.

Physicians' desk reference (2002). Medical Economics Co Inc, Montvale, NJ.

Pollo A, Vighetti S, Rainero I and Benedetti F (2003). Placebo analgesia and the heart. *Pain*, **102**, 125–33.

Powell DA (1994). Rapid associative learning: conditioned bradycardia and its central nervous system substrates. *Integrative Physiological and Behavioral Sciences*, **29**, 109–33.

Powell DA, Chachich M, Murphy V, McLaughlin J, Tebbutt D and Buchanan SL (1997). Amygdala-prefrontal interactions and conditioned bradycardia in the rabbit. *Behavioral Neuroscience*, **111**, 1056–74.

Prager G, Klein P, Schmitt M and Prager R (1994). Antihypertensive efficacy of cilazapril 2.5 and 5.0 mg once-daily versus placebo on office blood pressure and 24-hour blood pressure profile. *Journal of Cardiovascular Pharmacology*, **24**(Suppl. 3), S93–9.

Preston RA, Materson BJ, Reda DJ and Williams DW (2000). Placebo-associated blood pressure response and adverse effects in the treatment of hypertension. Observations from a Department of Veterans Affairs Cooperative Study. *Archives of Internal Medicine*, **160**, 1449–54.

Rana JS, Mannam A, Donnell-Fink L, Gervino EV, Sellke FW and Laham RJ (2005). Longevity of the placebo effect in the therapeutic angiogenesis and laser myocardial revascularization trials in patients with coronary heart disease. *American Journal of Cardiology*, **95**, 1456–9.

Redwine K, Howard L, Simpson P, *et al.* (2012). Effect of placebo on ambulatory blood pressure monitoring in children. *Pediatric Nephrology*, **27**, 1937–42.

Robinson DS, Campbell D and Barnes PJ (2001). Addition of leukotriene antagonists to therapy in chronic persistent asthma: a randomized double-blind placebo-controlled trial. *Lancet*, **357**, 2007–11.

Sacchetti B, Scelfo B and Strata P (2005). The cerebellum: synaptic changes and fear conditioning. *Neuroscientist*, **11**, 217–27

Sacchetti B, Scelfo B, Tempia F and Strata P (2004). Long-term synaptic changes induced in the cerebellar cortex by fear conditioning. *Neuron*, **42**, 973–82.

Sandberg S, Jarvenpaa S, Penttinen A, Paton JY and McCann DC (2004). Asthma exacerbations in children immediately following stressful life events: a Cox's hierarchical regression. *Thorax*, **59**, 1046–51.

Sassano P, Chatellier G, Corvol P and Ménard J (1987). Influence of observer's expectation on the placebo effect in blood pressure trials. *Current Therapy Research*, **41**, 304–12.

Schroeder K and Fahey T (2001). Over-the-counter medications for acute cough in children and adults in ambulatory setting. *Cochrane Database of Systematic Reviews*, **3**, CD001831.

Schroeder K and Fahey T (2002). Systematic review of randomized controlled trials of over the counter cough medicines for acute cough in adults. *British Medical Journal*, **324**, 1–6.

Supple WF Jr and Kapp BS (1993). The anterior cerebellar vermis: essential involvement in classically conditioned bradycardia in the rabbit. *Journal of Neuroscience*, **13**, 3705–11.

Wechsler ME, Kelley JM, Boyd IO, *et al.* (2011). Active albuterol or placebo, sham acupuncture, or no intervention in asthma. *New England Journal of Medicine*, **365**, 119–26.

Weiss RJ (1991). Effects of antihypertensive agents on sexual function. *American Family Physician*, **44**, 2075–82.

Weiss RJ, Stapff M and Lin Y (2013). Placebo effect and efficacy of nebivolol in patients with hypertension not controlled with lisinopril or losartan: a phase IV, randomized, placebo-controlled trial. *American Journal of Cardiovascular Drugs*, **13**, 129–40.

Zhang AZ and Pasternak GW (1981). Opiates and enkephalins: a common binding site mediates their analgesic actions in rats. *Life Sciences*, **29**, 843–57.

Zimmermann-Viehoff F, Meissner K, Koch J, Weber CS, Richter S and Deter HC (2013). Autonomic effects of suggestive placebo interventions to increase or decrease blood pressure: A randomized controlled trial in healthy subjects. *Journal of Psychosomatic Research*, **75**, 32–5.

Chapter 9

Gastrointestinal and genitourinary disorders

Summary points

- Irritable bowel syndrome (IBS) is one of the best models of gastro-intestinal disorders for understanding placebo mechanisms.
- Several brain regions are inhibited by a placebo treatment in people suffering from IBS.
- Gastrointestinal symptoms can be conditioned, which indicates that learning may play an important role.
- Subjective symptoms are more affected than objective symptoms in genitourinary disorders.
- Expectations are crucially involved in sexual functions.

9.1 Gastrointestinal disorders

9.1.1 Reduction in gastrointestinal symptoms is common in patients who receive placebo treatments

Several gastrointestinal disorders show substantial improvements following placebo treatments. This occurs with functional bowel disorders like functional dyspepsia and IBS (Box 9.1), and organic gastrointestinal diseases like duodenal ulcer and inflammatory conditions (Enck and Klosterhalfen, 2005; Bernstein, 2006; Musial et al., 2007). Symptom reduction in placebo groups of clinical trials of functional dyspepsia ranges from 6–72% (Mearin et al., 1999; Allescher et al., 2001), whereas it ranges from 3–84% for IBS (Klein, 1988; Jackson et al., 2000; Poynard et al., 2001; Cremonini et al., 2003; Spanier et al., 2003). Likewise, symptom reduction in placebo groups of clinical trials of ulcerative colitis was as high as 40% for subjective measures, about 30% for endoscopic examination, and 25% for histological remission in a study by Ilnyckyj et al. (1997), whereas it was 18% for remission in Crohn's disease (Su et al., 2004). It should be noted, however, that neither spontaneous remission nor regression to the mean could be ruled out in all these studies. Indeed, Enck and Klosterhalfen (2005) re-analyzed the data from the study by Spiller (1999), with particular regard to the relationship between the magnitude of remission in placebo groups and the duration of the studies. They found that with longer treatment

Box 9.1 Irritable bowel syndrome

Irritable bowel syndrome (IBS) is a good model to study placebo and nocebo effects because the psychological component seems to play an important role in many circumstances. Its main symptoms are chronic abdominal pain, discomfort, bloating, and alteration of bowel habits. IBS is estimated to affect about 10–15% of the population younger than 45 years and about twice as many women as men. Many hypotheses have been put forward about its pathophysiology, including altered communication between brain and gut, gastrointestinal motor disorders, hypersensitivity to pain, bacterial gastroenteritis, food sensitivity, and genetics. Interestingly, IBS is often associated with mental or psychological disorders, such as anxiety, depression, and post-traumatic stress disorder. Probably, its pathophysiology is multifactorial, and a combination of many factors is likely to lead to IBS emergence and maintenance. Accordingly, different treatments have been found to affect the course of the disease, for example, all those interventions that reduce stress, anxiety, and depression. These include pharmacotherapy with anxiolytics and/or antidepressants, relaxation techniques, and psychotherapy.

duration the improvement in placebo groups stabilized at around 40%. In addition, if the sample size comprised more than 500 people with IBS, a similar stabilization of 40% improvement was found. This suggests that regression to the mean may contribute to symptom remission in placebo groups.

Although none of these studies allow definitive conclusions to be made on the relative contribution of natural history, regression to the mean, and real placebo responses in gastrointestinal disorders such as IBS and ulcerative colitis, some of their findings are interesting. For example, some showed that the rate of remission in placebo groups with ulcerative colitis depended on the number of visits; three or fewer visits were less likely to induce large remissions in patients who received the placebo (compared to four or more visits) (Ilnyckyj et al., 1997). Similarly, the number of study visits during the trial, as well as the duration of the study and the severity of disease at entry, were good predictors of remission in the placebo groups in clinical trials on Crohn's disease (Su et al., 2004). However, some contrasting results have also been found regarding the relationship between the number of visits and the placebo response rate (Patel et al., 2005; Pitz et al., 2005).

Overall, placebo response rates in functional bowel disorders trials, for example, functional dyspepsia and IBS, are similar to those in nonintestinal pain conditions and are comparable with other organic gastrointestinal diseases, such as duodenal ulcer and inflammatory bowel diseases (Enck et al., 2012). In more recent studies that used different methodologies, ranging from meta-analyses and re-analyses to a variety of experimental setups, placebos have been confirmed to produce positive therapeutic outcomes, although no clear mechanism can be identified (Garud et al., 2008; Enck et al., 2009; Meissner, 2009; Cremonini et al., 2010; Ford and Moayyedi, 2010; Gallahan et al., 2010; Capurso et al., 2012; Weimer et al., 2012).

It is interesting to note that the characteristics of both doctor and patient can influence the response to placebos. Kelley et al. (2009) performed an analysis of videotape and psychometric data from a clinical trial of patients with IBS who were treated with placebo acupuncture in either a warm empathic interaction (Augmented), a neutral interaction (Limited), or a waitlist control (Waitlist). The relationships between the placebo response and (1) patient personality and demographics, (2) treating practitioner, and (3) the patient–practitioner interaction (from videotape analysis) were examined. The investigators found that patient extraversion, agreeableness, openness to experience, and female gender were associated with placebo response, but these effects held only in the augmented group. Regression analyses controlling for all other independent variables suggested that only extraversion is an independent predictor of placebo response. Therefore, as already discussed in section 2.3.4, personality may influence the placebo response, but only in the warm, empathic, augmented group.

9.1.2 Increasing the frequency of placebo administration increases clinical improvement

In support of the relationship between the number of visits and the increased improvement in placebo groups in ulcerative colitis (Ilnyckyj et al., 1997) and in Crohn's disease (Su et al., 2004), analysis of duodenal ulcer clinical trials suggests that the number of placebos that the patient receives increases the healing rate. It has long been known that the healing rates of duodenal ulcer in patients who take a placebo treatment varies substantially across randomized controlled trials (Gudjonsson and Spiro, 1978; Moerman, 1983; Poynard and Pignon, 1989; Dobrilla and Scarpignato, 1994). In 1999, a systematic literature review was published by de Craen et al. (1999), in which 79 randomized placebo-controlled clinical trials were analyzed by considering the frequency of administration of placebos. In 51 trials with a total of 1821 patients, placebos were given on the basis of a four-times-a-day regimen, whereas in 28 trials with a total of 1504 patients they were given twice a day. It was found that the healing rate in the four-times-a-day regimen was 44.2%; it dropped significantly to 36.2% in the twice-a-day regimen.

Similar findings have been obtained in IBS. In another systematic review of 84 placebo-controlled trials in patients with IBS, Pitz et al. (2005) found that higher rates of global improvement correlated with the frequency of placebo administration, the duration of the study and overall treatment effect of the active agent. Likewise, higher rates of decreased abdominal pain correlated with the frequency of placebo administration and the overall treatment effect. Interestingly, Pitz et al. (2005) also found that decreased abdominal pain in placebo groups was different in studies performed between 1999 and 2004 (a mean decrease rate of 20.6%) compared with studies before 1999 (a mean decrease rate of 31.2%). In fact, the average frequency of placebo administration was found to be 2.0 per day in the period between 1999 and 2004 and 2.7 times per day in studies before 1999, thus further supporting the relationship between frequency of placebo administration and clinical improvement (Fig. 9.1).

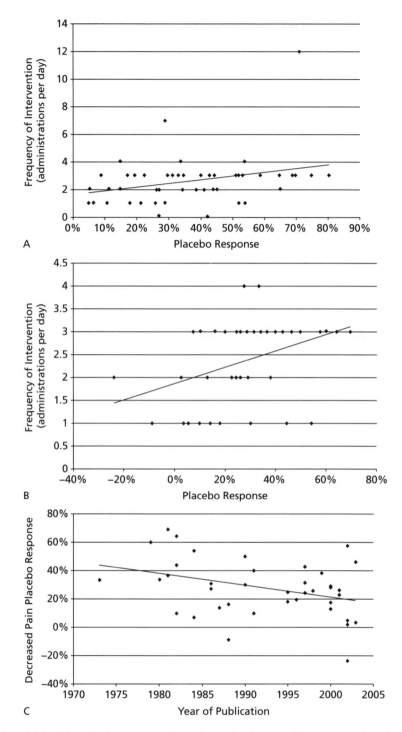

Fig. 9.1 (A) Global placebo response plotted against frequency of intervention showing higher placebo response rates (%) with increasing frequency of intervention (p = 0.03). (B) Decreased pain placebo response plotted against frequency of intervention showing

9.1.3 The placebo responses in irritable bowel syndrome can be imaged in the brain

IBS is one of the gastrointestinal disorders, and actually one of the painful conditions, in which the placebo effect has been studied in detail. It is a functional disorder of the bowel, mainly characterized by abdominal pain, and with no abnormalities seen on routine clinical testing. The abdominal pain may be associated with either diarrhea or constipation and may be the result of a previous infectious episode. Although no specific cause is known for the disorder, many factors may contribute, such as stress, infections, and biochemical changes (e.g., cytokines). The treatment is based on either diet, pharmacological agents (e.g., antispasmodics), or even psychotherapy.

Verne et al. (2003) and Vase et al. (2003) performed two similar studies in which patients suffering from IBS were exposed to rectal distension by means of a balloon barostat, a type of visceral stimulation that simulates their clinical pain. A no-treatment group, a rectal placebo group, and a rectal lidocaine group were studied. A study by Verne et al. (2003) was conducted according to a double-blind crossover design in which the patients were told that they "may receive an active pain-reducing medication or an inert placebo agent." There was a significant pain-relieving effect of rectal lidocaine as compared to rectal placebo, and a significant pain-relieving effect of rectal placebo as compared to no-treatment. In the study by Vase et al. (2003), patients were told that the agent they had just been given was known to significantly reduce pain in some people. A much larger placebo analgesic effect was found in this second study and it did not significantly differ from that of rectal lidocaine. Both of these studies show that adding an overt suggestion for pain relief can increase placebo analgesia to a magnitude that matches that of an active agent (see Fig. 4.2A,B). In both studies, patients were also asked to rate their expected pain level and their desire for pain relief; it was found that both of these contribute to placebo analgesia. In addition, there was also a significant reduction in anxiety ratings in the two experiments (Vase et al., 2003; Verne et al., 2003). These findings were confirmed by a subsequent study showing that ratings of desire for pain reduction, expected pain, and anxiety all decreased over time as the placebo effect increased over time (Vase et al., 2005).

In the study by Vase et al. (2003) there appeared to be a consistent enhancement of pain intensity and unpleasantness in the predicted direction when a nocebo was administered, but the pain ratings in the nocebo condition were not significantly different from the natural history group. It should be noted, however, that the mean visceral pain intensity between the placebo and the nocebo condition was as large as 3.9 units

---

Fig. 9.1 (continued) increased placebo response rates with increasing frequency of intervention (p = 0.02). (C) Decreased pain placebo response plotted against year of publication showing higher placebo response rates in studies with earlier publication dates (p = 0.03). Reprinted from *Clinical Gastroenterology and Hepatology*, 3 (3), Marshall Pitz, Mary Cheang, and Charles N. Bernstein, Defining the predictors of the placebo response in irritable bowel syndrome, pp. 237–47, Copyright (2005), with permission from Elsevier.

on a 10-unit scale, which indicates a powerful modulation of visceral pain by opposing placebo–nocebo suggestions.

The strong placebo responses observed by Vase et al. (2003) led the same investigators to use brain imaging techniques to map the neural changes during the placebo response in IBS. As already described for placebo analgesia (section 4.1.9), Price et al. (2007) conducted a functional magnetic resonance imaging study in which brain activity of IBS patients was measured in response to rectal distension by a balloon barostat. A substantial placebo response was produced by verbal suggestions of improvement, and this was accompanied by reductions in neural activity in the thalamus, the primary and secondary somatosensory cortex, the insula and anterior cingulate cortex, as well as by increases in neural activity in the rostral anterior cingulate cortex, bilateral amygdala, and periaqueductal gray (see also Price et al., 2008) (Fig. 9.2). The study by Price et al. (2007) is important because it is one of the first neuroimaging placebo studies in the clinical setting, indicating that placebos act on the brain in a clinically relevant condition in the same way as they do in the experimental setting.

Overall, results from different studies suggest that pains associated with both visceral and widespread secondary cutaneous hyperalgesia are dynamically maintained

NATURAL HISTORY   **PLACEBO**

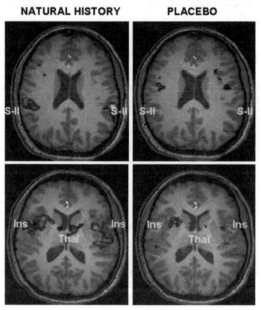

Fig. 9.2 Brain regions showing large reductions in pain-related brain activity during the placebo condition compared with untreated natural history or baseline condition in patients with irritable bowel syndrome. The thalamus (Thal), second somatosensory area (S-II) and insular cortical regions (Ins) show reduced activity. Reproduced from Donald D. Price, Damien G. Finniss, and Fabrizio Benedetti, A Comprehensive Review of the Placebo Effect: Recent Advances and Current Thought, Annual Review of Psychology, 59 (1), pp. 565–590 Copyright 2008, Annual Reviews. DOI: 10.1146/annurev. psych.59.113006.095941. Reproduced with permission of Annual Review http://www.annualreviews.org. (See Plate 12.)

by tonic impulse input from the noninflamed colon and/or rectum and by brain-to-spinal cord facilitation. Enhanced visceral and somatic pains are accompanied by enhanced pain-related brain activity in IBS patients as compared to normal control subjects; placebos can normalize both their hyperalgesia and enhanced brain activity (Price et al., 2009). That pain in IBS is likely to be at least partly maintained by peripheral impulse input from the colon/rectum is supported by results showing that local rectal-colonic anesthesia normalizes visceral and somatic hyperalgesia in IBS patients and visceral and somatic hypersensitivity in "IBS-like" rats (Price et al., 2009). These forms of hyperalgesia are also highly modifiable by placebo and nocebo factors, probably through synergistic interactions that occur between placebo/nocebo factors and enhanced afferent processing (Price et al., 2009).

It is interesting to note that perceived treatment group affects the response to placebo. By using functional magnetic resonance imaging, Kotsis et al. (2012) analyzed the behavioral and neural responses during expectation-mediated placebo analgesia in a rectal pain model. Brain responses during cued anticipation and painful stimulation were measured after participants were informed that they had a 50% chance of receiving either a potent analgesic drug or an inert substance (double-blind administration). In reality, all received placebo. Then, the researchers compared the responses in subjects who retrospectively indicated that they had received the drug and those who believed they had received placebo. Rectal pain-induced discomfort was significantly lower in the perceived drug treatment group, along with significantly reduced activation of the insular, the posterior and anterior cingulate cortices during pain anticipation, and of the anterior cingulate cortex during pain. Thus, perceived treatment constitutes an important aspect in placebo analgesia and can induce different brain responses, depending on personal beliefs and expectations.

In contrast to many studies on opioid-mediated placebo analgesia (section 4.1.6) the placebo analgesic effect in IBS has been found to be naloxone-insensitive, suggesting mediation by nonopioid mechanisms (Vase et al., 2005). In an attempt to identify possible mediators and predictors of the placebo response in IBS, Kokkotou et al. (2010) found an association between changes in serum levels of osteoprotegerin (OPG) and tumor necrosis factor (TNF)-related weak inducer of apoptosis (TWEAK) and placebo response. However, the exact meaning of these changes is not clear and further confirmation is necessary. As already mentioned in section 2.3.5, the catechol-O-methyltransferase (COMT) functional val158met polymorphism was found to be associated to the placebo effect in IBS. The strongest placebo response occurred in met/met homozygotes (Hall et al., 2012).

9.1.4 Salivary secretion can be conditioned

Salivation was the first physiological function to be conditioned in the experiments by Pavlov (1910) although the conditioned salivary response was not conceptualized in terms of a placebo effect. Salivary secretion is an important function of the digestive system, and several experiments show how neutral stimuli can induce conditioned placebo responses. For example, in 1925, Collins and Tatum (1925) performed an experiment whereby morphine was administered to dogs daily for about a week. Each injection produced copious salivation. The investigators soon realized that the dogs salivated copiously simply when the experimenter entered the laboratory with a syringe in his hands. Similar observations were made by Kleitman and Crisler (1927) and by Russian investigators such as Krylov (Pavlov, 1927). In all these cases, the ritual performed by the experimenter preparing the injection elicited salivary secretion in the dogs, in the same way as food did in Pavlov's original experiments. In conditioning research today, salivary secretion has been replaced with other physiological functions, but the conditioned salivary response is still a very good example of how a neutral stimulus (the placebo) can induce a conditioned response after many pairings with an unconditioned stimulus (food or drug).

9.1.5 **Gastrointestinal symptoms can be learned**

There are at least two important conditions that have been studied in detail and are very good examples of how learning can be important in gastrointestinal symptoms.

The first condition is anticipatory nausea and vomiting before a chemotherapy session for the treatment of cancer. In this case there is ample experimental evidence that conditioning may play a crucial role. Although it relates to the gastrointestinal apparatus, it will be discussed in more detail in section 10.1.2.

The second condition has to do with motion sickness. Several experimental approaches have used a rotating chair to induce motion-related nausea (Klosterhalfen et al., 2000, 2005; Rohleder et al., 2006). In general it is assumed that the conditioned stimulus is the rotation context, and the unconditioned stimulus is the rotation itself; the unconditioned response is the series of symptoms induced by the rotation such as nausea, the urge to vomit, dizziness, headache, tiredness, sweating, and general discomfort (Stockhorst et al., 2007). After repeated exposures to the rotation, the sight of the rotating chair sometimes induces anticipatory symptoms, like nausea and the urge to vomit, which themselves represent the conditioned response. This model is useful because rotation can also induce changes in the secretion of cortisol and other endogenous substances like TNF-α and interleukin-2β (Stockhorst et al., 2007).

The interest in the rotation model resides in the clear-cut analogy with anticipatory nausea and vomiting in cancer chemotherapy (see section 10.1.2). The conditioned stimulus "rotation context" is similar to the "chemotherapy context" and the unconditioned stimulus "rotation" can be compared to the "chemotherapy." Therefore, this model has been used to try to both simulate and reduce anticipatory nausea and vomiting. At least two experimental approaches have been used to prevent anticipatory rotation symptoms. The first is called latent inhibition and it consists of pre-exposing subjects to the rotation context several times before the rotation itself. The second is called overshadowing and it consists of pairing a couple of conditioned stimuli (rotation context plus a second stimulus) with the rotation itself (where the second conditioned stimulus is more salient than the rotation context). Using both procedures makes it is possible to reduce the strength of conditioning so that the conditioned response (in this case nausea and vomiting) has been found to be reduced (Klosterhalfen et al., 2005; Stockhorst et al., 2006, 2007).

It is also worth noting that in these studies some gender differences have been found. For example, habituation of the cortisol response after repeated rotations was found to be restricted to women (Rohleder et al., 2006) and in latent inhibition studies women showed lower cortisol increases after rotation than men (Klosterhalfen et al., 2005). There was also a higher responsiveness in women compared to men for both conditioning of anticipatory nausea and its modification by latent inhibition and overshadowing (Klosterhalfen et al., 2005).

Learning of gastrointestinal symptoms is therefore an interesting phenomenon and it is relevant to the understanding of placebo and placebo-related effects. This will be discussed further in the context of anticipatory nausea and vomiting in cancer chemotherapy (section 10.1.2). In this sense, nocebo learned phenomena that induce gastrointestinal symptoms can be managed by using a behavioral approach aimed at either preventing or reducing learning.

9.1.6 Placebo- and nocebo-induced expectations may lead to clinical improvement and worsening respectively

A number of studies have manipulated the patient's expectations in order to see whether gastric functions can be affected, but unfortunately these studies have produced contrasting and nondefinitive findings. One of the first studies to use this experimental approach was that by Sternbach (1964), who showed that inducing either positive or negative expectations influences gastric motility in the expected direction. In 1999, Mearin et al. (1999) performed a study in patients suffering from functional dyspepsia and who were treated with a placebo therapy for 8 weeks. Unfortunately, this study did not use a no-treatment control group, thus no definitive conclusions can be drawn. However, there are some interesting findings that are worthy of consideration (Fig. 9.3). After the 8 weeks of placebo treatment, 80% of patients reported an improvement in their global health status and their global symptom index decreased significantly. Although the mean group effect on postprandial gastroduodenal motility did not show significant changes, a significant improvement in antral motility was observed in a subset of patients with antral hypomotility. There was also an increase in the number of gastric phases III which represent a specific subtype of gastric motility. In addition, after 8 weeks of placebo treatment, no change was observed in gastric sensitivity to distension, despite the clinical improvement. Mearin and colleagues concluded that since the clinical improvement is constant and remarkable while gastric function improvement is variable, clinical improvement in patients who receive a placebo treatment for functional dyspepsia seems to occur independently of detectable changes in both gastroduodenal motility and hypersensitivity to distension.

Another study performed by Levine et al. (2006) showed that positive and negative expectations affected both subjective symptoms and gastric motor activity, but in the unexpected direction. A nausea-inducing rotating optokinetic drum was used, and 75 patients were subdivided into three groups. The first was given placebo pills that they believed to be an agent protecting them against nausea and motion sickness; the second was given the same inert substance but they believed it increased nausea and motion sickness; the third (control) group knew that the placebo pills contained an inert substance. In contrast to the studies by Sternbach (1964) and Mearin et al. (1999) it was found that subjective symptoms of motion sickness were significantly lower in the negative-expectation group compared with those in the positive-expectation group.

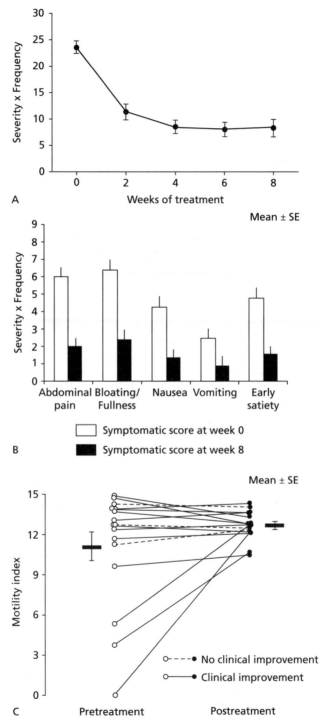

Fig. 9.3 Dissociation between clinical improvement and changes in gastric motility after placebo treatment. (A) Dyspeptic symptoms, expressed as the global symptom score

Likewise, the abnormal gastric activity induced by the rotating optokinetic drum was reduced by the nocebo suggestions compared to placebo. A possible explanation for this somehow unexpected positive effect of nocebo suggestions could be explained, at least in part, by the fact that the negative-expectation subjects anticipated a sickening experience which was far more innocuous than they had expected. The opposite explanation might hold true for the positive-expectation group.

Vernia et al. (2010) studied lactose intolerance in patients who performed a standard 25 g lactose tolerance test, which is based on a "positive" H_2 breath test associated with abdominal symptoms. A total of 27 patients reporting symptoms despite a negative H_2 breath test underwent a sham breath test following ingestion of 1 g of glucose (well below the standard dose of 25 g). Twelve out of these 27 patients (44.4%) presented abdominal symptoms during the sham test, which indicates that symptoms reported by patients during the test can sometimes be attributable to a nocebo effect.

It appears clear that several studies have found expectations will consistently affect both gastric/abdominal symptoms and gastric motor activity. The exact mechanisms and meaning behind these changes are somewhat contrasting and still unclear across these studies by Sternbach (1964), Mearin et al. (1999), Levine et al. (2006), and Vernia et al. (2010).

9.2 Genitourinary disorders

9.2.1 Reductions of subjective lower urinary tract symptoms are larger than reductions of objective symptoms in placebo groups

As for other systems, a few data—if any—are available on placebo and placebo-related effects in the genitourinary system. The main reason for this is that all the clinical trials that have been performed do not discriminate real placebo responses from other factors. In fact, a large number of clinical trials have been performed across many genitourinary disorders, yet there is very little information on the magnitude and possible mechanisms of the placebo response. Here a couple of examples are presented in order to give an idea of the possible nature of both placebo and nocebo effects in the genitourinary apparatus.

Fig. 9.3 (continued) (severity × frequency), significantly improve after placebo treatment. The symptomatic response, already present at 2 weeks of treatment, was sustained during the 8-week follow-up period. (B) Improvement occurs in all five dyspeptic symptoms evaluated during the 8 weeks of placebo treatment. (C) Despite the clinical improvement, no significant changes in postprandial antral motility are observed after placebo treatment. However, in patients with severe antral hypomotility, placebo treatment significantly improves motility. Data are expressed as mean ± SEM. Reprinted by permission from Macmillan Publishers Ltd: *The American Journal of Gastroenterology*, 94 (1), Fermin Mearin, Agustin Balboa, Natalia Zarate, Mercedes Cucala, Juan-R Malagelada et al., Placebo in functional dyspepsia: symptomatic, gastrointestinal motor, and gastric sensorial responses, pp. 116–25 Copyright 1999, Nature Publishing Group.

Lower urinary tract symptoms are represented by storage symptoms such as urinary incontinence, voiding symptoms (slow and/or intermittent stream), and post-micturition symptoms like a feeling of incomplete emptying. They are good examples of how patients who receive a placebo report large subjective improvements accompanied by small objective changes (Moyad, 2002; van Leeuwen et al., 2006). For example, an overactive bladder and urinary urge incontinence are likely to be mediated by activation of acetylcholine muscarinic receptors; there is a response to antimuscarinic agents that ranges from 45–77% and to placebos from 32–64% when urge incontinence episodes are assessed. However, more objective assessment (mean voided volume per micturition) shows that placebo groups show a 5–6% increase, whereas the active treatment groups show a 10–22% increase (van Leeuwen et al., 2006).

A similar discrepancy in subjective and objective improvements in placebo groups has been found in bladder outlet obstruction and benign prostatic enlargement, which are characterized by reduced flow of stream and a feeling of incomplete emptying (van Leeuwen et al., 2006). In clinical trials with drugs such as α1-adrenoreceptor antagonists and 5 α-reductase inhibitors, decreases in symptom scores are seen in placebo-treated patients of 9–34%, compared with 22–45% in patients who received active treatment. When more objective measurements were undertaken, such as peak urinary flow rate, increases of flow rate of 2–9% were observed in placebo groups against 17–33% in active treatment groups. In addition, trials with finasteride and dutasteride (5 α-reductase inhibitors that suppress the formation of dihydrotestosterone from testosterone and prevent prostate growth) show a reduction in prostate volume of 18–27% in the active treatment groups, and an increase in prostate size of 2–14% in the placebo groups (van Leeuwen et al., 2006).

There are some studies on the duration of symptom reduction in placebo groups but, as we have already seen for other conditions, the absence of a no-treatment control group means spontaneous remission cannot be ruled out. Take, for example, trials on bladder outlet obstruction and benign prostatic enlargement in which tamsulosin was compared to placebo. These show that the placebo effect can be maintained for over a year, although spontaneous remission could not be ruled out (Nickel, 1998). Likewise a trial comparing finasteride with placebo showed the placebo effect lasted for 8 months, although no control group was run to rule out spontaneous remission (McConnell et al., 1998). Interestingly, Nickel (1998) found that placebo treatment did not change the need for prostate surgery, suggesting once again that the placebo effect is related in this case to self-reported urinary symptoms, rather than to objective changes.

Overall, a review of placebo-controlled, randomized trials in overactive bladder syndrome by Mangera et al. (2011), shows statistically significant improvements in three patient-reported outcomes after placebo treatment: incontinence episodes per day, micturition episodes per day and mean micturition volume from baseline. However, no mechanism can be inferred from this and other studies (Lee et al., 2009; Staskin et al., 2012).

9.2.2 Sexual function may improve after placebo and worsen after nocebo

Since sex requires a complex interaction between psychological and physiological factors (Box 9.2), not surprisingly placebo responses are common. There are several examples of improvements in placebo groups of clinical trials on sexual dysfunction, although unfortunately no mechanism can be inferred from these studies. Some of the best examples are trials that assess the efficacy of sildenafil citrate for treating male erectile dysfunction. In a meta-analysis by Fink et al. (2002) on 27 trials (a total of 6659 men), sildenafil was more likely than placebo to lead to successful sexual intercourse. However the percentage of successful intercourse attempts in the placebo groups was 21% versus 57% in the sildenafil groups. Likewise, the percentage of men experiencing at least one successful intercourse during treatment was 45% in the placebo groups versus 83% in the sildenafil groups. Interestingly, improvements in placebo groups also occur in people with spinal cord injury. One study focused on the efficacy and tolerability of vardenafil in 418 men with erectile dysfunction due to traumatic spinal cord injury (Giuliano et al., 2006). They found that over 12 weeks of treatment the mean per-patient penetration was 76% for vardenafil versus 41% for placebo, maintenance of erection was 59% for vardenafil versus 22% for placebo, and ejaculation was 19% for vardenafil versus 10% for placebo.

Box 9.2 Sex and the brain

Masters and Johnson (1966) have identified four phases of sexual activity. First, excitation is a period of increasing attention that aims to prepare the sexual act. Second, a plateau is reached, in which sexual attention is constantly high. Third, orgasm is that short-lasting phase where the peak of pleasure is reached. Fourth, resolution occurs, whereby attention decreases. These four phases are followed by a refractory period that may last minutes, hours, and even days, depending on the individual. Interestingly, whereas the intensity of other motivated behaviors, like hunger and thirst, depends on the time lag from the latest meal or drink, the temporal factor in sex is not as important as for hunger and thirst. Sensory stimuli (visual, auditory, or tactile) play a much more important role to initiate another sexual act. In addition, the refractory period can be shortened in males if the partner changes, the so-called Coolidge effect. During the Coolidge effect, dopamine is released in the nucleus accumbens when the male copulates with the first female, then decreases to normal levels, but it is released again at high levels in the presence of a new female.

Many brain regions take part in the sexual act and these have been analyzed in great detail, particularly in animals. The medial preoptic area of the hypothalamus and the medial amygdala have been found to be hyperactive when animals make sex spontaneously, and the stimulation of the medial preoptic area increases the frequency of the sexual intercourses in rodents whereas the stimulation of the medial amygdala induces dopamine release. Gender-specific regions have also been found. For example, the sexually dimorphic nucleus of the hypothalamus is important for sexual activity in males, whereas the ventromedial nucleus of the hypothalamus is crucial for sexual behavior in females. Given the important role of dopamine in reward mechanisms (see section 3.3), it is interesting to note that dopaminergic activity increases during the sexual act and that dopamine blockade in the medial preoptic area by means of antagonists reduces sexual activity. In humans, dopaminergic drugs have been found to stimulate sexual behavior.

De Araujo et al. (2009) performed a prospective, controlled, single-blind study in which 123 patients with erectile dysfunction were randomly assigned to three groups: group 1 was informed that they were receiving a substance for erectile dysfunction treatment; group 2 was informed that they could be receiving an active drug or placebo; group 3 was aware that they were receiving a placebo. Placebo capsules were dispensed to all patients. After 8 weeks of the intervention, erectile dysfunction severity improved in all three groups and no difference was found among groups, whereas improvement in quality of erection was only significant in group 2.

Changes in sexual function during placebo treatment have also been found in women in clinical trials for the management of sexual dysfunction. For example, Bradford and Meston (2007) studied 16 women with sexual arousal and orgasmic dysfunction after randomization to receive placebo treatment for 8 weeks. In this study, their age, length of relationship, psychological symptoms, and scores on self-report measures were tested. The researchers found a significant improvement in sexual function scores after 8 weeks of treatment with placebo. They also found that age and length of relationship predicted the magnitude of change in sexual function. In general, as stressed by Bradford and Meston (2009) and Bradford (2013) and as occurs in other medical conditions, the placebo response in sexual dysfunction is a complex phenomenon that represents cognitive, behavioral, motivational, and relational mediating factors. Instructions given to trial participants, behavioral changes required to participate in a trial, changes in partner behavior, and interactions with study staff may influence participants' expectations of benefit and therefore their responses to placebo treatment.

Sexual function can be affected by nocebos as well although, yet again, the underlying mechanisms are totally unknown. One of the most natural situations for observing nocebo effects involves the information about possible side effects of drugs. In the genitourinary apparatus there is a nice example. The drug finasteride is used to treat prostatic hyperplasia and it is known to cause sexual side effects such as erectile dysfunction, loss of libido and ejaculation disorders, with a frequency of 15% after 1 year of treatment. Mondaini et al. (2007) studied 107 patients with a diagnosis of benign prostatic hyperplasia, randomly subdivided into two groups. The first group received finasteride for 1 year and the possible side effects were described to them in detail by the physician; the second group received the same dose of finasteride but was not informed about the possible side effects. The second (noninformed) group reported one or more sexual side effects with a frequency of 15.3%, and the first (informed) group showed a frequency as large as 43.6%. In particular, the incidence of erectile dysfunction, decreased libido, and ejaculation disorders were 9.6%, 7.7%, and 5.7%, respectively, in the noninformed group; they were 30.9%, 23.6%, and 16.3%, respectively, in the informed group. Thus, the patient's knowledge about the possible side effects of finasteride may have a dramatic psychological impact on sexual function.

Another example is represented by the side effects of combined oral contraceptives. Placebo-controlled, randomized trials document that nonspecific side effects are not significantly more common with combined oral contraceptives than with inert pills. These reported nonspecific side effects may be attributable to nocebo effects (Grimes and Schulz, 2011).

9.3 **Points for further discussion**

1   A detailed investigation of the placebo effect has been performed in IBS, including brain imaging studies. This analysis should be extended to other gastrointestinal pathologies, such as Crohn's disease, ulcerative colitis, and functional dyspepsia. For example, in inflammatory conditions (Crohn's disease and ulcerative colitis) it would be interesting to study mediators of inflammation after placebo treatment.

2   The physiology and biochemistry of the gastrointestinal system is well understood, and both hormones and the autonomic nervous system have been found to modulate gastric and intestinal functions. Therefore, placebo responsiveness in gastrointestinal disorders might involve both the endocrine and the nervous system.

3   Many clinical trials have been carried out in the genitourinary system; however, why some placebo groups improve is not known. Diseases of the kidney and of the genital apparatus deserve more attention and, in particular, we need to know whether placebos affect only subjective symptoms or objective physiological parameters as well.

4   As the psychological component is very important in sexual function, both in men and in women, a more detailed analysis of the biological mechanisms of the placebo effect is necessary. For example, the effects of placebos on pleasure and orgasm could be analyzed from a neuroendocrine perspective.

References

Allescher HD, Bockenhoff A, Knapp G, Wienbeck M and Hartung J (2001). Treatment of non-ulcer dyspepsia: a meta-analysis of placebo-controlled prospective studies. *Scandinavian Journal of Gastroenterology*, **36**, 934–41.

Bernstein CN (2006). The placebo effect for gastroenterology: tool or torment. *Clinical Gastroenterology and Hepatology*, **4**, 1302–8.

Bradford A (2013). Listening to placebo in clinical trials for female sexual dysfunction. *Journal of Sexual Medicine*, **10**, 451–9.

Bradford A and Meston C (2007). Correlates of placebo response in the treatment of sexual dysfunction in women: a preliminary report. *Journal of Sex Medicine*, **4**, 1345–51.

Bradford A and Meston CM (2009). Placebo response in the treatment of women's sexual dysfunctions: a review and commentary. *Journal of Sex and Marital Therapy*, **35**, 164–81.

Capurso G, Cocomello L, Benedetto U, Cammà C and Delle Fave G (2012). Meta-analysis: the placebo rate of abdominal pain remission in clinical trials of chronic pancreatitis. *Pancreas*, **41**, 1125–31.

Collins KH and Tatum AL (1925). A conditioned reflex established by chronic morphine poisoning. *American Journal of Physiology*, **74**, 14–15.

Cremonini F, Delgado-Aros S and Camilleri M (2003). Efficacy of alosetron in irritable bowel syndrome: a meta-analysis of randomized controlled trials. *Neurogastroenterology and Motility*, **15**, 79–86.

Cremonini F, Ziogas DC, Chang HY, *et al.* (2010). Meta-analysis: the effects of placebo treatment on gastro-oesophageal reflux disease. *Alimentary Pharmacology and Therapeutics*, **32**, 29–42.

de Araujo AC, da Silva FG, Salvi F, Awad MC, da Silva EA and Damião R (2009). The management of erectile dysfunction with placebo only: does it work? *Journal of Sexual Medicine*, **6**, 3440–8.

De Craen AJM, Moerman DE, Heisterkamp SH, Tytgat GNJ, Tijssen JGP and Kleijnen J (1999). Placebo effect in the treatment of duodenal ulcer. *British Journal of Clinical Pharmacology*, **48**, 853–60.

Dobrilla G and Scarpignato C (1994). Placebo and placebo effects: their impact on the evaluation of drug response in patients. *Digestive Diseases*, **12**, 368–77.

Enck P, Horing B, Weimer K and Klosterhalfen S (2012). Placebo responses and placebo effects in functional bowel disorders. *European Journal of Gastroenterology and Hepatology*, **24**, 1–8.

Enck P and Klosterhalfen S (2005). The placebo response in functional bowel disorders: perspectives and putative mechanisms. *Neurogastroenterology and Motility*, **17**, 325–31.

Enck P, Vinson B, Malfertheiner P, Zipfel S and Klosterhalfen S (2009). The placebo response in functional dyspepsia—reanalysis of trial data. *Neurogastroenterology and Motility*, **21**, 370–7.

Fink HA, MacDonald R, Rutks IR, Nelson DB and Wilt TJ (2002). Sildenafil for male erectile dysfunction: a systematic review and meta-analysis. *Archives of Internal Medicine*, **162**, 1349–60.

Ford AC and Moayyedi P (2010). Meta-analysis: factors affecting placebo response rate in the irritable bowel syndrome. *Alimentary Pharmacology and Therapeutics*, **32**, 144–58.

Gallahan WC, Case D and Bloomfeld RS (2010). An analysis of the placebo effect in Crohn's disease over time. *Alimentary Pharmacology and Therapeutics*, **31**, 102–7.

Garud S, Brown A, Cheifetz A, Levitan EB and Kelly CP (2008). Meta-analysis of the placebo response in ulcerative colitis. *Digestive Diseases and Sciences*, **53**, 875–91.

Giuliano F, Rubio-Aurioles E, Kennelly M *et al.* (2006). Efficacy and safety of vardenafil in men with erectile dysfunction caused by spinal cord injury. *Neurology*, **66**, 210–16.

Grimes DA and Schulz KF (2011). Nonspecific side effects of oral contraceptives: nocebo or noise? *Contraception*, **83**, 5–9.

Gudjonsson B and Spiro HM (1978). Response to placebos in ulcer disease. *American Journal of Medicine*, **65**, 399–402.

Hall KT, Lembo AJ, Kirsch I *et al.* (2012). Catechol-O-methyltransferase val158met polymorphism predicts placebo effect in irritable bowel syndrome. *PLoS One*, **7**, e48135.

Ilnyckyj A, Shanahan F, Anton PA, Cheang M and Bernstein CN (1997). Quantification of the placebo response in ulcerative colitis. *Gastroenterology*, **112**, 1854–8.

Jackson JL, O'Malley PG, Tomkins G, Balden E, Santoro J and Kroenke K (2000). Treatment of functional gastrointestinal disorders with antidepressant medications: a meta-analysis. *American Journal of Medicine*, **108**, 65–72.

Kelley JM, Lembo AJ, Ablon JS *et al.* (2009). Patient and practitioner influences on the placebo effect in irritable bowel syndrome. *Psychosomatic Medicine*, **71**, 789–97.

Klein KB (1988). Controlled treatment trials in the irritable bowel syndrome: a critique. *Gastroenterology*, **95**, 232–41.

Kleitman N and Crisler G (1927). A quantitative study of the salivary conditioned reflex. *American Journal of Physiology*, **79**, 571–614.

Klosterhalfen S, Kellermann S, Stockhorst U *et al.* (2005). Latent inhibition of rotation chair-induced nausea in healthy male and female volunteers. *Psychosomatic Medicine*, **67**, 335–40.

Klosterhalfen S, Ruttgers A, Krumrey E *et al.* (2000). Pavlovian conditioning of taste aversion using a motion sickness paradigm. *Psychosomatic Medicine*, **62**, 671–7.

Kokkotou E, Conboy LA, Ziogas DC *et al.* (2010). Serum correlates of the placebo effect in irritable bowel syndrome. *Neurogastroenterology and Motility*, **22**, 285–e81.

Kotsis V, Benson S, Bingel U *et al.* (2012). Perceived treatment group affects behavioral and neural responses to visceral pain in a deceptive placebo study. *Neurogastroenterology and Motility*, **24**, 935–e462.

Lee S, Malhotra B, Creanga D, Carlsson M and Glue P (2009). A meta-analysis of the placebo response in antimuscarinic drug trials for overactive bladder. *BMC Medical Research Methodology*, **9**, 55.

Levine ME, Stern RM and Koch KL (2006). The effects of manipulating expectations through placebo and nocebo administration on gastric tachyarrhythmia and motion-induced nausea. *Psychosomatic Medicine*, **68**, 478–86.

Mangera A, Chapple CR, Kopp ZS and Plested M (2011). The placebo effect in overactive bladder syndrome. *Nature Reviews Urology*, **8**, 495–503.

Masters W and Johnson V (1966). *The human sexual response.* Little Brown, Boston, MA.

McConnell JD, Briskewitz R, Walsh P *et al.* (1998). The effect of finasteride on the risk of acute urinary retention and the need for surgical treatment among men with benign prostatic hyperplasia. Finasteride long-term efficacy and safety study group. *New England Journal of Medicine*, **338**, 557–63.

Mearin F, Balboa A, Zarate N, Cucala M and Malagelada JR (1999). Placebo in functional dyspepsia: symptomatic, gastrointestinal motor, and gastric sensorial responses. *American Journal of Gastroenterology*, **94**, 116–25.

Meissner K (2009). Effects of placebo interventions on gastric motility and general autonomic activity. *Journal of Psychosomatic Research*, **66**, 391–8.

Moerman DE (1983). General medical effectiveness and human biology: placebo effects in the treatment of ulcer disease. *Medical Anthropology*, **14**, 13–6.

Mondaini N, Gontero P, Giubilei G et al. (2007). Finasteride 5 mg and sexual side effects: how many of these are related to a nocebo phenomenon? *Journal of Sex Medicine*, **4**, 1708–12.

Moyad MA (2002). The placebo effect and randomized trials: analysis of conventional medicine. *Urological Clinic of North America*, **29**, 125–33.

Musial F, Klosterhalfen S and Enck P (2007). Placebo responses in patients with gastrointestinal disorders. *World Journal of Gastroenterology*, **13**, 3425–9.

Nickel JC (1998). Placebo therapy of benign prostatic hyperplasia: a 25-month study. Canadian PROSPECT Study Group. *British Journal of Urology*, **81**, 383–7.

Patel SM, Stason WB, Legedza A *et al.* (2005). The placebo effect in irritable bowel syndrome trials: a meta-analysis. *Neurogastroenterology and Motility*, **17**, 332–40.

Pavlov IP (1910). *The work of the digestive glands.* Charles Griffin, London.

Pavlov IP (1927). *Conditioned reflexes.* Oxford University Press, London.

Pitz M, Cheang M and Bernstein CN (2005). Defining the predictors of the placebo response in irritable bowel syndrome. *Clinical Gastroenterology and Hepatology*, **3**, 237–47.

Poynard T and Pignon JP (1989). *Acute treatment of duodenal ulcer. Analysis of 293 randomized clinical trials.* John Libbey Eurotext, Paris.

Poynard T, Regimbeau C and Benhamou Y (2001). Meta-analysis of smooth muscle relaxants in the treatment of irritable bowel syndrome. *Alimentary Pharmacology and Therapeutics*, **15**, 355–61.

Price DD, Craggs J, Verne GN, Perlstein WM, Robinson ME (2007). Placebo analgesia is accompanied by large reductions in pain-related brain activity in irritable bowel syndrome patients. *Pain*, **127**, 63–72.

Price DD, Craggs JG, Zhou Q, Verne GN, Perlstein WM and Robinson ME (2009). Widespread hyperalgesia in irritable bowel syndrome is dynamically maintained by tonic visceral impulse input and placebo/nocebo factors: evidence from human psychophysics, animal models, and neuroimaging. *NeuroImage*, **47**, 995–1001.

Price DD, Finniss DG and Benedetti F (2008). A comprehensive review of the placebo effect: recent advances and current thought. *Annual Review of Psychology*, **59**, 565–90.

Rohleder N, Otto B, Wolf JM *et al.* (2006). Sex-specific adaptation of endocrine and inflammatory responses to repeated nauseogenic body rotation. *Psychoneuroendocrinology*, **31**, 226–36.

Spanier JA, Howden CW and Jones MP (2003). A systematic review of alternative therapies in the irritable bowel syndrome. *Archives of Internal Medicine*, **163**, 265–74.

Spiller RC (1999). Problems and challenges in the design of irritable bowel syndrome clinical trials: experience from published trials. *American Journal of Medicine*, **107**, 91S–97S.

Staskin DR, Michel MC, Sun F, Guan Z and Morrow JD (2012). The effect of elective sham dose escalation on the placebo response during an antimuscarinic trial for overactive bladder symptoms. *Journal of Urology*, **187**, 1721–6.

Sternbach RA (1964). The effects of instructional sets on autonomic responsivity. *Psychophysiology*, **62**, 67–72.

Stockhorst U, Enck P and Klosterhalfen S (2007). Role of classical conditioning in learning gastrointestinal symptoms. *World Journal of Gastroenterology*, **13**, 3430–7.

Stockhorst U, Steingrueber HJ, Enck P and Klosterhalfen S (2006). Pavlovian conditioning of nausea and vomiting. *Autonomic Neuroscience*, **129**, 50–7.

Su C, Lichtenstein GR, Krok K, Brensinger CM and Lewis JD (2004). A meta-analysis of the placebo response rates of remission and response in clinical trials of active Crohn's disease. *Gastroenterology*, **126**, 1257–69.

van Leeuwen JHS, Castro R, Busse M and Bemelmans BLH (2006). The placebo effect in the pharmacologic treatment of patients with lower urinary tract symptoms. *European Urology*, **50**, 440–52.

Vase L, Robinson ME, Verne GN and Price DD (2003). The contributions of suggestion, expectancy and desire to placebo effect in irritable bowel syndrome patients. An empirical investigation. *Pain*, **105**, 17–25.

Vase L, Robinson ME, Verne GN and Price DD (2005). Increased placebo analgesia over time in irritable bowel syndrome (IBS) patients is associated with desire and expectation but not endogenous opioid mechanisms. *Pain*, **115**, 338–47.

Verne GN, Robinson ME, Vase L and Price DD (2003). Reversal of visceral and cutaneous hyperalgesia by local rectal anesthesia in irritable bowel syndrome (IBS) patients. *Pain*, **105**, 223–30.

Vernia P, Di Camillo M, Foglietta T, Avallone VE and De Carolis A (2010). Diagnosis of lactose intolerance and the "nocebo" effect: the role of negative expectations. *Digestive and Liver Disease*, **42**, 616–9.

Weimer K, Schulte J, Maichle A, *et al.* (2012). Effects of ginger and expectations on symptoms of nausea in a balanced placebo design. *PLoS One*, **7**, e49031.

Chapter 10

Special medical conditions and therapeutic interventions

Summary points

- Cancer progression is not affected by placebo treatments; however, symptoms can be reduced by placebos.

- Nocebo effects are crucially involved in anticipatory nausea and vomiting before a cancer chemotherapy session, with a basic mechanism of classical conditioning.

- Placebo surgery may induce improvement in surgical clinical trials, but it also raises many ethical questions.

- Some alternative and complementary therapies, like acupuncture, have both a specific effect and a placebo component.

- Placebo and placebo-related effects are a good model to better understand the mechanisms underlying the patient–provider interaction.

10.1 Oncology

10.1.1 Placebos may induce symptom reduction but not cancer regression

Several randomized, double-blind, placebo-controlled clinical trials have been run in cancer patients. Many of these trials have not so much to do with cancer per se but rather with symptoms associated with the neoplasm. For example, in clinical trials of antiemetics for the control of chemotherapy-induced nausea and vomiting, positive results in patients who receive a placebo have been found with a frequency of approximately 15% (Beck et al., 1993). This percentage is quite low compared to trials of analgesics for the control of malignant pain. In fact, Moertel et al. (1976) performed a review of four analgesic trials for cancer pain and found that 39% of those patients who received a placebo experienced a satisfactory reduction (more than 50% decrease) in pain. Boureau et al. (1988) performed a randomized, double-blind, placebo-controlled trial in patients with pain from bone metastases and found that 51% of those who received a twice-daily intramuscular injection of placebo experienced a satisfactory reduction of pain that lasted up to 7 days.

In a subsequent review of randomized clinical trials, Chvetzoff and Tannock (2003) performed an interesting and informative comparison between subjective symptoms and cancer progression in patients who received placebo treatment. They found that the percentage of patients in placebo groups who reported pain decreases ranged from 0% to approximately 21%, whereas the percentage of patients who showed improvement in appetite ranged from 8–27%. The results obtained for weight gain showed that 7–17% of patients in placebo groups gained weight. Likewise, performance status, as assessed by a physician, improved in 6–14% of patients in placebo groups. By contrast, quality of life did not improve in any placebo group. In a different study in which anxiety and depression were assessed in placebo versus alprazolam groups, a satisfactory reduction (more than 50%) in anxiety was found in 39% of patients who received a placebo compared to 50% of those who received the active medication, whereas 39% of patients in both the placebo and medication groups showed improvement in depressive symptoms (Wald et al., 1993).

Chvetzoff and Tannock (2003) also reviewed studies that analyzed cancer progression in placebo groups, as assessed by measuring neoplasm size (according to the World Health Organization criteria). The overall rate in tumor size reduction in placebo groups was 2.7% and the rate of a serum marker reduction was 1.7%. Overall, these studies suggest that placebo administration is associated with improved control of symptoms such as pain, appetite, anxiety, and depression, but rarely with reduced progression of the tumor. The precise nature of this improvement in symptoms is not known, as there are no natural history control groups in these trials and spontaneous remission cannot be ruled out. In this regard, it should be pointed out that the 2.7% rate in reduction of tumor size seen in placebo groups might be nothing more than spontaneous remission (Box 10.1). In fact, if one trial on renal cell cancer—which is known to undergo spontaneous regression—is excluded from the analysis, the percentage drops to 1.4% (Chvetzoff and Tannock, 2003).

A variety of symptoms have been reported to undergo robust placebo as well as nocebo effects (Garg, 2011). For example, de la Cruz et al. (2010) conducted a retrospective study to determine the frequency and predictors of placebo and nocebo effects in patients with cancer-related fatigue. The analysis of 105 patients showed that 56% had a placebo response, whereas insomnia (79%), anorexia (53%), nausea (38%), and restlessness (34%) represented the most common reported nocebo effects.

10.1.2 Cancer chemotherapy induces conditioned nocebo responses

Anticipatory responses in cancer chemotherapy, like nausea and vomiting, represent an example of conditioned nocebo effects, and have been labeled "a natural laboratory" for the study of conditioning in humans by Andrykowski and Otis (1990). Nesse et al. (1980) had already described the case of a patient who was being treated with nausea-inducing chemotherapy (mechlorethamine, vincristine, procarbazine, and prednisone) for Hodgkin's disease (a type of lymphoma). After a number of chemotherapy sessions, the patient reported nausea and sometimes vomiting when in the presence of an odor in the clinic before the chemotherapy session. Nesse et al. (1980)

Box 10.1 Spontaneous regression of cancer

The spontaneous remission of cancer has always been the subject of many controversies, from both a scientific and a more popular viewpoint. For example, in the latter case spontaneous remission has often been misinterpreted in a variety of ways, ranging from miracles to mysterious healing and from quackery to the power of mind. From a strict scientific standpoint, spontaneous regression of cancer is a well-documented phenomenon that may occur in a number of cancers, such as the embryonal tumors in children, carcinoma of the female breast, chorionepithelioma, adenocarcinoma of the kidney, neuroblastoma, malignant melanoma, sarcomas, and carcinoma of the bladder and skin. Everson and Cole (1968) defined spontaneous regression as "the partial or complete disappearance of a malignant tumor in the absence of treatment or in the presence of therapy considered inadequate to exert a significant influence on the disease," along with the requirement that the original presence of cancer was proven by the microscopic examination of tissues. Although "spontaneous" means "without any apparent cause," it is interesting to note that regression is usually associated with acute infections, fever, and immunostimulation (Jessy, 2011). Indeed, in 1891 the surgeon William Coley faced the problem of an extensive postoperative wound after the removal of a sarcoma. The wound became severely infected and the patient developed high fever. However, after each attack of fever the tumor shrank more and more, and finally disappeared completely. Suspecting that the infection was somehow responsible for the regression, Coley himself developed a cure, a sort of vaccine called "Coley's toxins," which was successfully used in many countries for different types of cancer. Coley was considered to have treated more sarcoma patients than any other physician up to that time (Jessy, 2011). This approach slowly declined over the following years for a number of reasons. First, surgery became a sterile procedure with fewer postsurgical infections. Second, radiotherapy and chemotherapy slowly gained widespread consensus. Third, the advent of antibiotics and antipyretics further reduced the incidence of postsurgical infections and fever, respectively (Jessy, 2011). Therefore, today we have to consider some spontaneous remissions of different types of cancer as the result of an infection.

found this pretreatment nausea in 44% of their patients, and suggested it was a classically conditioned response. The conditioned stimulus is represented in this case by contextual cues present in the chemotherapy environment, for example, an odor, whereas the unconditioned stimulus is the chemotherapy itself; the unconditioned response is the chemotherapy-induced nausea and vomiting (Fig. 10.1A). Many other studies have confirmed anticipatory nausea and vomiting in chemotherapy sessions (Bernstein, 1991; Jacobson et al., 1993; Stockhorst et al., 1993, 1998, 2006). Thus, as explained in section 9.1.5, gastrointestinal symptoms can be learned.

Nocebo effects in chemotherapy are mainly represented by anticipatory nausea and vomiting, for which prevalence ranges from 10–63% (Stockhorst et al., 2000) and can

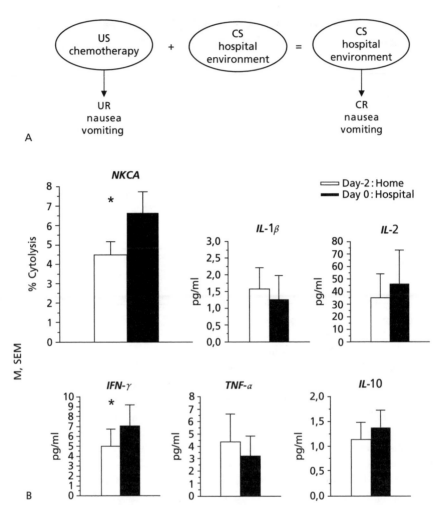

Fig. 10.1 (A) The classical conditioning model in cancer chemotherapy. CR, conditioned response; CS, conditioned stimulus; UR, unconditioned response; US, unconditioned stimulus. (B) Examples of anticipatory immune responses to a cancer chemotherapy session 2 days before hospital admission (at home; white bars) and on the first day in the hospital (black bars). Note the significant increase of natural killer cell activity (NKCA) and interferon-gamma (IFN-γ) in the presence of chemotherapy-related CS in the hospital environment compared to a lower level in the relatively CS-free home environment. Interleukin IL-1β, IL-2, tumor necrosis factor (TNF)-α, and IL-10 do not show significant anticipatory changes. Reprinted from *Brain, Behavior, and Immunity*, 14 (3), Ursula Stockhorst, Simone Spennes-Saleh, Dieter Körholz, Ulrich Göbel, Marion E. Schneider, Hans-Joachim Steingrüber, and Sibylle Klosterhalfen, Anticipatory Symptoms and Anticipatory Immune Responses in Pediatric Cancer Patients Receiving Chemotherapy: Features of a Classically Conditioned Response?, pp. 198–218, Copyright (2000), with permission from Elsevier.

be as high as 59% even with antiemetic treatment (Tyc et al., 1997). It should be noted that anticipatory food aversion and immunomodulation have also been described (Jacobson et al., 1993; Stockhorst et al., 2000). Stockhorst et al. (1993) asked 55 cancer patients to record several symptoms, like nausea, vomiting, dizziness, sweating, and headache, after a session of chemotherapy treatment and just before a subsequent treatment. An association was found between the occurrence of the post-treatment symptoms and the occurrence of subsequent pretreatment symptoms. Interestingly, Stockhorst and colleagues also showed a chemotherapy-related food aversion, whereby food items that were consumed prior to a chemotherapy cycle were judged to be of lower hedonic quality when tasted in a subsequent test.

In an interesting study of pediatric cancer patients receiving chemotherapy, Stockhorst et al. (2000) assessed both anticipatory nausea and vomiting and anticipatory immunomodulation (Fig. 10.1B) and found that natural killer cell activity was increased predominantly in those children with anticipatory nausea and vomiting. These responses, particularly the duration and occurrence of anticipatory nausea and vomiting, correlated positively with those induced by the chemotherapy. Overall, the results obtained by Stockhorst et al. are important because they show multiple conditioned nocebo responses, involving both symptom reports and immune responses.

The likelihood of anticipatory nausea and vomiting increases according to the following factors: emetogenicity of the chemotherapy protocol (the intensity of the unconditioned stimulus), the intensity of post-treatment symptoms (the magnitude of the unconditioned response), and the number of pairings between the chemotherapy context and chemotherapy itself (Bovbjerg, 2006; Stockhorst et al., 2007). In addition, anticipatory nausea has been shown to affect the severity of subsequent post-treatment nausea or, in other words, anticipatory nausea developed during early chemotherapy cycles may add to post-treatment nausea (Bovbjerg, 2006).

10.2 Surgery

10.2.1 Patients undergoing placebo surgery show a high rate of improvement

Due to ethical constraints, placebo groups in different types of surgery are rare and difficult to investigate. In fact, placebo surgery is problematic from an ethical standpoint and is the focus of lively debates and discussions when a surgical procedure needs to be evaluated for its effectiveness (see section 11.1.2). However, when placebo surgery trials have been done, patients who underwent placebo surgery showed a high rate of clinical improvement, even though in most of these trials it is not possible to distinguish between the real placebo effects, natural history of the disease, and regression to the mean.

For example, in the 1950s some placebo surgery trials were performed that are often cited as good examples of the placebo effect. However, no natural history group was run as a control in these trials, thus spontaneous remission could not be ruled out. In these studies, placebo surgery was performed for treatment of angina pectoris, a condition whereby there is inadequate blood supply of the heart (Dimond et al., 1958; Cobb et al., 1959). This approach was rationalized because in the 1950s angina pectoris was treated frequently by ligation of the internal mammary arteries—it was believed that blood could find alternative routes into the heart, thus improving heart circulation, but several years later it was found that no new blood vessel could be detected in the heart, thus making the validity of the procedure questionable. Therefore, Dimond et al. (1958) and Cobb et al. (1959) decided to perform sham surgery whereby patients underwent the same surgical procedures for mammary artery ligation, but without actual ligation of the internal mammary arteries. Some patients showed an improvement in terms of pain, physical performance, and electrocardiogram results. Overall, there was a substantial improvement in those that received real surgery, in 67% of the patients; a substantial improvement in the placebo group was present in 83% of the patients.

Other examples of cardiovascular surgery were provided in section 8.1, such as laser myocardial revascularization in people with coronary heart disease (Rana et al., 2005). Once more, it is uncertain that these are true placebo effects as no information about the natural course of the disease is available.

Another case of placebo surgery that is often taken as an example of a powerful placebo effect is sham arthroscopic surgery for osteoarthritis of the knee. In a trial by Moseley and colleagues (Moseley et al., 2002) 165 patients who completed the study were randomly assigned to receive either arthroscopic debridement, arthroscopic lavage, or placebo surgery. For the placebo, skin incisions were made and debridement was simulated, but the arthroscope was not inserted. The investigators found no differences in pain ratings and knee function between the three groups either at 1 year or 2 years after surgery. Again, no definitive conclusions can be drawn because no natural history group was used as a control.

Rosseland et al. (2004) studied the effects of intra-articular injections of saline into the knee. These investigators compared the analgesic effects of a 10-mL dose and a 1-mL dose and found that both were effective in relieving pain. This is important because it rules out the possibility that a high dose of saline is capable of affecting pain, for example, by cooling or by diluting algogenic substances. In this sense, a 1-mL dose can indeed be considered a placebo.

Some neurosurgical trials of deep-brain stimulation for the treatment of Parkinson's disease have been performed under strictly controlled conditions, with a no-treatment group that rules out possible confounding factors like natural history. These studies are described in sections 5.1 and 5.2, particularly those performed by Pollo et al. (2002), Benedetti et al. (2003), and Mercado et al. (2006). In fact these studies show that expectations may affect Parkinsonian symptoms, particularly bradykinesia. In another study on deep-brain stimulation for treatment of pain, sham stimulation of the thalamus induced a decrease in pain intensity of 28% and in unpleasantness of 24% (Marchand et al., 2003). These findings confirm the notion that surgical treatments have an important placebo component which, in this case, is mediated by the expectation of benefit.

10.2.2 Improvement may occur in those who believe they have received transplantation

Studies on transplantation of embryonic cells for the treatment of Parkinson's disease give us further insight into the role of expectation in placebo surgery. Some clinical

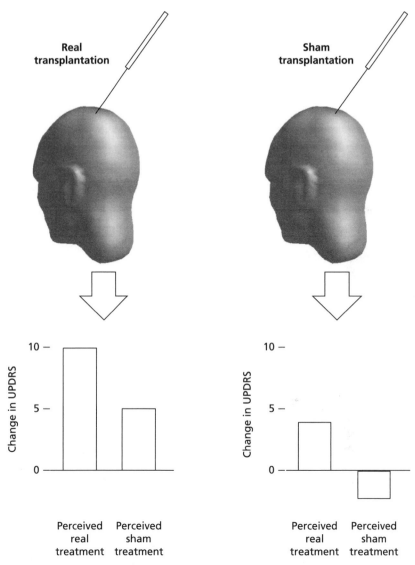

Fig. 10.2 Patients who received real transplantation show larger improvement when they believe they underwent real treatment. Conversely, if they believe they underwent sham treatment, the improvement is much smaller. This also holds true for patients who underwent sham treatment. UPDRS = Unified Parkinson's Disease Rating Scale.

trials have tried to demonstrate the efficacy of grafting embryonic cells, but genuine placebo effects cannot be identified due to the lack of appropriate control groups (Freed et al., 2001; Freeman et al., 2002; Olanow et al., 2003). However, a more recent study clearly shows that expectations matter in the therapeutic outcome of surgical interventions, as already partially described earlier (section 5.1.2). In this study, McRae et al. (2004) assessed the patient's perceived assignment to either the true transplantation or sham transplantation procedure. They found improvements in both the transplant and the sham surgery groups on several outcome measures, such as physical and quality of life scores. However, perceived assignment to the true transplantation group had a beneficial impact on the overall outcome and this effect lasted approximately 1 year (Fig. 10.2). In fact, patients who believed they had received the transplanted tissue showed significant improvements regardless of whether they received sham surgery or fetal tissue implantations.

10.3 Physical therapies

10.3.1 It is difficult to devise placebo physical therapies

Understanding placebo effects in physical therapy is difficult for the same reasons as for psychotherapy. In reality, it is difficult to devise placebo treatments that are similar to real physical therapies in all respects. A physical therapy is based on the manipulation of some body parts and/or the application of physical (e.g., mechanical or thermal) agents on the body. For example, how should we devise a placebo treatment that is similar to a real physiotherapeutic manipulation (e.g., a massage) of the body? As this is almost impossible, no good placebo control exists.

A good example is transcutaneous electrical nerve stimulation (TENS), which is usually applied to painful areas of the body. In order to stimulate the afferent fibers of the peripheral nerves it is necessary to increase the intensity of stimulation until the patient feels a tingling sensation. For this reason, no good placebo exists for TENS—the tingling sensation is not compatible with a sham stimulation and vice versa, because a sham stimulation that does not evoke a tingling sensation is considered by the patient to be ineffective. Many trials have compared TENS and placebo but most of them are flawed due to the lack of a satisfactory placebo control and, in addition, contrasting results have been obtained (Simmonds and Kumar, 1994). In general, pain reduction in patients who received placebo TENS is large. For example, Langley et al. (1984) found placebo TENS caused a 37% effect on resting pain, but the effect of placebo TENS reached 72% when pain was assessed during "gripping." A study by Deyo and colleagues (Deyo et al., 1990) found a 47% improvement in the active TENS group, whereas the improvement in the placebo group was as large as 42%. No definitive conclusions can be drawn from these as well as from most clinical trials on TENS, as spontaneous remission cannot be ruled out.

It is interesting to note that in one study on helium–neon laser treatment of osteoarthritis, Basford et al. (1987) found no specific effects of the laser and the rate of pain reduction and strength improvement in the placebo groups was as large as 100%. In general, clinical improvement in patients who receive a placebo physical therapy is high, and many interventions such as static magnets and ultrasound in osteoarthritic knee pain do not show significant differences compared to placebo interventions (Bjordal et al., 2007). Certainly one of the major difficulties in these clinical trials is to have satisfactory placebo control groups. In most trials there are no untreated groups, thus it is not possible to rule out spontaneous remission and regression to the mean.

However, in this regard, one study that used a no-treatment group is worth mentioning. Hashish et al. (1988) assessed the effects of real ultrasound and placebo ultrasound on pain and swelling following bilateral surgical extraction of lower third molar teeth. There was a significant reduction of swelling in the placebo group, in the range of 30–35%, compared to the untreated group, and this was accompanied by a reduction of C-reactive protein (CRP) levels in the placebo group of 25–38% compared with the untreated group. These placebo responses were independent of plasma cortisol levels and the subject's anxiety state. Here is a strong suggestion that this is a genuine placebo response to sham ultrasound therapy, because inflammatory parameters are objectively affected.

10.4 **Complementary and alternative therapies**

10.4.1 **Do complementary and alternative therapies work through placebo effects?**

Many clinical trials have attempted to assess the effectiveness of diverse complementary and alternative therapies, but the mechanisms underlying the effects of both the treatments and the placebos are not known. Perhaps the same mechanisms described throughout this book are at work here. For example, alternative treatments for pain certainly induce expectations of analgesia, the mechanisms for which are described in Chapter 4. Likewise, alternative therapies for other conditions (such as motor disorders) induce expectations of motor improvement, as described in Chapter 5.

A study performed by Link et al. (2006) on sham administration of herbal supplements is indicative of the frequency of placebo–nocebo symptom reporting. Participants were given placebos that they believed to be herbs which enhanced mental performance, along with a list of possible beneficial and adverse effects. As far as the placebo responses are concerned, 33.3% of the participants experienced elevated mood, 36.1% improved memory, 61.1% clearer thinking, 52.8% increased mental alertness, 27.8% enhanced sensory perception, and 30.6% increased energy levels. As to the nocebo symptoms, 5.6% experienced sensitivity to bright lights, 22.2% dry mouth, 8.3% headache, 16.7% fatigue, and 5.6% mild gastrointestinal disturbance. It is interesting that 89% of the participants reported at least one symptom.

In a systematic review and meta-analysis of randomized placebo-controlled clinical trials of different complementary and alternative therapies for irritable bowel syndrome, Dorn et al. (2007) assessed the magnitude of clinical improvement in the placebo groups of 19 trials. The mean effect of placebo treatments on global symptom improvement was 42.6%, with a range of 15–72.2%. There was correlation with both the duration of the trial and the number of office visits. Interestingly, the authors noted that the magnitude of the improvement in placebo groups in complementary and alternative medicine trials is similar to that seen in conventional medicine, which suggests that complementary and alternative therapies do not particularly enhance the improvement in placebo groups.

The important role of expectation in complementary and alternative treatments is shown again by a study on aromatherapy (Howard and Hughes, 2008). Lavender aroma and expectations were tested in a model of post-stress relaxation according to a double-blind design, whereby 96 healthy women were exposed to lavender, placebo, or no aroma after exposure to an arousing cognitive task. Where an aroma was presented, different verbal suggestions were delivered in order to manipulate participants' expectations about the aroma's impact on their relaxation. The researchers found no effect of aroma on their galvanic skin response during relaxation, whereas the verbal instructions were associated with a given pattern of relaxation. When the women expected an inhibitory effect of the aroma, they relaxed more, but when they expected a facilitatory effect, they relaxed less. These effects were independent of ratings of attitudes towards aromatherapy.

Overall, we should consider complementary and alternative interventions like other interventions that induce expectations of clinical benefit. Pills, syrups, injections, acupuncture needles, magnets, and herbs may all induce expectation of improvement in pain, motor performance, anxiety, or respiratory function. Thus, the neurobiological mechanisms are likely to be the same as those described throughout this book.

10.4.2 Acupuncture is likely to work through both specific and placebo effects

For understanding the role and mechanisms of placebos in complementary and alternative treatments, acupuncture (Box 10.2) represents the best known intervention (Dhond et al., 2007). In 2005, a brain imaging study was performed that clearly showed the relative contributions of specific and placebo mechanisms of acupuncture (Pariente et al., 2005). In a single-blind, randomized crossover study in 14 patients suffering from painful osteoarthritis, three interventions were compared by positron emission tomography scans: (1) real acupuncture, (2) placebo Streitberger needle acupuncture (whereby the needle is pushed against the skin but it actually moves into the handle, giving the impression that it has pierced the skin), and (3) overt placebo (whereby subjects are told the needle will not pierce the skin and that it has no therapeutic effectiveness). As shown in Fig. 10.3, real acupuncture was found to activate the ipsilateral insula to a greater extent than placebo. Interestingly, both real acupuncture and placebo Streitberger needle, in which there is the same expectation of effect, produced a more powerful effect than overt placebo, in which there is no expectation; this was seen in the right dorsolateral prefrontal cortex, anterior cingulate cortex, and midbrain. Therefore, acupuncture seems to have both specific effects in the insula and placebo effects in the dorsolateral and cingulate cortices, and in the midbrain—these are the very same regions described in other brain imaging studies of placebo analgesia (Petrovic et al., 2002; Wager et al., 2004; Zubieta et al., 2005) (see also section 4.1.9). Although the study by Pariente et al. (2005) is interesting, note that there were no analgesic effects

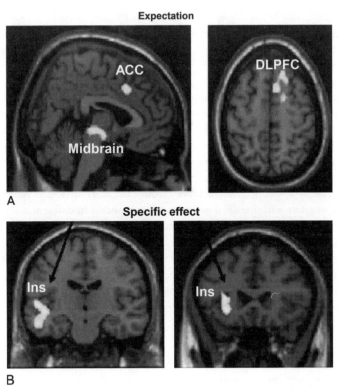

Fig. 10.3 Acupuncture has a placebo component in the dorsolateral prefrontal cortex (DLPFC), the anterior cingulate cortex (ACC) and the midbrain, activated by expectation of analgesia (A) and a specific effect in the insula (Ins), which is activated by real acupuncture (B). Reprinted from *Neurolmage*, 4 (7), Jérémie Pariente, Peter White, Richard SJ Frackowiak, and George Lewith, Expectancy and belief modulate the neuronal substrates of pain treated by acupuncture, pp. 1161–67, Copyright (2005), with permission from Elsevier. (See Plate 13.)

of any of the three treatments on experimental or ongoing pain—whether the insula activity is related to acupuncture effectiveness is still not clear.

In another neuroimaging study of experimental pain processing in healthy subjects with functional magnetic resonance, Kong et al. (2006) found that placebo needle-induced analgesia was associated with increased activity during a painful stimulation. These increases occurred within multiple pain-related regions, including the bilateral rostral anterior cingulate cortex, lateral prefrontal cortex, right anterior insula, supramarginal gyrus, and left inferior parietal lobe. In addition, pain ratings correlated negatively with the bilateral prefrontal cortex, rostral anterior cingulate cortex, cerebellum, right fusiform, parahippocampus, and pons. Kong et al. (2006) suggest that placebo needling may evoke different types of brain responses from those typically seen in studies utilizing creams and pills.

Box 10.2 Traditional Chinese versus Western interpretation of acupuncture

Many medical concepts change completely across different cultures worldwide. There are many medical approaches that neglect, completely or in part, the Western approach. One of the most popular examples is represented by traditional Chinese medicine, which uses medical concepts in opposition to the Western medical world. For example, the concept of Qi (vital energy) is crucial in many medical practices such as acupuncture. Qi is said to flow along different channels of the body, which are called meridians, and many therapeutic approaches are aimed at interfering with Qi by restoring its normal flow through the body meridians. Acupuncture aims to interfere with the Qi flow by inserting a needle in different points of the skin. The fundamental difference between the traditional Chinese approach and the Western medical approach resides in the explanation of the underlying mechanism and in the interpretation of acupuncture within a scientific and philosophical context (Fig. 10.4).

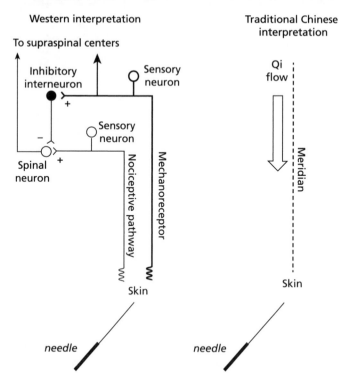

Fig. 10.4 The Western and Traditional Chinese interpretations of the possible mechanism of action of acupuncture.

> **Box 10.2 Traditional Chinese versus Western interpretation of acupuncture (continued)**
>
> The effects, if any, that follow the insertion of an acupuncture needle into the skin can be seen within a Western context, which is based on key anatomical-physiological concepts, or within a traditional Chinese context, which is mainly based on philosophical foundations. According to the first mechanistic interpretation, when the needle pierces the skin, it stimulates mechanoreceptors which activate inhibitory interneurons. These, in turn, inhibit pain transmission along the nociceptive pathway. According to the Chinese philosophical explanation, when the needle pierces the skin, it interferes with the Qi flow in a given meridian of the body. This induces a restoration of Qi flow, which had been lost and had caused illness. Whether or not acupuncture is really effective, either interpretation does not make a big difference from the perspective of the patient. What matters is the efficacy of acupuncture, be it a mechanoreceptor inhibition or a Qi restoration or merely a placebo effect.

10.4.3 Expectations in acupuncture clinical trials can make a big difference

We have already seen in sections 4.1.3, 5.1.2, and 10.2.2 that in clinical trials of acupuncture for the management of pain and in clinical trials of the surgical treatment of Parkinson's disease, expectations play an important role. Bausell et al. (2005) conducted a study on acupuncture in which patients were asked which group they believed they belonged to (either placebo or real acupuncture). They found that those patients who believed they belonged to the real treatment group experienced a greater clinical improvement than those who believed they belonged to the placebo group.

In a different study, Linde et al. (2007) performed four randomized controlled trials in which real acupuncture was compared to placebo acupuncture in migraine, tension-type headache, chronic low back pain and osteoarthritis of the knee. This study examined the effects of 864 patients' expectations on the therapeutic outcome, irrespective of which group the patients belonged to. The patients were asked whether they considered acupuncture to be an effective therapy in general and what they personally expected from it. In addition, after three acupuncture sessions they were asked how confident they were that they would benefit from the treatment. The investigators found that those with higher expectations about acupuncture experienced larger clinical improvements than those with lower expectations, irrespective of the allocation to real acupuncture or placebo acupuncture. Thus it did not really matter whether the patients actually received the real or the sham procedure. What mattered was whether they believed in acupuncture and expected a benefit from it. Not only did the authors find a significant difference between patients with low and high expectations in the 8 weeks of treatment, but also in a follow-up at 6 months.

These findings on the role of expectations in acupuncture clinical trials for the control of pain highlight the importance of considering expectations as a potential variable that needs to be controlled in clinical trials (Benedetti, 2005, 2007). This can be done by assessing the patient's perceived assignment to an experimental group (either placebo or active treatment).

10.5 Doctor–patient interaction

10.5.1 The interaction of patients with their doctors may be therapeutic per se

This section is useful to reiterate what we have already discussed in Chapter 3, and to stress that the mere doctor–patient interaction may be therapeutic per se. The provider, be it a doctor or nurse or caregiver, represents an essential and powerful context around a therapy, and the patient–provider interaction can include many placebo and placebo-related effects (Benedetti, 2002). In fact, as the expectation of therapeutic benefit is mainly induced by words, it is not surprising that interactions with medical personnel may per se be therapeutic. Balint (1955) talked about the whole atmosphere around the treatment, and that includes doctors and nurses. They can transmit a lot of information to the patient through their words, attitudes, and behavior. Physicians have long known the powerful effect of their relationship with their patients and, accordingly, have used appropriate words and attitudes with them. For example, Kaplan et al. (1989) found that blood pressure, blood sugar, functional status, and overall health status were consistently related to specific aspects of physician–patient communication.

There are a number of studies that have shown that the doctor–patient relationship plays an important role in the outcome of illness (Stewart et al., 1979; Starfield et al., 1981; Gracely et al., 1985; Greenfield et al., 1985; Bass et al., 1986; Stewart, 1995), and it has also been found that diagnostic tests, which have nothing to do with therapy, may induce clinical improvement (Sox et al., 1981).

Although the underlying mechanisms are not always understood, many factors could be at work here. For example, besides expectations of improvement, it is possible that a better interaction between the doctor and the patient might lead to a better compliance with the drug regimens (Inui et al., 1976). In this regard, it is worth mentioning the Coronary Drug Project (1980). This was a randomized double-blind placebo-controlled trial evaluating the efficacy of lipid lowering drugs in the long-term treatment of coronary heart disease. The 5-year mortality rate in 1103 men treated with clofibrate was 20%. Similarly, 2789 treated with placebo showed a mortality of 20.9%. Patients who were found to take at least 80% of their prescribed medication (good adherers) had significantly lower mortality (15%) than poor adherers (24.6%). Virtually identical findings occurred in those assigned to the placebo group, in which good adherers had 15.1% mortality and poor adherers 28.3% mortality. This suggests that placebo may be quite powerful, and its effects may be intertwined with other phenomena, such as compliance and adherence.

The importance of the patient–provider interaction had already been shown in the 1960s in a series of studies on the emotional impact that the anesthetist has upon his or her patient (Egbert et al., 1963, 1964). Egbert et al. (1964) found a reduction in postoperative pain in patients who had been informed about the course of their postoperative pain and encouraged to overcome it. Moreover, their requirement for narcotics was much lower than the control group. In more recent years, a similar approach has been used in more controlled conditions in which the patient–provider interaction has been eliminated through hidden administration of medical treatments. In this situation, a computer-controlled infusion pump delivers a drug automatically, without a doctor or nurse in the room, and the patient remains completely unaware that an analgesic treatment has been started. As previously discussed in detail, for example, in section 4.1.4, a hidden medical treatment delivered by a computer is less effective than a treatment delivered openly by a doctor.

In some conditions the number of the doctor visits is also a good predictor of clinical improvement. This issue was discussed in section 9.1 with respect to ulcerative colitis and Crohn's disease, whereby the number of visits had a varying effect on remissions—three or fewer visits were less likely to induce large remissions in patients who received placebo, compared with four or more visits (Ilnyckyj et al., 1997). Good predictors of remission in the placebo groups in these trials were the number of study visits during the trial, the length of the study, and the severity of the disease at entry (Su et al., 2004).

The opposite is also true. The words and attitudes of the provider that induce negative expectations in the patient may lead to clinical worsening and nocebo effects; this has been noted many times throughout this book (see also Benedetti et al., 2007). It is also interesting to remember that the primary reason for law suits in the United States is not medical injury itself, but the failure of communication between doctors and their patients (Beckman et al., 1994; Levinson, 1994). Again, this emphasizes the important role of the patient–provider interaction.

10.5.2 Using the appropriate words may change the therapeutic outcome

Subtle differences in communication with the patient have been found to affect the outcome of a therapy. Thomas (1987) conducted either positive or negative general-practice consultations in patients with different kinds of pain, cough, giddiness, nasal congestion, or tiredness. In the positive consultations, patients were given a firm diagnosis and therapeutic assurance. If no prescription was to be given they were told that they required none, and if a prescription was to be given they were told that the therapy would certainly make them better. In the negative consultations, no firm assurance was given; for example, if no prescription was to be given the doctor said: "I cannot be certain what your problem is, therefore I will give you no treatment." Conversely if a prescription was to be given the patients were told: "I am not sure that the treatment I am going to give you will have an effect." In all cases, the treatment was a placebo. Two weeks after consultation there was a significant difference in recovery between the positive and negative groups, but not between the treated and untreated groups, which indicates that the words the doctor used were crucial for recovery.

These findings are supported by both nonclinical and clinical studies. For example, Kirsch and Weixel (1988) showed that different verbal instructions produce different outcomes. In this study, caffeinated and decaffeinated coffee were administered following different verbal suggestions. In one case, the usual double-blind design was used, so the subjects knew either real or decaffeinated coffee was being administered.

In the other, decaffeinated coffee was deceptively presented as real coffee. The researchers found that the placebo response was more robust following deceptive administration than the double-blind paradigm, which suggests that the double-blind administration induces less certain expectations about the outcome compared with the deceptive administration.

We have seen in section 4.1.2 that this paradigm (double-blind versus deceptive administration) can be reproduced in the clinical setting. In fact, Pollo et al. (2001) treated several postoperative patients with buprenorphine on request for 3 days consecutively and a basal infusion of saline solution. However, the symbolic meaning of the saline infusion varied in three different groups of patients. The first group was told nothing (the natural history or no-treatment group), the second was told that the infusion could be either a potent analgesic or a placebo (classic double-blind administration), and the third was told that the infusion was a potent painkiller (deceptive administration). During the 3-day treatment, the doses of buprenorphine requested were recorded to assess the placebo effect of the saline infusion. The reduction of requests in the deceptive administration group was larger than that in the double-blind group. Therefore, the uncertainty of verbal instructions and attitudes leads to different results, indicating that subtle differences in the doctor's words may have a significant impact on therapeutic outcomes.

10.6 Other conditions with no available data

There are many conditions for which clinical trial data do not allow any conclusion or speculation. Although in these conditions a large number of clinical trials have been performed, no direct investigation of placebo responses or placebo groups has been done. After all, many of the conditions described in this book could be included here. For example, we do not know anything about the genitourinary apparatus or physical therapies, although sometimes just a single study allows some sort of speculation (see more about the genitourinary apparatus in section 9.2 and physical therapies in section 10.3).

A good example of these issues is seen in pediatrics. Nothing can be inferred from clinical trials in children, and there is no clear indication that placebo effects are different in children and adults. Unfortunately, only a few trials have attempted to address this issue, and one of the reasons for this is ethics (Weimer et al., 2013). For instance, some studies show some differences in placebo groups of adults and children, such as clinical trials on children who receive placebo for migraine. In general, adolescents and children show higher rates of clinical improvement than adults when treated with placebos (Loder et al., 2005), and their responses are as large as 48.5% for improvement and 32.3% for adverse events (average of two studies) (Hamalainen et al., 1997; Winner et al., 2002). However, the exact nature of this difference is unknown.

Other systems like the skin, eyes, and ears have not been investigated in detail, and only little information is available on them. Take, for example, the study by Klinger et al. (2007) on the role of classical conditioning and expectation in patients with atopic dermatitis; what they actually investigated was not the dermatitis itself but the pain arising from the damaged cutaneous tissue. On the other hand, an attempt to understand the psychobiological underpinnings of the placebo response in a dermatological condition was performed by Ader et al. (2010), who used behavioral conditioning in patients suffering from psoriasis. Initially, lesions were treated with 0.1% acetonide triamcinolone under standard treatment conditions. Thereafter, a standard therapy group continued on continuous reinforcement (active drug every treatment) with 100% of the initial dose; partial reinforcement patients received a full dose 25–50% of the time and placebo medication other times; control patients received continuous reinforcement with 25–50% of the initial dose. The frequency of relapse under partial reinforcement (26.7%) was lower than in control patients (61.5%) and did not differ from full-dose treatment (22.2%). Therefore, a partial schedule of pharmacotherapeutic reinforcement could maintain psoriasis patients with a cumulative amount of corticosteroid that was relatively ineffective when administered under standard treatment conditions. Ader et al. (2010) concluded that corticosteroid doses can be dramatically reduced by using this paradigm.

Another example is seen in itch, whereby both placebo and nocebo effects have been described, but the underlying mechanisms are unknown (van Laarhoven et al., 2011). A similar situation is present in Meniere's disease, where pathology of the inner ear is characterized by unpredictable dizziness, tinnitus, hearing loss, and pain, due to the increased fluid in the inner ear. Thomsen et al. (1981) conducted a trial in which some patients were implanted with tubes to drain off the fluid from the inner ear, and some patients were not implanted. Up to 70% of patients in both groups were found to improve, and the improvement in the placebo group was still present 9 years later (Bretlau et al., 1989; Welling and Nagaraja, 2000). Yet again, the very nature of that improvement is not known.

The occurrence, magnitude, and nature of placebo and placebo-related effects in other conditions (infectious diseases, pregnancy, childbirth, or injury by external causes such as trauma and poisoning) are completely unknown, and the clinical trials on them do not contribute to any firm conclusions. Therefore, all these medical conditions present an exciting challenge for future research, even though ethical constraints limit the study of the placebo effect in many of them.

10.7 **Points for further discussion**

1 We need to better understand whether anticipatory nausea and vomiting (considered as a conditioned nocebo effect) before cancer chemotherapy can be blocked by behavioral techniques that are aimed at preventing conditioning.

2 Better understanding of the natural history of different types of cancer would be valuable, so that a clear-cut distinction between spontaneous remissions and real placebo responses in oncology can be made.

3 The issues regarding the need for and ethics of performing placebo surgery must be resolved.

4 Are placebo responses in complementary and alternative therapies larger than in conventional treatments? Although this question should be quite easy to answer, there have been no systematic investigations in this direction to date.

5 The placebo effect is a good model for studying the doctor–patient relationship. However difficult from a methodological point of view, many experiments conducted in the laboratory setting should be repeated for real interactions between the doctor and his or her patient.

6 Many medical disciplines including pediatrics, dermatology, ophthalmology, and others should be investigated in detail, because we know nothing about genuine placebo effects in these medical fields.

References

Ader R, Mercurio MG, Walton J *et al.* (2010). Conditioned pharmacotherapeutic effects: a preliminary study. *Psychosomatic Medicine*, **72**, 192–7.

Andrykowski MA and Otis ML (1990). Development of learned food aversions in humans: investigation in a "natural laboratory" of cancer chemotherapy. *Appetite*, **14**, 145–58.

Balint M (1955). The doctor, his patient, and the illness. *Lancet*, **1**, 683–8.

Basford JR, Sheffield CG, Mair SD and Ilstrup DM (1987). Low energy helium neon laser treatment of thumb osteoarthritis. *Archives of Physical Medicine and Rehabilitation*, **68**, 794–7.

Bass MJ, Buck C, Turner L, Dickie G, Pratt G and Campbell Robinson H (1986). The physician's actions and the outcome of illness in family practice. *Journal of Family Practice*, **23**, 43–7.

Bausell RB, Lao L, Bergman S, Lee WL and Berman BM (2005). Is acupuncture analgesia an expectancy effect? Preliminary evidence based on participants' perceived assignments in two placebo-controlled trials. *Evaluation & the Health Professions*, **28**, 9–26.

Beck TM, Ciociola AA, Jones SE *et al.* (1993). Efficacy of oral ondansetron in the prevention of emesis in out-patients receiving cyclophosphamide-based chemotherapy. *Annals of Internal Medicine*, **118**, 407–13.

Beckman HB, Markakis KM, Suchman AL and Frankel RM (1994). The doctor-patient relationship and malpractice: lessons from plaintiff depositions. *Archives of Internal Medicine*, **154**, 1365–70.

Benedetti F (2002). How the doctor's words affect the patient's brain. *Evaluation & the Health Professions*, **25**, 369–86.

Benedetti F (2005). The importance of considering the effects of perceived group assignment in placebo-controlled trials. *Evaluation & the Health Professions*, **28**, 5–6.

Benedetti F (2007). What do you expect from this treatment? Changing our mind about clinical trials. *Pain*, **128**, 193–4.

Benedetti F, Lanotte M, Lopiano L and Colloca L (2007). When words are painful—unraveling the mechanisms of the nocebo effect. *Neuroscience*, **147**, 260–71.

Benedetti F, Pollo A, Lopiano L, Lanotte M, Vighetti S *et al.* (2003). Conscious expectation and unconscious conditioning in analgesic; motor and hormonal placebo/nocebo responses. *Journal of Neuroscience*, **23**, 4315–23.

Bernstein IL (1991). Aversion conditioning in response to cancer and cancer treatment. *Clinical Psychology Reviews*, **11**, 185–91.

Bjordal JM, Johnson MI, Lopes-Martins RA, Bogen B, Chow R and Ljunggren AE (2007). Short-term efficacy of physical interventions in osteoarthritic knee pain. A systematic review and meta-analysis of randomised placebo controlled trials. *Biomed Central Musculoskeletal Disorders*, **8**, 51.

Boureau F, Leizorovicz A and Caulin F (1988). Placebo effect on bone metastasis pain. *Presse Médicale*, **17**, 1063–6.

Bovbjerg DH (2006). The continuing problem of post chemotherapy nausea and vomiting: contribution of classical conditioning. *Autonomic Neuroscience*, **129**, 92–8.

Bretlau P, Thomsen J, Tos M and Johnsen NJ (1989). Placebo effect in surgery for Meniere's disease: nine-year follow-up. *American Journal of Otology*, **10**, 259–61.

Chvetzoff G and Tannock IF (2003). Placebo effects in oncology. *Journal of the National Cancer Institute*, **95**, 19–29.

Cobb LA, Thomas GI, Dillard DH, Merendino KA and Bruce RA (1959). An evaluation of internal mammary artery ligation by double blind technique. *New England Journal of Medicine*, **260**, 1115–18.

Coronary Drug Project (1980). Influence of adherence to treatment and response of cholesterol on mortality in the coronary drug project. *New England Journal of Medicine*, **303**, 1038–41.

de la Cruz M, Hui D, Parsons HA and Bruera E (2010). Placebo and nocebo effects in randomized double-blind clinical trials of agents for the therapy for fatigue in patients with advanced cancer. *Cancer*, **116**, 766–74.

Deyo RA, Walsh NE, Martin DC, Scoenfeld LS and Ramamurthy S (1990). A controlled trial of transcutaneous electrical nerve stimulation (TENS) and exercise for chronic low back pain. *New England Journal of Medicine*, **322**, 1627–34.

Dhond RP, Kettner N and Napadow V (2007). Do the neural correlates of acupuncture and placebo effects differ? *Pain*, **128**, 8–12.

Dimond EG, Kittle CF and Crockett JE (1958). Evaluation of internal mammary ligation and sham procedure in angina pectoris. *Circulation*, **18**, 712–13.

Dorn SD, Kaptchuk TJ, Park JB *et al.* (2007). A meta-analysis of the placebo response in complementary and alternative clinical trials of irritable bowel syndrome. *Neurogastroenterology Motility*, **19**, 630–7.

Egbert LD, Battit GE, Turndorf H and Beecher HK (1963). The value of the preoperative visit by an anesthetist. *Journal of the American Medical Association*, **185**, 553–5.

Egbert LD, Battit GE, Welch CE and Bartlett MK (1964). Reduction of postoperative pain by encouragement and instruction of patients. *New England Journal of Medicine*, **270**, 825–7.

Everson T and Cole W (1968). *Spontaneous regression of cancer*. Saunders, Philadelphia, PA.

Freed C, Greene P, Breeze R *et al.* (2001). Transplantation of embryonic dopamine neurons for severe Parkinson's disease. *New England Journal of Medicine*, **344**, 710–19.

Freeman T, Watts R, Hauser R *et al.* (2002). A prospective, randomized, double-blind, surgical placebo-controlled trial of intrastriatal transplantation of fetal porcine ventral mesencephalic tissue (neurocell-PD) in subjects with Parkinson's disease. *Experimental Neurology*, **175**, 426.

Garg AK (2011). Nocebo side-effects in cancer treatment. *Lancet Oncology*, **12**, 1181–2.

Gracely RH, Dubner R, Deeter WR and Wolskee PJ (1985). Clinicians' expectations influence placebo analgesia. *Lancet*, **1**, 43.

Greenfield S, Kaplan S and Ware JE (1985). Expanding patient involvement in care. *Annals of Internal Medicine*, **102**, 520–8.

Hamalainen ML, Hoppu K and Santavuori P (1997). Sumatriptan for migraine attacks in children: a randomized placebo-controlled study. *Neurology*, **48**, 1100–3.

Hashish I, Hai HK, Harvey W, Feinmann C and Harris M (1988). Reduction of postoperative pain and swelling by ultrasound treatment: a placebo effect. *Pain*, **33**, 303–11.

Howard S and Hughes BM (2008). Expectancies, not aroma, explain impact of lavender aromatherapy on psychophysiological indices of relaxation in young healthy women. *British Journal of Health Psychology*, **13**, 603–17.

Ilnyckyj A, Shanahan F, Anton PA, Cheang M and Bernstein CN (1997). Quantification of the placebo response in ulcerative colitis. *Gastroenterology*, **112**, 1854–8.

Inui TS, Yourtee EL and Williamson JW (1976). Improved outcomes in hypertension after physician tutorials. *Annals of Internal Medicine*, **84**, 646–51.

Jacobson PB, Bovbjerg DH, Schwartz MD *et al.* (1993). Formation of food aversions in cancer patients receiving repeated infusions of chemotherapy. *Behavioral Research and Therapy*, **31**, 739–48.

Jessy T (2011). Immunity over inability: the spontaneous regression of cancer. *Journal of Natural Science, Biology and Medicine*, **2**, 43–9.

Kaplan SH, Greenfield S and Ware JE Jr. (1989). Assessing the effects of physician-patient interactions on the outcomes of chronic disease. *Medical Care*, **27**(Suppl 3), S110–27.

Kirsch I and Weixel LJ (1988). Double-blind versus deceptive administration of a placebo. *Behavioral Neuroscience*, **102**, 319–23.

Klinger R, Soost S, Flor H and Worm M (2007). Classical conditioning and expectancy in placebo hypoalgesia: a randomized controlled study in patients with atopic dermatitis and persons with healthy skin. *Pain*, **128**, 31–9.

Kong J, Gollub RL, Rosman IS *et al.* (2006). Brain activity associated with expectancy-enhanced placebo analgesia as measured by functional magnetic resonance imaging. *Journal of Neuroscience*, **26**, 381–8.

Langley GB, Sheppeard H, Johnson M and Wigley RD (1984). The analgesic effects of transcutaneous electrical nerve stimulation and placebo in chronic pain patients. *Rheumatology International*, **4**, 119–23.

Levinson W (1994). Physician-patient communication: a key to malpractice prevention. *Journal of the American Medical Association*, **272**, 1619–20.

Linde K, Witt CM, Streng A *et al.* (2007). The impact of patient expectations on outcomes in four randomized controlled trials of acupuncture in patients with chronic pain. *Pain*, **128**, 264–71.

Link J, Haggard R, Kelly K and Forrer D (2006). Placebo/nocebo symptom reporting in a sham herbal supplement trial. *Evaluation & the Health Professions*, **29**, 394–406.

Loder E, Goldstein R and Biondi D (2005). Placebo effects in oral triptan trials: the scientific and ethical rationale for continued use of placebo controls. *Cephalalgia*, **25**, 124–31.

Marchand S, Kupers RC, Bushnell MC and Duncan GH (2003). Analgesic and placebo effects of thalamic stimulation. *Pain*, **105**, 481–8.

McRae C, Cherin E, Yamazaki G *et al.* (2004). Effects of perceived treatment on quality of life and medical outcomes in a double-blind placebo surgery trial. *Archives of General Psychiatry*, **61**, 412–20.

Mercado R, Constantoyannis C, Mandat T *et al.* (2006). Expectation and the placebo effect in Parkinson's disease patients with subthalamic nucleus deep brain stimulation. *Movement Disorders*, **21**, 1457–61.

Moertel CG, Taylor WF, Roth A and Tyce FA (1976). Who responds to sugar pills? *Mayo Clinic Proceedings*, **51**, 96–100.

Moseley JB, O'Malley K, Petersen NJ *et al.* (2002). A controlled trial of arthroscopic surgery for osteoarthritis of the knee. *New England Journal of Medicine*, **347**, 81–8.

Nesse RM, Carli T, Curtis GC and Kleinman PD (1980). Pretreatment nausea in cancer chemotherapy: a conditioned response? *Psychosomatic Medicine*, **42**, 33–6.

Olanow C, Goetz C, Kordower J *et al.* (2003). A double-blind controlled trial of bilateral nigral transplantation in Parkinson's disease. *Annals of Neurology*, **54**, 403–14.

Pariente J, White P, Frackowiak RSJ and Lewith G (2005). Expectancy and belief modulate the neuronal substrates of pain treated by acupuncture *NeuroImage*, **25**, 1161–7.

Petrovic P, Kalso E, Petersson KM and Ingvar M (2002). Placebo and opioid analgesia—imaging a shared neuronal network. *Science*, **295**, 1737–40.

Pollo A, Amanzio M, Arslanian A, Casadio C, Maggi G and Benedetti F (2001). Response expectancies in placebo analgesia and their clinical relevance. *Pain*, **93**, 77–84.

Pollo A, Torre E, Lopiano L *et al.* (2002). Expectation modulates the response to subthalamic nucleus stimulation in Parkinsonian patients. *NeuroReport*, **13**, 1383–6.

Rana JS, Mannam A, Donnell-Fink L, Gervino EV, Sellke FW and Laham RJ (2005). Longevity of the placebo effect in the therapeutic angiogenesis and laser myocardial revascularization trials in patients with coronary heart disease. *American Journal of Cardiology*, **95**, 1456–9.

Rosseland LA, Helgesen KG, Breivik H and Stubhaug A (2004). Moderate-to-severe pain after knee arthroscopy is relieved by intraarticular saline: a randomized controlled trial. *Anesthesia and Analgesia*, **98**, 1546–51.

Simmonds MJ and Kumar S (1994). Pain and the placebo in rehabilitation using TENS and laser. *Disability and Rehabilitation*, **16**, 13–20.

Sox HC, Margulies I and Sox CH (1981). Psychologically mediated effects of diagnostic tests. *Annals of Internal Medicine*, **95**, 680–5.

Starfield B, Wray C, Hess K, Gross R, Birk PS and D'Lugoff BC (1981). The influence of patient-practitioner agreement on outcome of care. *American Journal of Public Health*, **71**, 127–32.

Stewart MA (1995). Effective physician-patient communication and health outcomes: a review. *Canadian Medical Association Journal*, **152**, 1423–33.

Stewart MA, McWhinney IR and Buck CW (1979). The doctor-patient relationship and its effect upon outcome. *Journal of Royal College of General Practice*, **29**, 77–82.

Stockhorst U, Enck P and Klosterhalfen S (2007). Role of classical conditioning in learning gastrointestinal symptoms. *World Journal of Gastroenterology*, **13**, 3430–7.

Stockhorst U, Klosterhalfen S, Klosterhalfen W, Winkelmann M and Steingrueber HJ (1993). Anticipatory nausea in cancer patients receiving chemotherapy: classical conditioning etiology and therapeutical implications. *Integrative Physiological and Behavioral Sciences*, **23**, 177–81.

Stockhorst U, Spennes-Saleh S, Koerholz D *et al.* (2000). Anticipatory symptoms and anticipatory immune responses in pediatric cancer patients receiving chemotherapy: features of a classically conditioned response? *Brain, Behavior and Immunity*, **14**, 198–218.

Stockhorst U, Steingrueber HJ, Enck P and Klosterhalfen S (2006). Pavlovian conditioning of nausea and vomiting. *Autonomic Neuroscience*, **129**, 50–7.

Stockhorst U, Wiener JA, Klosterhalfen S, Klosterhalfen W, Aul C and Steingrueber HJ (1998). Effects of overshadowing on conditioned nausea in cancer patients: an experimental study. *Physiology and Behavior*, **64**, 743–53.

Su C, Lichtenstein GR, Krok K, Brensinger CM and Lewis JD (2004). A meta-analysis of the placebo response rates of remission and response in clinical trials of active Crohn's disease. *Gastroenterology*, **126**, 1257–69.

Thomas KB (1987). General practice consultations: is there any point in being positive? *British Medical Journal*, **294**, 1200–2.

Thomsen J, Bretlau P, Tos M and Johnsen NJ (1981). Placebo effect in surgery for Meniere's disease. A double-blind, placebo-controlled study on endolymphatic sac shunt surgery. *Archives of Otolaryngology*, **107**, 271–7.

Tyc VL, Mulhem RK, Barclay DR, Smith BF and Bieberich AA (1997). Variables associated with anticipatory nausea and vomiting in pediatric cancer patients receiving ondansetron antiemetic therapy. *Journal of Pediatric Psychology*, **22**, 45–58.

van Laarhoven AI, Vogelaar ML, Wilder-Smith OH, van Riel PL, van de Kerkhof PC *et al.* (2011). Induction of nocebo and placebo effects on itch and pain by verbal suggestions. *Pain*, **152**, 1486–94.

Wager TD, Rilling JK, Smith EE *et al.* (2004). Placebo-induced changes in fMRI in the anticipation and experience of pain. *Science*, **303**, 1162–6.

Wald TG, Kathol RG, Noyes R Jr, Carroll BT and Clamon GM (1993). Rapid relief of anxiety in cancer patients with both alprazolam and placebo. *Psychosomatics*, **34**, 324–32.

Weimer K, Gulewitsch MD, Schlarb AA, Schwille-Kiuntke J, Klosterhalfen S and Enck P (2013). Placebo effects in children: a review. *Pediatric Research*, **74**, 96–102.

Welling DB and Nagaraja HN (2000). Endolymphatic mastoid stunt: a re-evaluation of efficacy. *Otolaryngology–Head and Neck Surgery*, **122**, 340–5.

Winner P, Lewis D, Visser WH, Jiang K, Ahrens S and Evans JK (2002). Rizatriptan 5 mg for the acute treatment of migraine in adolescents: a randomized, double-blind, placebo-controlled study. *Headache*, **42**, 49–55.

Zubieta JK, Bueller JA, Jackson LR *et al.* (2005). Placebo effects mediated by endogenous opioid activity on μ-opioid receptors. *Journal of Neuroscience*, **25**, 7754–62.

Part 4

Clinical, ethical, and methodological considerations

Several implications, and possibly applications, emerge from the recent insights into the mechanisms of the placebo effect. These include the possible use of placebos in medical practice, at least in some circumstances, although many ethical constraints must be considered. This holds true both in routine medical practice and in the clinical trial setting. In addition, what we have learned over the past few years is that the mechanisms of different placebo responses can be unraveled only by designing complex experiments, in order to identify real psychobiological placebo effects and to differentiate them from other confounding factors, such as spontaneous remissions. In this Part 4, all these aspects are considered and described in detail.

Chapter 11

Clinical–ethical implications and applications

Summary points

- The recent neurobiological advances in placebo research can stimulate the development of new clinical trial designs for the validation of new treatments.

- The recent neurobiological advances in placebo research lead to an uncertainty principle, whereby it is not possible to fully understand the action of a therapeutic agent.

- One of the main implications of the recent advances in placebo research is the possibility of inducing drug-like effects without drugs, thus opening up the potential of reducing drug intake.

- As social stimuli may activate the same biochemical and receptorial pathways on which drugs act, several cognitive and affective factors can modulate the action of drugs.

11.1 Assessing the effectiveness of new therapies

11.1.1 The debate of using placebos in clinical trials is still open

Although placebos are routinely administered in clinical trials, a lively discussion surrounds their use. This discussion focuses on at least two aspects. The first is an ethical one, and the second is more technical and methodological. As far as the ethical issue is concerned, the World Medical Association Declaration of Helsinki (World Medical Association, 2000) contains a paragraph (Paragraph 29) that states:

> The benefits, risks, burdens and effectiveness of a new method should be tested against those of the best current prophylactic, diagnostic, and therapeutic methods. This does not exclude the use of placebo, or no treatment, in studies where no proven prophylactic, diagnostic or therapeutic method exists.

Thus the Declaration of Helsinki maintains that it is unethical to assign patients to receive a placebo when effective treatment exists. However, it should be noted that the World Medical Association added a footnote to Paragraph 29 in October 2002, with the title "Note of clarification on Paragraph 29 of the World Medical Association Declaration of Helsinki." This footnote reads (World Medical Association, 2002):

The World Medical Association hereby reaffirms its position that extreme care must be taken in making use of a placebo-controlled trial and that in general this methodology should only be used in the absence of existing proven therapy. However, a placebo-controlled trial may be ethically acceptable, even if proven therapy is available, under the following circumstances: —Where for compelling and scientifically sound methodological reasons its use is necessary to determine the efficacy or safety of a prophylactic, diagnostic or therapeutic method; or —Where a prophylactic, diagnostic or therapeutic method is being investigated for a minor condition and the patients who receive placebo will not be subject to any additional risk of serious or irreversible harm. All other provisions of the Declaration of Helsinki must be adhered to, especially the need for appropriate ethical and scientific review.

This revision has been criticized by many authors. For example, Michels and Rothman (2003) consider this clarification to be a step backward in bioethics. The positions of official organizations, such as the US Food and Drug Administration (FDA), the American Medical Association (AMA), the European Committee for Proprietary Medicinal Products (CPMP), and the World Health Organization (WHO) are contrasting. For example, the FDA has always defended placebo-controlled studies for the development of new treatments, even if effective therapies exist (Temple, 2002). According to Rothman and Michels (1994), this violates Paragraph 29 of the Declaration of Helsinki. The AMA supports the position of the FDA, and asserts that the existence of an accepted therapy does not necessarily preclude the use of controls (Council on Ethical and Judicial Affairs of the American Medical Association, 1996; Michels and Rothman, 2003). By contrast, the WHO states that placebos are not justified if there is already an approved and accepted treatment for the condition that a candidate therapy is designed to treat (Council for International Organizations of Medical Sciences, 1993). The European CPMP takes a more ambiguous position, as it affirms that in principle placebo-controlled trials are required to show effectiveness of a new product, but it is recognized that suitable alternative designs may be developed (Committee for Proprietary Medicinal Products, 1998). The latest version of the Declaration of Helsinki is shown in Box 11.1.

As discussed in detail by Califf and Al-Khatib (2002), Levine (2002), Pocock (2002), Rothman and Michels (2002), and Temple (2002) in the book *The Science of the Placebo* (Guess et al., 2002), placebo defenders, in general, often use the utilitarian argument, such that exposing subjects to placebo treatment is justified by the knowledge gained for future patients. Conversely, placebo opponents reply that ethical obligations to the single individual take precedence over science and society. Placebo defenders also affirm that the approval of institutional review boards and local ethics committees and the patient's informed consent are sufficient, but placebo opponents contend that most informed consent forms are incomprehensible, thus making the patient unable to judge the experimental situations. Another argument raised by placebo defenders is about the use of placebos for symptomatic treatments and not for curative therapies, but placebo opponents contend that there is no justification even for minor discomfort. Of course, omitting standard treatment is not acceptable in many circumstances, such as cancer, congestive heart failure and epilepsy. In such cases, add-on studies (in which all patients receive standard therapy and then are randomized to added new treatment or added placebo) may be useful as they establish the value of the addition.

Box 11.1 World Medical Association Declaration of Helsinki—Ethical Principles for Medical Research Involving Human Subjects

Adopted by the 18th WMA General Assembly, Helsinki, Finland, June 1964 and amended by the:

29th WMA General Assembly, Tokyo, Japan, October 1975

35th WMA General Assembly, Venice, Italy, October 1983

41st WMA General Assembly, Hong Kong, September 1989

48th WMA General Assembly, Somerset West, Republic of South Africa, October 1996

52nd WMA General Assembly, Edinburgh, Scotland, October 2000

53rd WMA General Assembly, Washington DC, USA, October 2002 (Note of Clarification added)

55th WMA General Assembly, Tokyo, Japan, October 2004 (Note of Clarification added)

59th WMA General Assembly, Seoul, Republic of Korea, October 2008

64th WMA General Assembly, Fortaleza, Brazil, October 2013.

Preamble

1 The World Medical Association (WMA) has developed the Declaration of Helsinki as a statement of ethical principles for medical research involving human subjects, including research on identifiable human material and data.

The Declaration is intended to be read as a whole and each of its constituent paragraphs should be applied with consideration of all other relevant paragraphs.

2 Consistent with the mandate of the WMA, the Declaration is addressed primarily to physicians. The WMA encourages others who are involved in medical research involving human subjects to adopt these principles.

General Principles

3 The Declaration of Geneva of the WMA binds the physician with the words, "The health of my patient will be my first consideration," and the International Code of Medical Ethics declares that, "A physician shall act in the patient's best interest when providing medical care."

4 It is the duty of the physician to promote and safeguard the health, well-being and rights of patients, including those who are involved in medical research. The physician's knowledge and conscience are dedicated to the fulfilment of this duty.

Box 11.1 World Medical Association Declaration of Helsinki—Ethical Principles for Medical Research Involving Human Subjects (continued)

5 Medical progress is based on research that ultimately must include studies involving human subjects.

6 The primary purpose of medical research involving human subjects is to understand the causes, development and effects of diseases and improve preventive, diagnostic and therapeutic interventions (methods, procedures and treatments). Even the best proven interventions must be evaluated continually through research for their safety, effectiveness, efficiency, accessibility and quality.

7 Medical research is subject to ethical standards that promote and ensure respect for all human subjects and protect their health and rights.

8 While the primary purpose of medical research is to generate new knowledge, this goal can never take precedence over the rights and interests of individual research subjects.

9 It is the duty of physicians who are involved in medical research to protect the life, health, dignity, integrity, right to self-determination, privacy, and confidentiality of personal information of research subjects. The responsibility for the protection of research subjects must always rest with the physician or other health care professionals and never with the research subjects, even though they have given consent.

10 Physicians must consider the ethical, legal and regulatory norms and standards for research involving human subjects in their own countries as well as applicable international norms and standards. No national or international ethical, legal or regulatory requirement should reduce or eliminate any of the protections for research subjects set forth in this Declaration.

11 Medical research should be conducted in a manner that minimises possible harm to the environment.

12 Medical research involving human subjects must be conducted only by individuals with the appropriate ethics and scientific education, training and qualifications. Research on patients or healthy volunteers requires the supervision of a competent and appropriately qualified physician or other health care professional.

13 Groups that are underrepresented in medical research should be provided appropriate access to participation in research.

14 Physicians who combine medical research with medical care should involve their patients in research only to the extent that this is justified by its potential preventive, diagnostic or therapeutic value and if the physician has good reason to believe that participation in the research study will not adversely affect the health of the patients who serve as research subjects.

15 Appropriate compensation and treatment for subjects who are harmed as a result of participating in research must be ensured.

Box 11.1 World Medical Association Declaration of Helsinki—Ethical Principles for Medical Research Involving Human Subjects (continued)

Risks, Burdens and Benefits

16 In medical practice and in medical research, most interventions involve risks and burdens.

17 All medical research involving human subjects must be preceded by careful assessment of predictable risks and burdens to the individuals and groups involved in the research in comparison with foreseeable benefits to them and to other individuals or groups affected by the condition under investigation.

Measures to minimise the risks must be implemented. The risks must be continuously monitored, assessed and documented by the researcher.

18 Physicians may not be involved in a research study involving human subjects unless they are confident that the risks have been adequately assessed and can be satisfactorily managed.

When the risks are found to outweigh the potential benefits or when there is conclusive proof of definitive outcomes, physicians must assess whether to continue, modify or immediately stop the study.

Vulnerable Groups and Individuals

19 Some groups and individuals are particularly vulnerable and may have an increased likelihood of being wronged or of incurring additional harm.

All vulnerable groups and individuals should receive specifically considered protection.

20 Medical research with a vulnerable group is only justified if the research is responsive to the health needs or priorities of this group and the research cannot be carried out in a non-vulnerable group. In addition, this group should stand to benefit from the knowledge, practices or interventions that result from the research.

Scientific Requirements and Research Protocols

21 Medical research involving human subjects must conform to generally accepted scientific principles, be based on a thorough knowledge of the scientific literature, other relevant sources of information, and adequate laboratory and, as appropriate, animal experimentation. The welfare of animals used for research must be respected.

22 The design and performance of each research study involving human subjects must be clearly described and justified in a research protocol.

The protocol should contain a statement of the ethical considerations involved and should indicate how the principles in this Declaration have been addressed.

Box 11.1 World Medical Association Declaration of Helsinki—Ethical Principles for Medical Research Involving Human Subjects (continued)

The protocol should include information regarding funding, sponsors, institutional affiliations, potential conflicts of interest, incentives for subjects and information regarding provisions for treating and/or compensating subjects who are harmed as a consequence of participation in the research study.

In clinical trials, the protocol must also describe appropriate arrangements for post-trial provisions.

Research Ethics Committees

23 The research protocol must be submitted for consideration, comment, guidance and approval to the concerned research ethics committee before the study begins. This committee must be transparent in its functioning, must be independent of the researcher, the sponsor and any other undue influence and must be duly qualified. It must take into consideration the laws and regulations of the country or countries in which the research is to be performed as well as applicable international norms and standards but these must not be allowed to reduce or eliminate any of the protections for research subjects set forth in this Declaration.

The committee must have the right to monitor ongoing studies. The researcher must provide monitoring information to the committee, especially information about any serious adverse events. No amendment to the protocol may be made without consideration and approval by the committee. After the end of the study, the researchers must submit a final report to the committee containing a summary of the study's findings and conclusions.

Privacy and Confidentiality

24 Every precaution must be taken to protect the privacy of research subjects and the confidentiality of their personal information.

Informed Consent

25 Participation by individuals capable of giving informed consent as subjects in medical research must be voluntary. Although it may be appropriate to consult family members or community leaders, no individual capable of giving informed consent may be enrolled in a research study unless he or she freely agrees.

26 In medical research involving human subjects capable of giving informed consent, each potential subject must be adequately informed of the aims, methods, sources of funding, any possible conflicts of interest, institutional affiliations of the researcher, the anticipated benefits and potential risks of the study and the discomfort it may entail, post-study provisions and any other relevant aspects

Box 11.1 World Medical Association Declaration of Helsinki—Ethical Principles for Medical Research Involving Human Subjects (continued)

of the study. The potential subject must be informed of the right to refuse to participate in the study or to withdraw consent to participate at any time without reprisal. Special attention should be given to the specific information needs of individual potential subjects as well as to the methods used to deliver the information.

After ensuring that the potential subject has understood the information, the physician or another appropriately qualified individual must then seek the potential subject's freely-given informed consent, preferably in writing. If the consent cannot be expressed in writing, the non-written consent must be formally documented and witnessed.

All medical research subjects should be given the option of being informed about the general outcome and results of the study.

27 When seeking informed consent for participation in a research study the physician must be particularly cautious if the potential subject is in a dependent relationship with the physician or may consent under duress. In such situations the informed consent must be sought by an appropriately qualified individual who is completely independent of this relationship.

28 For a potential research subject who is incapable of giving informed consent, the physician must seek informed consent from the legally authorised representative. These individuals must not be included in a research study that has no likelihood of benefit for them unless it is intended to promote the health of the group represented by the potential subject, the research cannot instead be performed with persons capable of providing informed consent, and the research entails only minimal risk and minimal burden.

29 When a potential research subject who is deemed incapable of giving informed consent is able to give assent to decisions about participation in research, the physician must seek that assent in addition to the consent of the legally authorised representative. The potential subject's dissent should be respected.

30 Research involving subjects who are physically or mentally incapable of giving consent, for example, unconscious patients, may be done only if the physical or mental condition that prevents giving informed consent is a necessary characteristic of the research group. In such circumstances the physician must seek informed consent from the legally authorised representative. If no such representative is available and if the research cannot be delayed, the study may proceed without informed consent provided that the specific reasons for involving subjects with a condition that renders them unable to give informed consent have been stated in the research protocol and the study has been approved by a research ethics committee. Consent to remain in the research must be obtained as soon as possible from the subject or a legally authorised representative.

> **Box 11.1 World Medical Association Declaration of Helsinki—Ethical Principles for Medical Research Involving Human Subjects (continued)**
>
> 31 The physician must fully inform the patient which aspects of their care are related to the research. The refusal of a patient to participate in a study or the patient's decision to withdraw from the study must never adversely affect the patient-physician relationship.
>
> 32 For medical research using identifiable human material or data, such as research on material or data contained in biobanks or similar repositories, physicians must seek informed consent for its collection, storage and/or reuse. There may be exceptional situations where consent would be impossible or impracticable to obtain for such research. In such situations the research may be done only after consideration and approval of a research ethics committee.
>
> ## Use of Placebo
>
> 33 The benefits, risks, burdens and effectiveness of a new intervention must be tested against those of the best proven intervention(s), except in the following circumstances:
>
> Where no proven intervention exists, the use of placebo, or no intervention, is acceptable; or
>
>   Where for compelling and scientifically sound methodological reasons the use of any intervention less effective than the best proven one, the use of placebo, or no intervention is necessary to determine the efficacy or safety of an intervention and the patients who receive any intervention less effective than the best proven one, placebo, or no intervention will not be subject to additional risks of serious or irreversible harm as a result of not receiving the best proven intervention.
>
>   Extreme care must be taken to avoid abuse of this option.
>
> ## Post-Trial Provisions
>
> 34 In advance of a clinical trial, sponsors, researchers and host country governments should make provisions for post-trial access for all participants who still need an intervention identified as beneficial in the trial. This information must also be disclosed to participants during the informed consent process.
>
> ## Research Registration and Publication and Dissemination of Results
>
> 35 Every research study involving human subjects must be registered in a publicly accessible database before recruitment of the first subject.
>
> 36 Researchers, authors, sponsors, editors and publishers all have ethical obligations with regard to the publication and dissemination of the results of research. Researchers have a duty to make publicly available the results of their

---

Box 11.1 World Medical Association Declaration of Helsinki—Ethical Principles for Medical Research Involving Human Subjects (continued)

research on human subjects and are accountable for the completeness and accuracy of their reports. All parties should adhere to accepted guidelines for ethical reporting. Negative and inconclusive as well as positive results must be published or otherwise made publicly available. Sources of funding, institutional affiliations and conflicts of interest must be declared in the publication. Reports of research not in accordance with the principles of this Declaration should not be accepted for publication.

Unproven Interventions in Clinical Practice

37 In the treatment of an individual patient, where proven interventions do not exist or other known interventions have been ineffective, the physician, after seeking expert advice, with informed consent from the patient or a legally authorised representative, may use an unproven intervention if in the physician's judgement it offers hope of saving life, re-establishing health or alleviating suffering. This intervention should subsequently be made the object of research, designed to evaluate its safety and efficacy. In all cases, new information must be recorded and, where appropriate, made publicly available.

© 2014 World Medical Association, Inc. All Rights reserved.

As for the technical and methodological argument, several points have been raised by statisticians and clinical researchers in favor of the use of placebos in clinical research, for example, establishment of a reference point by means of placebo groups, the lack of statistical significance tests for equivalence trials (new versus old therapy), and the much larger population required for an equivalence trial compared with placebo-controlled trials (Califf, Al-Khatib, 2002; Levine, 2002; Pocock, 2002; Rothman and Michels, 2002; Temple, 2002). Although an equivalence (or noninferiority) trial is undoubtedly more ethical (because a new treatment under test is compared to an old proven, effective one) some methodological and interpretative problems arise; for example, if the new treatment works better than the old one (Fig. 11.1A) then the results would be convincing and the interpretation quite easy. In fact, in this case the conclusion would be that the old treatment might be replaced by the new one. However, if the new treatment does not work as well as the old one (Fig. 11.1B) at least two conclusions could be drawn. First, the new treatment is less effective than the old one; or, second, the new treatment is not effective at all. Without a placebo group, it is not possible to distinguish between these two interpretations. In contrast, if a placebo group is run, and if the new treatment is better than the placebo, then it is less effective than the old one—but it is still effective (Fig. 11.1C); whereas if the new treatment is equivalent to the placebo, then it is completely ineffective (Fig. 11.1D). This difference could be very important whenever the old treatment induces severe side effects and the

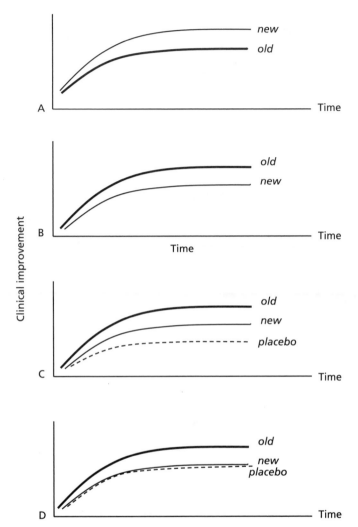

Fig. 11.1 Clinical trials in which a new treatment is compared to an old one. (A) If the new treatment is better than the old one, the interpretation of the results is quite easy, so that the old treatment can be replaced with the new one. (B) If the new treatment is worse than the old one, no conclusions can be drawn, as the new treatment can be either less effective than the new one or completely ineffective. To resolve this issue, a placebo group is necessary. If the new treatment is better than placebo (C) it can be considered less effective than the old one, but still effective. Conversely, if it does not differ from placebo (D), it can be considered to be completely ineffective.

new one induces fewer or no side effects at all. In such cases, it would be advisable to use a slightly less effective treatment with fewer side effects.

The main concern in the classical clinical trial approach is patient safety. In other words, no one wants to expose patients to possible risks that might result from depriving them of optimal treatment. In fact, in the classical clinical trial setting the ethical issue of placebo administration does not involve deception, as the patients are informed that they have a 50% chance of receiving either placebo or active treatment. However, in other clinical trial contexts the ethics of placebo administration have to do with deception. One of these contexts is the balanced placebo design (section 1.2.2) in which it is possible to manipulate expectations about the treatment being administered (see Fig. 1.2). For example, subjects might receive the placebo but be told it is the active drug, or they might receive active drug and be told it is a placebo. Similarly, they might receive the placebo and be told it is a placebo, or they might receive the active drug and be told they are receiving an active drug. It can be seen with this design that deception is unavoidable. Kirsch (2003) pointed out that this approach yields information that cannot be obtained from conventional clinical trials, as it provides direct assessment of drug effects and expectancy effects. Caspi (2002) has suggested that the balanced placebo design be used more frequently in clinical trials of drug efficacy. However, the deception inherent to this approach makes it scientifically problematic in many circumstances (Miller et al., 2005; Koshi and Short, 2007).

To resolve the ethical issue of deception, the American Psychological Association considers some situations in which deception is allowed (American Psychological Association, 1992): first, when the study is expected to have significant social and scientific value; second, when an equally effective nondeceptive approach is not available; third, when participants must not be deceived about any aspect of the study that would affect their willingness to participate; fourth, when deception must be explained to the participants at the end of the study. In a similar statement by the American Pain Society (Price, 2005; Sullivan et al., 2005) placebos are allowed when there is little harm to patients, or when the alternative active treatment is unproven, or when there is substantial benefit to future patients. In any case, placebos must not be used for punishment, deception, or long-term undertreatment of patients with pain. Wendler and Miller (2004) proposed to adopt a sort of authorized deception, whereby subjects are informed that they will be deceived but the exact nature of the deception is not revealed. In this way, the subjects give their informed consent, although they do not know how they will be deceived.

Despite all these ethical and methodological considerations, one very important issue remains difficult to resolve. It has to do with informed consent. The main problem is how it is understood by participants in the clinical trial. Most informed consent forms are incomprehensible, with many technical terms and a long list of beneficial and adverse effects. Certain populations of patients are unable even to understand simple procedures and instructions—a problem encountered at times in less developed countries (Bok, 2002); there are concerns about often nonexistent consent procedures and the poorly explained levels of risk for participants. In addition, the local institution review boards are at a great distance from the sponsoring institutions in the United States or Europe, thus not guaranteeing adequate control of the informed consent procedures.

The ethical issues in the field of placebo are far from being resolved, and might be worthy of more important discussion in bioethics (Miller and Colloca, 2011; Brody et al., 2012; Brody and Colloca, 2013). For example, as suggested by Bok (2002), it would make a difference if standard consent procedures required investigators to make sure subjects understood the precise difference between therapy and research. Similarly, it would make a big difference if subjects were fully informed about the risks, including those that might arise if they are in the placebo group.

11.1.2 Two examples of the ethics of placebo trials: surgery and schizophrenia

A special and particularly important situation in which placebos raise serious ethical questions is surgery. In fact, the use of sham surgical operations for validating surgical techniques is one of the most debated ethical issues of today. Placebo-controlled surgical trials are rare because surgery per se is dangerous, and simulation of a surgical operation, including anesthesia and infusion of different drugs, is often considered to be unnecessary and unsafe. However, we have seen throughout this book that the rate of improvement in placebo groups in surgical trials is high (see section 10.2.1) suggesting that many surgical procedures are based only on anecdotal evidence and weak scientific research.

There are several examples of placebo surgery with a clinical improvement. It is not always clear, however, whether such an improvement is a real placebo effect or a spontaneous remission. Several examples are presented in section 10.2, such as sham ligation of the mammary arteries in the 1950s by Dimond et al. (1958) and Cobb et al. (1959); sham arthroscopy of the knee by Moseley et al. (2002) and Rosseland et al. (2004); sham neurosurgical trials of deep-brain stimulation by Pollo et al. (2002), Benedetti et al. (2003a, 2003b), Marchand et al. (2003), and Mercado et al. (2006); and of fetal cells transplantation (e.g., McRae et al., 2004). These results strongly suggest the need to use placebo surgery in surgical trials in order to validate a surgical procedure with rigorous scientific evidence. It should be emphasized that in all these examples, the surgical risk ranges from minimal to high. For example, a small incision of the skin along with intravenous anesthesia for arthroscopy is no riskier than intravenous injection of a drug in phase 1 of a clinical trial. Conversely, drilling someone's skull for fetal cell transplantation is a more invasive and risky procedure. Are both these surgical procedures ethically acceptable? Or should we distinguish one surgical procedure from another, based on the degree of risk for the patient? The debate is still open and no clear answer is available today (Polgar and Ng, 2005; Boyle and Batzer, 2007; Horng and Miller, 2007). In fact, even minimally invasive procedures may be risky; these include catheter implantation for drug delivery, which is particularly risky if the catheter is inserted into a delicate part of the body, such as intracranially for treating Parkinson's disease (Nutt et al., 2003; Lang et al., 2006), where there is a continual risk of infection, hemorrhage, or dislodgement.

Despite the risks associated with invasive surgical procedures, by considering the number of patients who underwent completely ineffective ligation of their internal mammary arteries before the placebo-controlled trials by Dimond and Cobb's groups (Dimond et al., 1958; Cobb et al., 1959), the consequences of not conducting rigorous trials of surgery are evident for both patients (because mammary arterial ligation is a truly invasive procedure) and for society (because of the costs of such a procedure).

Another example of the ethical problems surrounding the use of placebos in clinical trials is presented by schizophrenia, especially one study of fluphenazine decanoate treatment (Streiner, 1999). In the first stage of the study, patients received a fixed dose of the medication for 1 year. After successfully completing this stage, patients were recruited onto a second much more controversial protocol. These chronic schizophrenic patients were randomized either to continue on the same dose of the active treatment or to receive a placebo. After 12 weeks, they were crossed over—those on placebo now received active treatment, and those on active treatment now received the placebo. Patients who were still stable then went through a withdrawal protocol, in order to identify the predictors of successful functioning without antipsychotic medication. During this withdrawal phase, one patient enrolled in the study committed suicide and another suffered a severe psychotic relapse. Although the Office for Protection from Research Risks did not find the study to be unethical, they considered the consent procedure to be flawed, and the family of one of the subjects sued the university concerned.

This trial shows how ethical problems relate to informed consent in schizophrenia. Is the capacity to understand the risks and benefits of a study compromised by the very nature of schizophrenia? It is this issue that often clouds the discussion of ethics of placebo-controlled trials in the case of the psychiatric disorder schizophrenia. This is a psychotic illness which, by definition, means that patients in the acute stage have a disturbed ability to interpret reality. Is it possible for someone who believes they are being controlled by voices or that they have supernatural powers to really appreciate the risks and benefits of a study? In general, there is no evidence that people with schizophrenia are not capable of consenting to research. However, it should be recognized that understanding the risks and benefits of treatment depends on many factors, and these may vary with the stage of the illness and the severity of symptoms. Whereas many of these patients have the capacity to participate in research studies, including placebo-controlled studies, there is always a substantial proportion of patients who are not capable (Zipursky and Darby, 1999).

As well as the problem of the informed consent in schizophrenic patients, several other ethical issues have been raised, such as the risk that the longer a psychotic patient remains untreated, the less well they are likely to do in the long run (Wyatt, 1991). Another concern is that psychotic patients may be at an increased risk of committing dangerous acts, such as violent and destructive behavior, including suicide. Therefore, many authors believe that the use of a placebo control may be acceptable in carefully defined circumstances, while in most cases the use of an active control in schizophrenia research is ethically and scientifically preferable (Weijer, 1999). In other words (and according to the Declaration of Helsinki) some claim that when an effective treatment exists, a new treatment must be compared with the old one. (For more on the methodological problems see the previous section 11.1.1 as well as Streiner, 1999). According to Streiner (1999), if a placebo arm is deemed necessary, then certain conditions must be met. These include: (1) setting very high requirements for informed consent; (2) using an external group to monitor adverse reactions; (3) requiring that attending physicians do not enroll their own patients into a trial; (4) not paying physicians on the basis of subjects completing the trial; (5) having a time limit for patients in the placebo condition; (6) using only drug-free or drug-resistant patients.

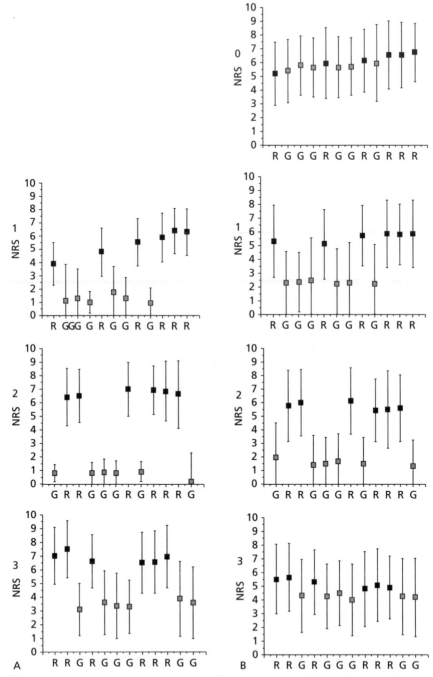

Fig. 11.2 (A) In blocks 1 and 2, the black squares represent painful stimuli associated with a red light (R) whereas the gray squares represent non-painful stimuli associated with a green light (G). In these two blocks, the stimulus intensity is surreptitiously reduced

11.1.3 **New designs can be envisaged that increase the sensitivity of the trial**

Throughout this book we have seen that many clinical trials show substantial improvements in placebo groups, although it is not always clear why such improvements occur (it can be because of spontaneous remission or regression to the mean or expectations of benefit). We have also seen that in many circumstances the placebo effect is a learning phenomenon which can be attributable to increased expectations, as occurs in pain and movement disorders (Chapters 4 and 5) or to classical conditioning, as occurs in the immune and endocrine systems (Chapter 7). For example, powerful placebo responses can be obtained after prior positive experience of effective treatments (Amanzio and Benedetti, 1999; Colloca and Benedetti, 2006). Therefore, it is also conceivable that the opposite situation (prior negative experience) may lead to small placebo responses. This would be very useful in clinical trials in order to increase the sensitivity of the assay, that is, the sensitivity of the trial.

Indeed it is possible to reduce placebo analgesic responses. This has been shown by Colloca and Benedetti (2006) who used electrical stimulation in healthy volunteers as an experimental pain model. Powerful placebo analgesic responses were obtained by means of a conditioning procedure, whereby a red light was associated with painful stimulation many times, and a green light was associated with nonpainful stimulation. After repeated associations of this kind, both the red and green light were presented in association with painful stimulation. Fig. 11.2 (left) shows the powerful placebo responses to the green light (bottom panel). This powerful conditioning-induced placebo analgesia could be dramatically reduced if, before the very same conditioning procedure, a sequence of red and green lights was associated with painful stimulation, in which the subjects did not experience any analgesia with the green light; this is shown in Fig. 11.2 (right). The potential to reduce placebo responses in this way might present an interesting approach for creating subjects with low placebo responsiveness, so they might be included in a clinical trial for comparison with active treatment. A procedure like this has never been carried out in a real clinical trial setting, but it is a promising approach for testing the efficacy of a new therapy.

◄──

Fig. 11.2 (continued) after placebo administration and associated with the green light. After this conditioning procedure, in block 3, despite all the stimuli being painful, the green light induces reduced pain reports (placebo analgesic responses) (NRS = numerical rating scale). Placebo analgesia is expressed as the difference between red-associated and green-associated pain reports. (B) In block 0 all the stimuli are painful but the red light anticipates pain while the green light anticipates analgesia. In this condition, no analgesic responses are elicited. Blocks 1 and 2 are the same as in (A). Although this conditioning procedure is identical to that on the left column, the placebo responses in block 3 are dramatically reduced, due to the negative experience of block 0. Reproduced from Luana Colloca and Fabrizio Benedetti, How prior experience shapes placebo analgesia, *Pain*, 124 (1), pp. 126–33 Copyright 2006, The International Association for the Study of Pain, with permission. DOI: http://dx.doi.org/10.1016/j.pain.2006.04.005

Another design worth considering for future trials is the open–hidden paradigm. As described in Chapters 4 and 5, the best evidence for a role of expectation in the therapeutic outcome is the decreased effectiveness of covert therapies. It is possible to eliminate the placebo (psychosocial) component and analyze the pharmacodynamic effects of the treatment, free of any psychological contamination, by making the patient completely unaware that a medical therapy is being carried out. To do this, drugs are administered through hidden infusions by machines (Levine et al., 1981; Gracely et al., 1983; Levine and Gordon, 1984; Amanzio et al., 2001; Benedetti et al., 2003a; Colloca et al., 2004). This approach might have an important impact on the design of clinical trials. In order to overcome the ethical constraints of the hidden administration of a treatment, the experimental design might consist of an unknown temporal sequence of drug administration, in which subjects know that a pharmacological agent will be administered but they do not know "when." If the drug really is effective, pain reduction correlates with the timing of drug administration.

Figure 11.3 shows a totally ineffective drug (metamizole) and an effective drug (buprenorphine) which were tested using this approach (Colloca and Benedetti, 2005). Whereas a straightforward difference between open and hidden administration is present for metamizole (a hidden injection is completely ineffective in reducing pain), a small difference is present for buprenorphine, which indicates that buprenorphine is effective, regardless of whether it is given overtly or covertly. The open–hidden paradigm might serve to decrease the debate on the use of placebos in clinical trials, as no placebo is administered in this paradigm (Price, 2001; Kirsch, 2003). This would provide a good alternative to placebo-controlled trials, therefore keeping within the ethical guidelines of the Declaration of Helsinki.

There are important limitations to the open–hidden paradigm. One of these is its applicability in only some circumstances. For example, to test the outcome following hidden administration of an oral medication is problematic from a methodological point of view—it is not easy to devise a protocol in which a pill is administered covertly. By contrast, intravenous infusions or intrathecal or intraspinal administration of drugs and electrical stimulations of the peripheral or central nervous system are amenable to hidden paradigms. Another limitation is the fact the injected drug should not produce perceptible side effects, otherwise the patient would realize that something is being administered.

Many other designs have been developed (Box 11.2), but the risk of sequence effects, whereby learning may confound the interpretation of the trial, is always lurking around the corner. As shown in Fig. 11.2 in the experiment by Colloca and Benedetti (2006), the previous exposure to either positive or negative treatments may have a dramatic influence on the therapeutic outcome.

11.1.4 The new insights into placebo mechanisms lead to an uncertainty principle

Today, the gold standard in clinical trial designs is the randomized, double-blind, placebo-controlled study with two arms (Kaptchuk, 1998, 2001). One arm of the trial consists of a group of randomized patients who receive the active treatment, whereas

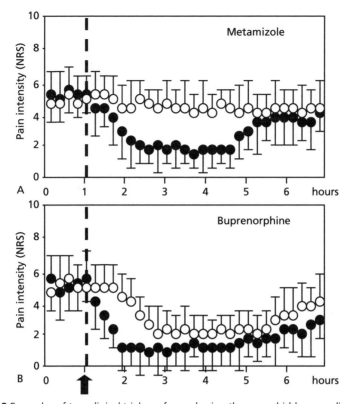

Fig. 11.3 Examples of two clinical trials performed using the open–hidden paradigm, revealing an ineffective and an effective treatment. In a clinical trial of this type, the larger the difference between the open and hidden administration, the larger the placebo component and, therefore, the smaller the effect of the active treatment being investigated. Conversely, the smaller the difference, the greater the specific effects of the treatment. (A) A 300-mg dose of metamizole was tested in ten patients to investigate whether it was effective in relieving post-thymectomy pain. One group of patients received an open injection (black circles) of metamizole combined with the information that the pain would soon subside. The patients in the other group knew that metamizole was going to be administered, but they did not know when (white circles). To do this, a computer-controlled infusion pump was preprogrammed to deliver the drug at the desired time, out of view of the patients. Note that a hidden injection was totally ineffective in reducing pain, thereby indicating that the positive outcome of the open administration was only a placebo effect. (B) A 0.2-mg dose of buprenorphine was tested in 12 patients to investigate whether it was effective in relieving post-thoracoscopy pain. The figure shows that the difference between the open (black circles) and hidden (white circles) conditions was small, thus indicating that buprenorphine was an effective analgesic. Note, however, the slower reduction in pain in the hidden patient group compared to the open one, which indicates that most of the initial benefit in the open group was attributable to a placebo effect. By using this approach, the real pharmacodynamic effect of the drug and the placebo component can be assessed without administration of a placebo. NRS, numerical rating scale. The arrow and the dashed lines show the time of drug administration. Reprinted by permission from Macmillan Publishers Ltd: *Nature Reviews Neuroscience*, 6 (7), Luana Colloca & Fabrizio Benedetti, Placebos and painkillers: is mind as real as matter?, pp. 545–552 Copyright 2005, Nature Publishing Group.

Box 11.2 The sequential parallel comparative design

An example of interesting new approach to clinical trials is represented by the sequential parallel comparative design (SPCD) (Fava et al., 2003). In the first part of the trial, a randomization is performed across patients to either drug or placebo. However, differently from other designs, more than half of patients are assigned to the placebo group. After the first part is finished, placebo responders and nonresponders are identified. The patients who did not respond to placebo are re-randomized to another trial with half receiving the drug and half the placebo (Fig. 11.4). The advantage of this design is that a large amount of patients are maintained in the second part of the trial, thus the statistical power is not lost. SPCD is particularly advantageous in trials that involve subjective outcome measures, such as those of antidepressants and analgesics. By using this design in a trial of major depressive disorder, Fava et al. (2012) were able to reduce the placebo effect from 17% in the first part of the trial to 8% in the second part.

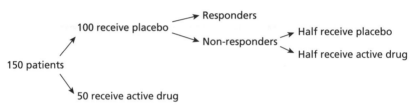

Fig. 11.4 The sequential parallel comparative design.

Another design, the two-way enrichment design (TED), goes a step further and also re-randomizes drug responders between drug and placebo (Ivanova and Tamura, 2011). As emphasized many times throughout this book, these are pragmatic clinical trials whose goal is only to find a difference between drug and placebo. Why some people respond to placebo is not the objective of these experimental designs.

the second arm takes the placebo. This is done according to the double-blind design, in which the patients are told that they could receive either the active treatment or the placebo, with a 50% chance of getting either. In order to conclude that the active treatment is effective, the outcome following its administration must be better than that of the placebo. On the basis of the placebo mechanisms described in this book, two important questions arise: Is this design appropriate for concluding that a therapy is effective? Can the tested drug interfere with all the biochemical mechanisms of the placebo?

In 1995, a clinical trial in postoperative pain was performed by Benedetti et al. (1995). In this study, the cholecystokinin (CCK) antagonist proglumide was better than placebo, and placebo was better than no-treatment for relief of postoperative pain (Fig. 11.5A). According to the methodology used in classical clinical trials, these results indicate that proglumide is a good analgesic that acts on the pain pathways, whereas placebo reduces pain by inducing expectations of analgesia, thus activating expectation pathways (Fig. 11.5A). However, this conclusion proved to be erroneous, as a hidden injection of proglumide was totally ineffective (Fig. 11.5B). Therefore, the likely interpretation of proglumide's mechanism of action is that it does not act on pain pathways at all, but rather on expectation pathways, thus enhancing the placebo analgesic response (Fig. 11.5B; see also section 4.1.6). In other words, proglumide induces a reduction of pain if, and only if, it is associated with a placebo procedure. Now we know that proglumide is not a painkiller, but it acts on placebo-activated opioid mechanisms (section 4.1.6).

This is the best example for showing why we need to understand the neurobiological mechanisms of the placebo response better. Borrowing Heisenberg's uncertainty principle from the field of physics, which imposes limits on the precision of a measurement (Wheeler and Zurek, 1983), we can apply a similar principle to the outcomes of clinical trials. Colloca and Benedetti (2005) noted—as per the uncertainty principle—that a dynamical disturbance is necessarily induced on a system by a measurement, so in clinical trials a dynamical disturbance might be induced on the brain by virtually any kind of drug. The very nature of this disturbance is the interference of the injected drug with the expectation pathways, which affects both the outcome measures and the interpretation of data. Therefore, as with Heisenberg's principle, the disturbance is the cause of the uncertainty. For example, a pharmacological analgesic agent has its own specific pharmacodynamic effect on pain pathways, but interference with the mechanisms of top-down control of pain might occur (Fig. 11.5C). We have no a priori knowledge about which substances act on pain pathways and which act on expectation mechanisms. Indeed, virtually all drugs might interfere with the top-down mechanisms, thus this uncertainty cannot be solved with the standard clinical trial design. The only way to partially resolve this problem is to make the expectation pathways, so to speak, silent. To do this, the treatment has to be given covertly (unexpectedly) so that the subject does not have any expectations (see section 4.1.4). In this way, a drug may be really given, at least in part, in a vacuum, free of any psychologically induced activation of biochemical pathways.

Therefore, several social stimuli within the context around the treatment can activate neurotransmitters and modulators that bind to the same receptors to which drugs bind, and these can trigger biochemical pathways that are similar to those activated by pharmacological agents. A summary of the receptor and biochemical pathways involved in these psychosocial responses is shown in Fig. 11.6. On the basis of the experimental evidence presented throughout this book, we now know that whenever a medical treatment is carried out, a complex biochemical matrix is activated by several social stimuli. This biochemical cascade of events inevitably interferes with any drug that is given. In other words, drugs are not administered in a vacuum, but rather in a complex biochemical environment which varies according to the patient's cognitive/affective state and to previous exposure to other pharmacological agents (conditioning). Fig. 11.6 shows that any drug, which will eventually be given for a specific condition, may act on a set of receptors that might have been modified by the therapeutic context. It appears clear that if we want to test

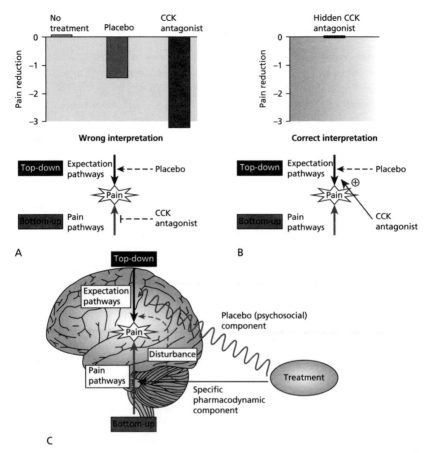

Fig. 11.5 An emerging uncertainty principle imposes limitations on our understanding of the effects of a therapeutic agent. (A) A clinical trial with three arms shows that a placebo is better than no treatment and that the cholecystokinin (CCK) antagonist, proglumide, is better than a placebo in relieving pain. According to the interpretation of a classical clinical trial, this leads to the erroneous belief that the CCK antagonist acts specifically on pain pathways (the bottom-up action) whereas the placebo acts on expectation pathways (the top-down control). (B) The interpretation in (A) is incorrect because if the same CCK antagonist is given by hidden injection, so that the patient is completely unaware that a drug is being administered and thus has no expectations, the drug is completely ineffective. As the drug has analgesic effects only in association with a placebo procedure, its action is not directed specifically to the pain pathways, but rather to the expectation pathways, which enhances the placebo analgesic response. (C) Any analgesic treatment consists of two components—the specific pharmacodynamic component and the placebo component. The latter is induced by the psychosocial context in which the treatment is given and elicits expectations of improvement. The uncertainty principle in a clinical trial is represented by the fact that a drug might act on expectation pathways (broken arrows) rather than pain pathways, which makes it extremely difficult to conclude whether or not a pharmacological substance is a real painkiller. The only way in which this uncertainty can be partially resolved, and the real pharmacodynamic effect of a painkiller established, is through the elimination of the placebo component, and, therefore, of the expectation

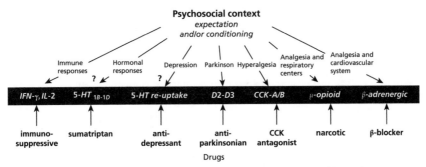

Fig. 11.6 The psychosocial context surrounding the therapy activates (through expectation and/or conditioning mechanisms) a number of biochemical/receptor pathways in different diseases and therapeutic interventions; the involvement of serotonin (5-HT) receptors in hormonal responses and depression is not definitive. These receptors are the same to which different drugs bind, thus indicating that cognitive and affective factors are capable of modulating the action of drugs. This interference between psychosocial context and drug action has profound implications for our understanding of drug action—when a drug is given, the very act of administering it (the psychosocial context) may perturb the system and change the response to the drug. CCK, cholecystokinin; 5-HT, 5-hydroxytryptamine; IL, interleukin; IFN, interferon. Reproduced from Fabrizio Benedetti, Mechanisms of placebo and placebo-related effects across diseases and treatments, *Annual Review of Pharmacology and Toxicology*, 48, pp. 33–60 Copyright 2008, Annual Reviews.

a new drug for relieving pain, the act of its administration may interfere with its real pharmacodynamic effects. Negative expectations may, for example, activate CCK-ergic systems (see section 4.2.3) or, conversely, positive expectations may activate opioid receptors (see section 4.1.6) and thus may modify the overall action of the drug under test.

On the basis of all these issues, complex cognitive/affective factors are capable of modulating the action of drugs through activation of the very same receptors to which drugs bind. Therefore, a drug that is tested according to the classical methodology of clinical trials can (paradoxically) be better than a placebo—even though it has no analgesic properties (Fig. 11.5). This should be taken into account whenever a new treatment is tested, because the very act of its administration may interfere with its real pharmacodynamic effects.

Fig. 11.5 (continued) pathways, by hidden treatments. Reprinted by permission from Macmillan Publishers Ltd: *Nature Reviews Neuroscience*, 6 (7), Luana Colloca & Fabrizio Benedetti, Placebos and painkillers: is mind as real as matter?, pp. 545–552 Copyright 2005, Nature Publishing Group. Data in (A) and (B) from Benedetti F, Amanzio M and Maggi G, Potentiation of placebo analgesia by proglumide, *Lancet*, 346, page 1231. (See Plate 14.)

11.2 **Harnessing placebo and placebo-related effects in the clinic**

11.2.1 **Drug-like effects can be obtained without drugs**

The debate on the use of placebos in medical practice is as important as that about their use in the clinical trial setting. The same arguments for and against the use of placebos can be applied to routine clinical practice as well, with the notable exception of deception. In fact, while no deception is present in the classical clinical trial, it is a necessary condition in routine medical practice. In this regard, an influential paper was published in the 1970s by Bok (1974). On the one hand, the administration of a placebo is seen as unethical as it necessarily involves some degree of deception, thus damaging the institution of medicine and contributing to the erosion of confidence and trust in medical staff and caregivers (see also Bok, 2002). On the other hand, the use of deception can sometimes be justified by invoking the concepts of both paternalism and benevolent deception, whereby the physician's purpose is not actually to deceive but to cure (Rawlinson, 1985). Sometimes the effect of illness is an undermining of the patient's autonomy, so that the physician must restore this loss, even through the use of benevolent paternalism and deception. However, if benevolent deception is applied to routine medical practice some rules are required, for example, it should never be employed for the convenience of the caregiver, it should only be used in cases where there is substantial evidence that it is necessary, and the doctor should determine whether any physical or psychological condition for which other treatments are indicated would be masked by the placebo itself (Rawlinson, 1985).

Price and collaborators (Vase et al., 2003; Verne et al., 2003) conducted a series of studies in which they tried to enhance placebo analgesia in patients suffering from irritable bowel syndrome. They found a potentiation of the placebo analgesic response when a placebo was given along with the verbal instructions: "The agent you have just been given is known to significantly reduce pain in some patients." There are at least two interesting aspects in these findings. First, no deception was present in this case, as indeed a placebo is known to reduce pain in some subjects. Second, these suggestions were enough to increase placebo analgesia to a magnitude that matched that of an active agent (in this case, rectal lidocaine) (Fig. 4.2A,B).

The ethical argument in favor of the use of placebos and deceptions in routine medical practice is strengthened by some studies that show the real positive effects of placebos in some circumstances. For example, we have seen (section 4.1.2) a reduction of narcotic intake for postoperative pain of about 30% obtained by simultaneous administration of saline solution that was deceptively stated to be a painkiller (Pollo et al. 2001). Likewise, we saw in section 4.2.1 (Fig. 4.12) that the hidden interruption of a narcotic in the postoperative phase prolonged the relapse of pain compared with an open interruption (Benedetti et al. 2003a). There are examples in fields other than pain. In section 7.2.2, a clinical case of a child with lupus was described, in whom a clinically successful outcome was achieved by providing only the conditioned stimuli on half the monthly chemotherapy sessions (Olness and Ader, 1992). Additional studies are certainly justified in this case, as the toxic effects of Cytoxan® are severe, and a placebo substitution therapy would reduce its intake.

Another example of placebo substitution therapy is given by a study performed in the 1960s in schizophrenic patients (Greenberg and Roth, 1966). Investigators reduced the amount of tranquillizers given to hospitalized schizophrenics on a daily basis, by replacing the amount of chlorpromazine with a placebo on 1 day of each week. There were no adverse effects in this study, so a regimen of drug on 5 days and placebo on 2 days was introduced, and one additional "placebo day" was added every 8 weeks. This gradual reduction of drug intake led to chlorpromazine being given only two to three times per week. Although there are a few studies of this kind, the question is: Should we abandon these therapeutic protocols that involve either deception or lack of information, even though they are beneficial to the patient?

For example, Fig. 11.7 shows data from the study by Pollo et al. (2001). If patients were treated with buprenorphine on request and, at the same time, a basal infusion of

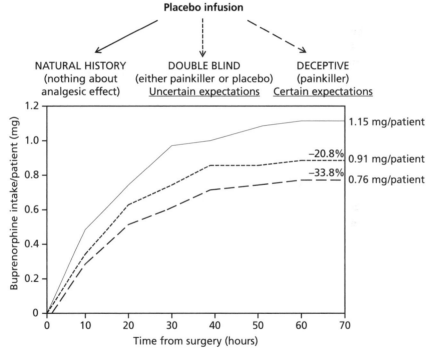

Fig. 11.7 Postoperative pain is treated with buprenorphine on request by patients in combination with a basal infusion of placebo (saline solution). However, the symbolic meaning of this saline basal infusion is changed in different groups of patients. In the natural history condition (solid lines), nothing is told about placebo; in the double-blind condition (dotted lines) patients are told it could be either a painkiller or a placebo; in the deceptive condition (dashed lines) patients are told it is a painkiller. Analgesia is represented by buprenorphine consumption. Patients who are given the saline solution deceptively ("It is a painkiller") show the lowest intake of buprenorphine. Reproduced from Pollo A., Amanzio M., Arslanian A., Casadio C., Maggi G. and Benedetti F., Response expectancies in placebo analgesia and their clinical relevance, Pain, 93, pp. 77–84 Copyright 2001, International Association for the Study of Pain.

saline solution was administered with different verbal instructions, then different outcomes were obtained. If nothing was said about analgesic effects (in the natural history or no-treatment group) the cumulative consumption of buprenorphine over a period of 3 days was 1.15 mg per patient. If the patients were told the infusion could be either a potent analgesic or a placebo (classic double-blind administration) the cumulative consumption of the narcotic dropped to 0.91 mg per patient; and if they were told it was a potent painkiller (deceptive administration) there was a further drop to 0.76 mg per patient (see also section 4.1.2). Despite these differences in doses, the time-course of pain was the same in all three groups over the 3-day period of treatment. In light of these results, the ethical debate on using placebos in clinical practice seems to be trivial, as in the study by Pollo et al. (2001) a dramatic reduction of narcotics was obtained by using deception.

Besides the possible additive effects of placebos and drugs that allow reduction of drug intake, one of the most practical implications of recent neurobiological advances in placebo research is the possibility to induce, at least in some circumstances, drug-like effects without the administration of drugs. Throughout this book we have seen that placebos can induce activation of endogenous opioids and dopamine, that placebo-conditioned responses of several immune mediators can be obtained through behavioral conditioning, and that nocebos activate the endogenous CCK-ergic systems. The obvious consequence of these findings is their exploitation both in the clinic and in other aspects of society, although important ethical constraints have so far limited the development of therapeutic paradigms with placebos.

It is conceivable today that many experimental protocols, so far carried out in animals and healthy volunteers, could be applied to real medical conditions. For example, there is compelling evidence that pharmacological conditioning can induce powerful placebo responses when the real drug is replaced with a placebo (Doering and Rief, 2012). This phenomenon is well documented in humans, for example, in pain (Amanzio and Benedetti, 1999), the immune (Goebel et al., 2002), endocrine, and motor systems (Benedetti et al., 2003b), although unfortunately no systematic investigation has been done in a real clinical setting. There are, however, some indications that application of placebo-induced drug-like effects without drugs is possible in the clinic. For example, Benedetti et al. (2004) conditioned Parkinson patients with repeated administrations of the anti-Parkinson drug, apomorphine, before the surgical implantation of electrodes for deep-brain stimulation (see also section 5.1.6). Apomorphine was then replaced with a placebo in the operating room; a powerful placebo reduction of muscle rigidity that mimicked the effects of apomorphine during the previous days was obtained. Although the effect was short-lasting (no longer than 20–30 minutes) it was useful from a clinical point of view because the patient improved and felt better for a while, thus making some surgical procedures easier and faster. These drug-mimicking effects could be particularly useful whenever a drug has important side effects. For example, Benedetti et al. (2004) found that presurgical apomorphine administration resulted in both clinical improvement and some side effects, like dyskinesia, whereas the placebo in the operating room induced improvement but not dyskinesia.

Outside the clinical setting, the practical implications of getting drug-like effects without drugs has been shown in sports medicine (section 13.1). Benedetti et al. (2007)

gave placebos in an experimental simulation of a sporting event. After repeated administrations of morphine in the training phase and replacement with a placebo on the day of the competition, an opioid-mediated increase in pain endurance and physical performance was induced even though no illegal drug was administered. This shows that athletes can be preconditioned with narcotics and then given a placebo just before the competition, thus avoiding administration of illegal drugs on the competition day. The ethical implications of placebo doping outside the clinic are discussed in section 13.1.2.

11.2.2 When doctors should treat their patients with placebos

There is widespread use of placebos in routine medical practice (see section 1.2.3). The main difference between the use of placebos in clinical trials and in clinical practice is that, according to the classical clinical trial methodology, patients know that they can receive either a placebo or an active treatment, thus there is no deception. In contrast, in routine medical practice, placebos are given deceptively. In fact, in clinics, wards, and doctor's offices, patients receive inert substances that they are told are real medications. Is this ethically acceptable? If so, when should doctors use placebos deceptively?

The answer is not very simple. The following case illustrates malpractice (Benedetti, 2004; Paice, 2004; Sullivan, 2004). A 52-year-old woman with a long history of chronic low back pain treated over time with various medications, including recent opioids, went to the emergency room for excruciating and paralyzing back pain. The doctor on duty working her up found that she just ran out of the pain medications she was previously on. She requested an intravenous painkiller for her pain, to which the doctor agreed verbally. However, instead of injecting the painkiller, he gave her intravenous placebo to see if it will work. Is this treatment acceptable?

To accept a placebo treatment in this situation would mean to be ready to accept a placebo trial before a medical intervention of any kind. In this case, there is no obvious justification for the use of a placebo and, indeed, its acceptance would lead to a dangerous generalization. In other words, the acceptance of this placebo intervention would lead to the generalization that a first attempt with a placebo is always acceptable and justified. There are many reasons why a placebo should not be given in this case. First, there is a total deception, as the woman requested a painkiller, and the doctor agreed, but then actually injected a placebo. It goes without saying that this is against any ethical principle. Even accepting the use of benevolent deception in routine medical practice (Rawlinson, 1985), some rules are necessary. For example, a placebo should never be employed for the convenience of a caregiver and it should only be used in cases where there is substantial evidence that it is necessary. Furthermore, the doctor should determine whether any physical or psychological condition for which other treatments are indicated would be masked by the placebo itself (Rawlinson, 1985). In this case, the doctor did not have any substantial evidence that a placebo was necessary; in fact, his diagnosis was that the woman just ran out of the pain medications she had been on previously. Therefore, the natural choice of the doctor should have been to reintroduce the interrupted therapy. In other words, taking both alternatives into consideration in this case (active drug versus placebo), the interrupted active treatment should have been considered the best choice with the highest likelihood of success (Benedetti, 2004).

In a different case, a physician decided to discontinue an opioid therapy in a 14-year-old boy complaining of intense headache, and in particular to replace morphine with a placebo (Rich, 2003). Although his rationale for switching from morphine to placebo was both a concern about addiction and the negative interactions of narcotics with other drugs, he informed neither the boy nor the mother. The outcome was positive and, indeed, the pain subsided and the boy was discharged from the hospital. This represents a good example of both efficacy of placebo therapy and its use to reduce the intake of narcotics. Nonetheless, the patient's mother discovered the deceptive use of the placebo and sued the doctor and three nurses for professional misconduct. Therefore, even though a positive outcome was obtained, when the boy's mother learned of the placebo, she was irate, and contacted a national patient advocacy organization claiming undertreated pain for his son. The ethical lesson of this case is that, even when doctors use placebos for a good reason and obtain good results, if patients and/or relatives discover the deception, this may damage the institution of medicine and may contribute to the erosion of trust in the medical personnel.

Such examples show it is not easy to find a general rule for use of placebos in clinical practice (Rich, 2003; Lichtenberg et al., 2004; Sullivan et al., 2005). As emphasized many times throughout the book (e.g., in section 11.2.1) perhaps the best evidence that placebos are ethically acceptable and justified in medical practice is the possibility of reducing the intake of toxic and dangerous drugs. It seems that all the uncertainties about the use of placebo in medical practice reflect our ignorance about a phenomenon that today is passing from the status of nuisance in clinical research to a target of scientific inquiry. As described in this book, there has been substantial progress in the neurobiological understanding of placebo and placebo-related effects in recent years. Following on from these new discoveries, our efforts should be directed towards developing new therapeutic protocols that exploit these mechanisms. Within the context of this new knowledge, we should be better able to approach the ethics of placebo administration. Therefore, fuller understanding of the placebo phenomenon across all medical conditions is necessary and essential, because it is likely to lead to new ways of thinking about therapies as well as to new ethical rules.

11.2.3 Patients with prefrontal impairment need larger doses of analgesics

In section 6.3.2, we can see that disruption of the prefrontal executive functions in people with Alzheimer's disease may affect placebo responsiveness. In fact, Benedetti et al. (2006) found that the magnitude of the placebo effect, as assessed by measuring the difference between open and hidden administration of an analgesic, was substantially reduced in Alzheimer's disease. This is in line with the involvement of frontal regions in placebo analgesia, such as the dorsolateral prefrontal cortex, which represents an important component of executive control (Wager et al., 2004; Zubieta et al., 2005). The loss or reduction of placebo responsiveness may have profound implications in routine clinical practice. In fact, in the same study by Benedetti et al. (2006) it was shown that a larger dose of analgesic could compensate for the loss of placebo and expectation mechanisms. By doubling the dose of the local anesthetic, lidocaine, from 1% to

2% to reduce post-venipuncture burning pain, no difference was found between open and hidden administrations, which indicates increased efficacy of hidden lidocaine at a dose of 2%. This may lead to the conclusion that probably some therapies need to be revised, if we take into consideration these findings. In other words, patients with pre-frontal impairment would need to be treated with higher doses of analgesics in order to compensate for the loss of the placebo effect. The study by Benedetti et al. (2006) is the first study to show disruption of placebo mechanisms in a clinical condition. It represents a natural situation in which a treatment is performed covertly. In fact, demented patients do not realize a therapy is being performed, so they do not expect anything, hence the psychological component of the therapy is lost.

The disruption of cognitive functions, such as prefrontal executive control, and the relation to decreased analgesic efficacy of some therapeutic interventions has profound implications that certainly need further investigation. In fact, epidemiological studies show that the number of people aged over 65 will increase substantially in the next decades all over the world, and that a considerable proportion of this population will develop dementia (Skoog, 2004) (see also Box 6.3). There is also ample evidence that ageing is associated with a high rate of painful conditions (Horgas and Elliott, 2004), thus the number of patients with dementia who will experience painful conditions is likely to increase. The implications are even greater if we consider that (as indicated in several studies) pain is undertreated in cognitively impaired elderly people. Fewer analgesics are prescribed for the oldest category of cancer patients (above 75 years) than for younger patients, and low cognitive performance is one of the predictors of this finding (Bernabei et al., 1998). Moreover, patients in advanced stages of dementia with hip fractures have been found to receive significantly less opioid analgesics than those who are cognitively intact (Morrison and Siu, 2000). These observations stress the importance of increasing our knowledge of the relationship between cognitive functioning, placebo responsiveness, and pain, and other symptoms as well.

11.2.4 **There is a danger around the corner**

Since the very ritual of the therapeutic act can change the patient's brain, anybody who performs a ritual can affect the physiology of the patient's brain and obtain positive effects. In the same way that a syringe filled with distilled water and handled by a doctor may induce expectations of benefit, the same expectations can be induced by talismans and eccentric rituals carried out by quacks and shamans. There is today a growing tendency to refer to the effects of placebos as real biological phenomena that need to be triggered and enhanced by a variety of odd, weird, and bizarre procedures. By exploring the Web, it is possible to find many websites that have taken the biological effects of placebos as a sort of justification for bizarre therapeutic rituals. Many claim that there is no difference between sugar pills and talismans if one wants to obtain positive responses, and it makes no difference if deception comes from a doctor or a quack or a shaman. According to this worrisome view, any healer would be justified to stimulate the release of endogenous chemicals by enhancing the patient's expectations. In this sense, science risks being exploited in the wrong way and, paradoxically, the neurobiological advances of placebo research can turn into a regression of medicine to past times, when the eccentricity and oddity of the therapies were the rule. It is crucial that we find a better way to communicate placebo research. This is not an easy task, for scientific advances will inevitably go against ethical concerns as we will learn more and more about the biology of a vulnerable aspect of mankind. The study of the biology of foibles and vulnerable aspects of mankind may unravel new mechanisms of how our brain works, but it may have a profound negative impact on our society as well. In particular, we need to better understand the ethical limits to increase expectations, as well as what to do if a patient trusts talismans more than pills and injections. In this way, we will avoid a worrisome future for medicine (Benedetti, 2012, 2014).

11.3 **Points for further discussion**

1 The ethics and methodology of clinical trials represent an important issue today that is the subject of lively debate. We should strive to develop new designs for validating new treatments, and these designs must be respectful of both ethical rules and rigorous scientific method.

2 The close interaction between the act of administering a drug (the psychosocial context) and the action of the drug itself needs to be disentangled. A better understanding of the expectation biochemical pathways and of the specific effects of pharmacological agents is in order.

3 The core concept of this book, that drug-like effects can be obtained without drugs, must be applied to a variety of clinical situations. Today we should start conceiving treatments in which placebos and drugs are given alternatively, so as to reduce the intake of drugs.

4 According to Barrett et al. (2006) there are several clinical actions that the physician must adopt in order to enhance placebo and placebo-related effects, such as speaking positively, giving encouragement, and providing reassurance, and so forth. Therefore, do we need to better educate physicians and nurses?

5 What are the rules regarding placebo administration in medical practice? Can a placebo be given as a therapy? Can it be given for diagnostic purposes?

6 Exploring clinical conditions with impaired prefrontal executive control may lead to re-elaboration of many therapies. In particular, when the expectation/placebo component is impaired, should we increase therapeutic doses in order to compensate for the loss of placebo mechanisms?

7 Good communication of placebo research is crucial and a good interaction between scientists, ethicists, and journalists is fundamental in order to avoid that quacks justify their practices by invoking the placebo effect.

References

Amanzio M and Benedetti F (1999). Neuropharmacological dissection of placebo analgesia: expectation-activated opioid systems versus conditioning-activated specific subsystems. *Journal of Neuroscience*, **19**, 484–94.

Amanzio M, Pollo A, Maggi G and Benedetti F (2001). Response variability to analgesics: a role for non-specific activation of endogenous opioids. *Pain*, **90**, 205–15.

American Psychological Association (1992). Ethical principles of psychologists and code of conduct. *American Psychologist*, **47**, 1597–611.

Barrett B, Muller D, Rakel D, Rabago D, Marchand L and Scheder J (2006). Placebo, meaning, and health. *Perspectives in Biology and Medicine*, **49**, 178–98.

Benedetti F (2004). Placebos and treatment of pain. *Pain Medicine*, **5**, 327–8.

Benedetti F (2012). The placebo response: science versus ethics and the vulnerability of the patient. *World Psychiatry*, **11**, 70–2.

Benedetti F (2014). Drugs and placebos: what is the difference?: understanding the molecular basis of the placebo effect could help clinicians to better use it in clinical practice. *EMBO Reports*, 17 March. [Epub ahead of print]

Benedetti F, Amanzio M and Maggi G (1995). Potentiation of placebo analgesia by proglumide. *Lancet*, **346**, 1231.

Benedetti F, Arduino C, Costa S et al. (2006). Loss of expectation-related mechanisms in Alzheimer's disease makes analgesic therapies less effective. *Pain* **121**, 133–44.

Benedetti F, Colloca L, Torre E et al. (2004). Placebo-responsive Parkinson patients show decreased activity in single neurons of subthalamic nucleus. *Nature Neuroscience*, **7**, 587–8.

Benedetti F, Maggi G, Lopiano L et al. (2003a). Open versus hidden medical treatments: the patient's knowledge about a therapy affects the therapy outcome. *Prevention & Treatment*, **6**(1).

Benedetti F, Pollo A and Colloca L (2007). Opioid-mediated placebo responses boost pain endurance and physical performance: is it doping in sport competitions. *Journal of Neuroscience*, **27**, 11934–9.

Benedetti F, Pollo A, Lopiano L et al. (2003b). Conscious expectation and unconscious conditioning in analgesic; motor and hormonal placebo/nocebo responses. *Journal of Neuroscience*, **23**, 4315–23.

Bernabei R, Gambassi G, Lapane K et al. (1998). Management of pain in elderly patients with cancer. *Journal of the American Medical Association*, **279**, 1877–82.

Bok S (1974). The ethics of giving placebos. *Scientific American*, **231**, 17–23.

Bok S (2002). Ethical issues in use of placebo in medical practise and clinical trials. In HA Guess, A Kleinman, JW Kusek and LW Engel, eds. *The science of the placebo: toward an interdisciplinary research agenda*, pp. 63–73. BMJ Books, London.

Boyle K and Batzer FR (2007). Is a placebo-controlled surgical trial an oxymoron? *Journal of Minimally Invasive Gynecology*, **14**, 278–83.

Brody H and Colloca L (2013). Patient autonomy and provider beneficence are compatible. *Hastings Center Report*, **43**, 6.

Brody H, Colloca L and Miller FG (2012). The placebo phenomenon: implications for the ethics of shared decision-making. *Journal of General Internal Medicine*, **27**, 739–42.

Califf RM, Al-Khatib SM (2002). Use of placebo in large-scale, pragmatic trials. In HA Guess, A Kleinman, JW Kusek and LW Engel, eds. *The science of the placebo: toward an interdisciplinary research agenda*, pp. 249–63. BMJ Books, London.

Caspi O (2002). When are placebo medication side effects due to the placebo phenomenon? *Journal of American Medical Association*, **287**, 2502.

Cobb LA, Thomas GI, Dillard DH, Merendino KA and Bruce RA (1959). An evaluation of internal mammary artery ligation by double blind technique. *New England Journal of Medicine*, **260**, 1115–18.

Colloca L and Benedetti F (2005). Placebos and painkillers: is mind as real as matter? *Nature Reviews Neuroscience*, **6**, 545–52.

Colloca L and Benedetti F (2006). How prior experience shapes placebo analgesia. *Pain*, **124**, 126–33.

Colloca L, Lopiano L, Lanotte M and Benedetti F (2004). Overt versus covert treatment for pain, anxiety and Parkinson's disease *Lancet Neurology*, **3**, 679–84.

Committee for Proprietary Medicinal Products (1998). *Note for guidance on the clinical investigation of medicinal products in the treatment of schizophrenia*. Committee for Proprietary Medicinal Products, London.

Council for International Organizations of Medical Sciences and World health Organization (1993). *International ethical guidelines for biomedical research involving human subjects*. CIOMS, Geneva.

Council on Ethical and Judicial Affairs of the American Medical Association (1996). Ethical use of placebo controls in clinical trials. *Proceedings of the House of Delegates of the American Medical Association*, **23–27 June**, 252–9.

Dimond EG, Kittle CF and Crockett JE (1958). Evaluation of internal mammary ligation and sham procedure in angina pectoris. *Circulation*, **18**, 712–13.

Doering BK and Rief W (2012). Utilizing placebo mechanisms for dose reduction in pharmacotherapy. *Trends in Pharmacological Sciences*, **33**, 165–72.

Fava M, Evins AE, Dorer DJ and Schoenfeld DA (2003). The problem of the placebo response in clinical trials for psychiatric disorders: culprits, possible remedies, and a novel study design approach. *Psychotherapy and Psychosomatics*, **72**, 115–27.

Fava M, Mischoulon D, Iosifescu D *et al.* (2012). A double-blind, placebo-controlled study of aripiprazole adjunctive to antidepressant therapy among depressed outpatients with inadequate response to prior antidepressant therapy (ADAPT-A Study). *Psychotherapy and Psychosomatics*, **81**, 87–97.

Goebel MU, Trebst AE, Steiner J *et al.* (2002). Behavioral conditioning of immunosuppression is possible in humans. *FASEB Journal*, **16**, 1869–73.

Gracely RH, Dubner R, Wolskee PJ and Deeter WR (1983). Placebo and naloxone can alter postsurgical pain by separate mechanisms. *Nature*, **306**, 264–5.

Greenberg LM and Roth S (1966). Differential effects of abrupt versus gradual withdrawal of chlorpromazine in hospitalized chronic schizophrenic patients. *American Journal of Psychiatry*, **123**, 221–6.

Guess HA, Kleinman A, Kusek JW and Engel LW, eds (2002). *The science of the placebo: toward an interdisciplinary research agenda*. BMJ Books, London.

Horgas AL and Elliott AF (2004). Pain assessment and management in persons with dementia. *Nursing Clinic of North America*, **39**, 593–606.

Horng SH and Miller FG (2007). Placebo-controlled procedural trails for neurological conditions. *Neurotherapeutics*, **4**, 531–6.

Ivanova A and Tamura RN (2011). A two-way enriched clinical trial design: combining advantages of placebo lead-in and randomized withdrawal. *Statistical Methods in Medical Research*, 4 December. [Epub ahead of print]

Kaptchuk TJ (1998). Powerful placebo: the dark side of the randomized controlled trial. *Lancet*, **351**, 1722–5.

Kaptchuk TJ (2001). The double-blind, randomized, placebo-controlled trial: gold standard or golden calf? *Journal of Clinical Epidemiology*, **54**, 541–9.

Kirsch I (2003). Hidden administration as ethical alternative to the balanced placebo design. *Prevention & Treatment*, **6**(1).

Koshi EB and Short CA (2007). Placebo theory and its implications for research and clinical practice: a review of the recent literature. *Pain Practice*, **7**, 4–20.

Lang AE, Gill S, Patel NK *et al.* (2006). Randomized controlled trial of intraputamenal glial cell line-derived neurotrophic factor infusion in Parkinson disease. *Annals of Neurology*, **59**, 459–66.

Levine RJ (2002). Placebo controls in clinical trials of new therapies for conditions for which there are known effective treatments. In HA Guess, A Kleinman, JW Kusek and LW Engel, eds. *The science of the placebo: toward an interdisciplinary research agenda*, pp. 264–80. BMJ Books, London.

Levine JD and Gordon NC (1984). Influence of the method of drug administration on analgesic response. *Nature*, **312**, 755–6.

Levine JD, Gordon NC, Smith R and Fields HL (1981). Analgesic responses to morphine and placebo in individuals with postoperative pain. *Pain*, **10**, 379–89.

Lichtenberg P, Heresco-Levy U and Nitzan U (2004). The ethics of the placebo in clinical practice. *Journal of Medical Ethics*, **30**, 551–4.

Marchand S, Kupers RC, Bushnell MC and Duncan GH (2003). Analgesic and placebo effects of thalamic stimulation. *Pain*, **105**, 481–8.

McRae C, Cherin E, Yamazaki G *et al.* (2004). Effects of perceived treatment on quality of life and medical outcomes in a double-blind placebo surgery trial. *Archives of General Psychiatry*, **61**, 412–20.

Mercado R, Constantoyannis C, Mandat T *et al.* (2006). Expectation and the placebo effect in Parkinson's disease patients with subthalamic nucleus deep brain stimulation. *Movement Disorders*, **21**, 1457–61.

Michels KB and Rothman KJ (2003). Update on unethical use of placebos in randomised trials. *Bioethics*, **17**, 188–204.

Miller FG and Colloca L (2011). The placebo phenomenon and medical ethics: rethinking the relationship between informed consent and risk-benefit assessment. *Theoretical Medicine and Bioethics*, **32**, 229–43.

Miller FG, Wendler D and Swartzman LC (2005). Deception in research on the placebo effect. *PLoS Medicine*, **2**, e262.

Morrison RS and Siu AL (2000). A comparison of pain and its treatment in advanced dementia and cognitively intact patients with a hip fracture. *Journal of Pain Symptom Management*, **19**, 240–8.

Moseley JB, O'Malley K, Petersen NJ *et al.* (2002). A controlled trial of arthroscopic surgery for osteoarthritis of the knee. *New England Journal of Medicine*, **347**, 81–8.

Nutt JG, Burchiel KJ, Comella CL *et al.* (2003). Randomized, double-blind trial of glial cell line-derived neurotrophic factor (GDNF) in PD. *Neurology*, **60**, 69–73.

Olness K and Ader R (1992). Conditioning as an adjunct in the pharmacotherapy of lupus erythematosus. *Journal of Developmental and Behavioral Pediatrics*, **13**, 124–5.

Paice JA (2004). Placebos and treatment of pain. *Pain Medicine*, **5**, 326.

Pocock SJ (2002). The pros and cons of non-inferiority (equivalence) trials. In HA Guess, A Kleinman, JW Kusek and LW Engel, eds. *The science of the placebo: toward an interdisciplinary research agenda*, pp. 236–48. BMJ Books, London.

Polgar S and Ng J (2005). Ethics, methodology and the use of placebo controls in surgical trials. *Brain Research Bulletin*, **67**, 290–7.

Pollo A, Amanzio M, Arslanian A, Casadio C, Maggi G and Benedetti F (2001). Response expectancies in placebo analgesia and their clinical relevance. *Pain*, **93**, 77–84.

Pollo A, Torre E, Lopiano L *et al.* (2002). Expectation modulates the response to subthalamic nucleus stimulation in Parkinsonian patients. *NeuroReport*, **13**, 1383–6.

Price DD (2001). Assessing placebo effects without placebo groups: an untapped possibility? *Pain*, **90**, 201–3.

Price DD (2005). New facts and improved ethical guidelines for placebo analgesia. *Journal of Pain*, **6**, 213–14.

Rawlinson MC (1985). Truth-telling and paternalism in the clinic: philosophical reflection on the use of placebo in medical practice. In L White, B Tursky and GE Schwartz, eds. *Placebo: theory, research, and mechanisms*, pp. 403–16. Guilford Press, New York.

Rich BA (2003). A placebo for the pain: a medico-legal case analysis. *Pain Medicine*, **4**, 366–72.

Rosseland LA, Helgesen KG, Breivik H and Stubhaug A (2004). Moderate-to-severe pain after knee arthroscopy is relieved by intraarticular saline: a randomized controlled trial. *Anesthesia and Analgesia*, **98**, 1546–51.

Rothman KJ and Michels KB (1994). The continuing unethical use of placebo controls. *New England Journal of Medicine*, **15**, 19–38.

Rothman KJ and Michels KB (2002). When is it appropriate to use a placebo arm in a trial? In HA Guess, A Kleinman, JW Kusek and LW Engel, eds. *The science of the placebo: toward an interdisciplinary research agenda*, pp. 227–35. BMJ Books, London.

Skoog I (2004). Psychiatric epidemiology of old age: the H70 study—the NAPE Lecture 2003. *Acta Psychiatrica Scandinavica*, **109**, 4–18.

Streiner DL (1999). Placebo-controlled trials: when are they needed? *Schizophrenia Research*, **35**, 201–10.

Sullivan M (2004). Placebos and treatment of pain. *Pain Medicine*, **5**, 325–6.

Sullivan M, Terman GW, Peck B *et al.* (2005). APS position statement on the use of placebos in pain management. *Journal of Pain*, **6**, 215–17.

Temple RJ (2002). Placebo controlled trials and active controlled trials: ethics and inference. In HA Guess, A Kleinman, JW Kusek and LW Engel, eds. *The science of the placebo: toward an interdisciplinary research agenda*, pp. 209–26. BMJ Books, London.

Vase L, Robinson ME, Verne GN and Price DD (2003). The contributions of suggestion, expectancy and desire to placebo effect in irritable bowel syndrome patients. *Pain*, **105**, 17–25.

Verne GN, Robinson ME, Vase L and Price DD (2003). Reversal of visceral and cutaneous hyperalgesia by local rectal anesthesia in irritable bowel syndrome (IBS) patients. *Pain*, **105**, 223–30.

Wager TD, Rilling, JK, Smith EE *et al.* (2004). Placebo-induced changes in fMRI in the anticipation and experience of pain. *Science*, **303**, 1162–6.

Weijer C (1999). Placebo-controlled trials in schizophrenia: are they ethical? Are they necessary? *Schizophrenia Research*, **35**, 211–8.

Wendler D and Miller FG (2004). Deception in the pursuit of science. *Archives of Internal Medicine*, **164**, 597–600.

Wheeler JA and Zurek H, eds (1983). *Quantum theory and measurement*. Princeton University Press, Princeton, NJ.

World Medical Association (2000). Declaration of Helsinki. Amended by the 52nd WMA General Assembly, Edinburgh, Scotland, October 2000. *Journal of American Medical Association*, **284**, 3043–5.

World Medical Association (2002). *Declaration of Helsinki. Note of clarification on Paragraph 29*. Word Medical Association, Washington, DC. Available at: <http://www.wma.net/e/home.html>.

Wyatt RJ (1991). Neuroleptics and the natural course of schizophrenia. *Schizophrenia Bulletin*, **17**, 325–51.

Zipursky RB and Darby P (1999). Placebo-controlled studies in schizophrenia—ethical and scientific perspectives: an overview of conference proceedings. *Schizophrenia Research*, **35**, 189–200.

Zubieta JK, Bueller JA, Jackson LR *et al.* (2005). Placebo effects mediated by endogenous opioid activity on μ-opioid receptors. *Journal of Neuroscience*, **25**, 7754–62.

Chapter 12

How to run a placebo study: a closer look into complex experimental designs

Summary points

- To study a placebo effect requires specific designs that cannot be performed in the classic clinical trial setting. Complex experimental designs are particularly necessary when one wants to investigate the neurobiological mechanisms, for example, by means of agonist and antagonist drugs.

- Complex pharmacological designs have used up to 12 experimental arms (groups) in order to answer specific questions.

- To study the role of learning in placebo effects, for example, conditioning, one needs to control the associations between conditioned and unconditioned stimuli both in the experimental and in the clinical setting.

- Several approaches are possible for hiding a therapy from the subject's view, so that he is totally unaware that a treatment is being performed.

12.1 What are we looking for?

The first question that should be asked when running a placebo study is "What are we looking for?" Although this seems quite obvious, in the large placebo literature this question is not always well posed. In this regard, we can go back to the Foreword of this book and to Chapters 1 and 2 in which the problem about the definition of placebo effect was described in detail. In other words, if we want to study the placebo effect, we cannot study classical pragmatic clinical trials because their experimental design is not appropriate for the analysis of placebo groups. What a pragmatic trial wants to look for is the superiority of the active treatment over the placebo, thus it is not interested in knowing what happens in the placebo group. Whether the improvement in the placebo group is due to a spontaneous remission or to a brain event of anticipation does not matter in a pragmatic clinical trial. Likewise, if no placebo is given, and the new treatment is compared with the old one, what matters is the superiority (superiority trials), the equivalence (equivalence trials), or the noninferiority (noninferiority trials) of the new treatment relative to the old one (see sections 1.2 and 11.1).

What is needed in a pragmatic clinical trial that wants to assess the efficacy of a therapy is the comparison between two groups, or arms—the active treatment arm versus the placebo arm. Otherwise, other designs do exist. For example, in crossover trials one group first receives the active treatment and then the placebo, whereas a second group first receives the placebo and then the active treatment (see sections 1.2 and 11.1 for further details). As no conclusion can be drawn about what is going on in the placebo arm by using these approaches, clinical trials are not informative at all and do not tell us anything about real placebo responses.

The simplest way to study the real placebo effect is to compare a placebo arm with a no-treatment arm, as we have seen many times throughout this book (e.g., Chapters 2 and 4). The difference between the no-treatment arm, which assesses the natural course of the disease, and the placebo arm, which assesses the outcome of the placebo treatment, represents the true placebo effect. This experimental approach is simple, as it requires the comparison between two groups only, but it merely tells us whether or not a placebo effect is present and what its magnitude is. Thus, within the context of modern placebo research, the comparison between a no-treatment arm and a placebo arm can be considered only the starting point for further investigation. In other words, first we want to assess whether a true placebo response occurs, and then we want to go on further to investigate the possible underlying mechanisms. If we want to study the biochemical and neurobiological mechanisms of the placebo effect, we need much more complex designs that can answer the many biological questions for a better comprehension of the phenomenon.

Box 12.1 The experimental design devised by James Lind

James Lind, a Scottish doctor, was probably one of the first physicians who devised a very simple experimental design to verify the therapeutic efficacy of several medicaments in scurvy. In 1747, while serving in the Royal Navy, he carried out a controlled experiment, which can be considered a rudimentary and oversimplified form of a 6-arms experiment. Lind selected 12 men suffering from scurvy from one ship. Interestingly, he limited his subjects to men who were as similar as possible, thus reducing variability due to extraneous factors. Then, he divided them into six pairs, giving each pair different supplements to their basic diet for 2 weeks. The treatments were all remedies that had been previously proposed by other physicians: (1) a quart of cider every day, (2) 25 drops of elixir vitriol (sulfuric acid) three times a day, (3) one half-pint of seawater every day, (4) a mixture of garlic, mustard, and horseradish, (5) two spoons of vinegar three times a day, (6) two oranges and one lemon every day. The men given citrus fruits recovered within 1 week, whereas the others experienced some improvement, but nothing compared to the subjects who consumed the citrus fruits. Therefore, Lind concluded that citrus fruit was substantially superior to the other treatments.

The following sections summarize several experimental designs performed in my laboratory, the results of which have been described throughout the book. It is not necessary to describe the results of the experiments here as they can be found in the other sections of the book. Rather, these examples illustrate how a placebo study should be designed and conducted, and which questions such designs can answer. This selection is mainly based on the complexity of the design, on the type of question needed to be answered, and the problem that one wants to look for. It is important to realize that these complex designs represent the very nature of placebo research, because they can uncover true placebo responses that are sometimes too small to be detected. Box 12.1 gives an example of a rudimentary form of 6-arms design performed in 1747.

12.2 **Many arms are better than two**

12.2.1 **The 12-arms experiment with placebo, naloxone, and proglumide**

In this experiment (Benedetti, 1996; see also sections 4.1.2 and 4.1.6), experimental ischemic arm pain was investigated to study the involvement of endogenous opioids and cholecystokinin (CCK) in placebo analgesia (Fig. 12.1). It was conducted according to a randomized double-blind paradigm on 340 healthy volunteers. The first 117 subjects were randomized to six control arms (or Groups).

Group 1 (n = 67) was the no-treatment, or natural history, arm and was used to furnish data on the normal changes in pain ratings; in this arm, when the subjects reached 7 on a numerical rating scale (NRS) ranging from 0 (no pain) to 10 (unbearable pain), a hidden injection of saline was performed. Arm 1 was used to show that it is safe to define a placebo responder in the following way: "A subject with pain rating of 7 or less at 15 minutes following administration of the placebo."

Group 2 (n = 10) was the "hidden naloxone" arm and was used to see whether 10 mg of naloxone produced an increase in pain. Therefore, this arm tells us whether naloxone per se has a hyperalgesic effect. In this arm, a hidden injection of naloxone was made at an NRS of 7.

Group 3 (n = 10) received hidden saline and Group 4 (n = 10) received hidden naloxone. They were used to monitor the possible effects of naloxone at low levels of pain intensity. A hidden injection of either saline (Group 3) or 10 mg of naloxone (Group 4) was performed 15 minutes before the beginning of pain, and the pain rating lasted until an NRS of 7 was reached.

Group 5 (n = 10) and *Group 6* (n = 10) were called "hidden proglumide" arms and were used to see whether proglumide per se produced a reduction in pain (Group 5, 0.05 mg; Group 6, 0.5 mg). In these arms, a hidden injection of proglumide was made at an NRS of 7.

The remaining 223 subjects received an injection of saline in full view (placebo) when an NRS of 7 was reached. If pain rating was 7 or less at 15 minutes following the open saline injection, a subject was considered to be a placebo responder. A percentage of 26.9% responders was found (n = 60) and these were randomized to Groups 7, 8, 9, or 10.

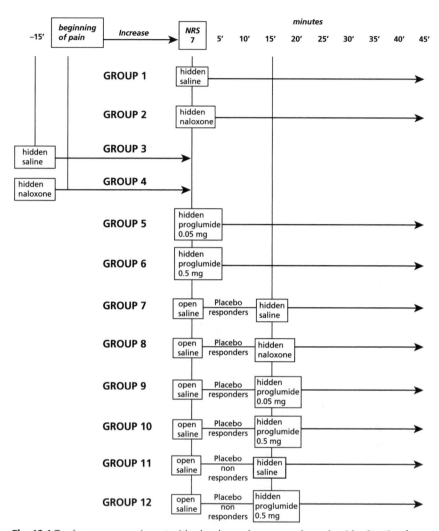

Fig. 12.1 Twelve-arms experiment with placebo, naloxone, and proglumide. Starting from a pain intensity numerical rating scale (NRS) of 7 (at time 0) the experimental conditions differed for each group. Subjects scored pain every 5 minutes up to 45 minutes. Groups 3 and 4 represent special cases whereby pain intensity was rated from the beginning of pain to NRS of 7. Reproduced from Fabrizio Benedetti, The opposite effects of the opiate antagonist naloxone and the cholecystokinin antagonist proglumide on placebo analgesia, *Pain*, 64 (3), pp. 535–543 Copyright 1996, The International Association for the Study of Pain, with permission.

Group 7 (n = 15) was defined the "placebo-saline" arm. In this arm, when the subjects reached 7 on the NRS, an injection of saline in full view of the subject (placebo) was performed. The subject was told that the injected substance was a potent painkiller acting within 20 minutes. After 15 minutes from the placebo injection, a hidden injection of saline was made, and this was compared with Groups 8, 9, and 10.

Group 8 (n = 15) was the "placebo-naloxone" arm. In this arm, when the subjects reached 7 on the NRS, an injection of saline in full view (placebo) was performed. As in Group 7, the subject was told that the substance was a powerful painkiller acting within 20 minutes. After 15 minutes from placebo injection, thus 5 minutes before the expected maximum effect, a hidden injection of 10 mg of naloxone was performed. This arm was used to see whether naloxone blocked the placebo analgesic response.

Group 9 (n = 15) and *Group 10* (n = 15) were called "placebo–proglumide" arms, and were the same as Group 8 but, after 15 minutes from the placebo injection, a hidden injection of 0.05 mg and 0.5 mg of proglumide, respectively, was made. These two arms were used to see whether proglumide enhanced the placebo analgesic response in a dose-dependent manner.

Most of the subjects (163 of 223) did not respond to the placebo. A nonresponder was defined as a subject with a pain rating of 8 or more at 15 minutes from the placebo injection; 30 of these 163 subjects were randomly chosen on the basis of previously as-signed numbers, and represented Groups 11 and 12.

Group 11 (n = 15) was defined as the "nonresponder saline" arm and was used as a control for comparison with Group 12. The procedure was the same as in Groups 7, 8, 9, and 10, but a hidden injection of saline was made in placebo nonresponders.

Group 12 (n = 15) was called the "nonresponder proglumide" arm and was used to see whether proglumide was effective in placebo nonresponders. The procedure was the same as in Group 11 but a hidden injection of 0.5 mg of proglumide was made in nonresponders after 15 minutes from the placebo injection.

It is important to point out that the subjects of Groups 1–6 did not know that any injection was performed, whereas those of Groups 7–12 were only aware of the first in-jection (placebo). Starting from the first score of 7, the subjects scored their pain every 5 minutes. After 45 minutes from the first injection, the experiment was discontinued even if pain ratings were still low, as the subjects usually reported being tired. Likewise, the subjects of Groups 3 and 4 rated their pain every 5 minutes, from the beginning of pain to NRS of 7.

In this experiment it was demonstrated that naloxone blocks placebo analgesia whereas proglumide enhances it. In addition it was shown that naloxone has no hyper-algesic effects on this type of pain, whereas proglumide has no analgesic effects. Also, proglumide was shown to have no effect in placebo nonresponders (Benedetti, 1996; see also sections 4.1.2 and 4.1.6).

12.2.2 The 12-arms experiment with placebo, naloxone, morphine, and ketorolac

In this experiment (Amanzio and Benedetti, 1999; see also section 4.1.6), experimental ischemic arm pain was studied to understand which conditions determine activation of endogenous opioids in placebo analgesia (Fig. 12.2). It was conducted according to a randomized double-blind paradigm on 229 healthy volunteers. To allow the double-blind administration of drugs and placebos, morphine or ketorolac or saline were given on days 2 and 3. On day 4, morphine or naloxone or saline were administered. To avoid a large number of subjects, only two or three subjects per Group received saline on days 2 and 3 and morphine or ketorolac on day 4. These subjects were not included in

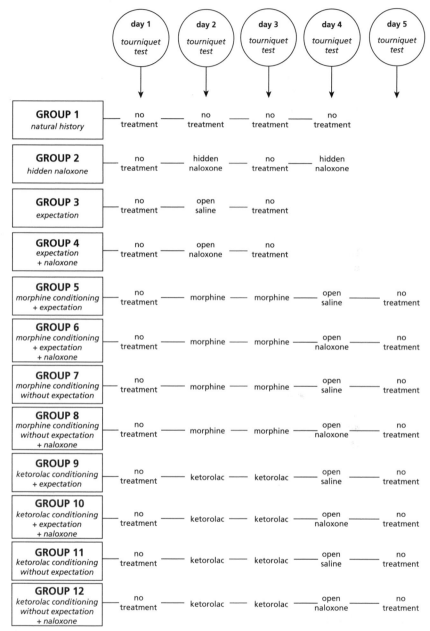

Fig. 12.2 Twelve-arms experiment with placebo, naloxone, morphine, and ketorolac. The experimental condition is specified for each group. The tourniquet test is used to induce ischemic arm pain. "No treatment" means that the tourniquet test was performed without the infusion of any drug. Reproduced from Martina Amanzio and Fabrizio Benedetti, Neuropharmacological Dissection of Placebo Analgesia: Expectation-Activated Opioid Systems versus Conditioning-Activated Specific Subsystems, *The Journal of Neuroscience*, 19 (1), pp. 484–494, figure 1 Copyright 1999, The Society for Neuroscience.

the study because they were used only to allow the double-blind design. All drugs were injected 10 minutes before the induction of the pain.

Group 1 (n = 56) was the no-treatment arm and the pain was induced for 4 days consecutively to assesses the natural course of pain over a 4-day period.

Group 2 (n = 25) received a hidden injection of naloxone on days 2 and 4 to ascertain whether naloxone per se affected this type of pain. These subjects did not know that any injection was being performed.

Group 3 (n = 16) received an open injection (in full view of the subject) of saline on day 2 and was told that it was a powerful painkiller. This arm was used to study the effect of expectation on pain relief.

Group 4 (n = 15) received an open injection of naloxone on day 2 and was told that it was a potent painkiller. In this way, the effect of naloxone on expectation-induced analgesia was tested.

Group 5 (n = 13) was treated with morphine (open injection) on days 2 and 3 (conditioning) and received an open injection of saline (placebo) on day 4, believing that it was morphine. Thus in this arm, the placebo response was tested after pharmacological conditioning.

Group 6 (n = 14) was treated with morphine (open injection) on days 2 and 3 (conditioning) and received an open injection of naloxone on day 4, believing that it was morphine. In this way, the effect of naloxone on placebo analgesia after pharmacological morphine conditioning was assessed.

Group 7 (n = 14) and *Group 8* (n = 16) received the same treatment as Groups 5 and 6. However, the open injections of saline or naloxone on day 4 were believed to be a nonanalgesic solution (antibiotic) used for sterility purposes. In these arms, the subjects did not expect any pain reduction, thus in this case the placebo analgesic response without expectation but with previous conditioning was tested.

Group 9 (n = 17), *Group 10* (n = 15), *Group 11* (n = 14), and *Group 12* (n = 14) were treated as Groups 5, 6, 7, and 8, with the exception that the pharmacological conditioning on days 2 and 3 was performed with the nonopioid analgesic, ketorolac.

This experiment demonstrated that morphine preconditioning induced placebo responses that were opioid-mediated, whereas nonopioid preconditioning with ketorolac induced placebo responses that were not mediated by endogenous opioids. In addition, it was shown that conditioning alone can produce placebo analgesia, even though no expectation is present. In general, expectation alone was shown to induce smaller placebo responses than expectation plus conditioning (Amanzio and Benedetti, 1999; see also section 4.1.6).

12.2.3 The 6-arms experiment on the somatotopic effects of placebo and naloxone

In this experiment (Benedetti et al., 1999; see also section 4.1.6) the aim was to induce local placebo responses in different parts of the body and to see whether naloxone specifically blocked these local placebo responses. Pain was induced by means of a subcutaneous injection of capsaicin simultaneously into the dorsal side of the right hand, left hand, right foot, and left foot. The experiments were performed in 173 subjects according to a randomized double-blind design (Fig. 12.3).

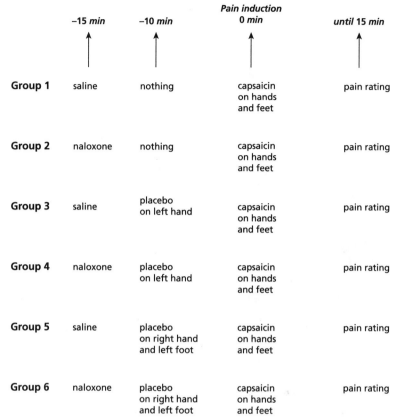

Fig. 12.3 Six-arms experiment on the somatotopic effects of placebo and naloxone. Starting from time 0 (induction of capsaicin pain) the same design was used for all the subjects, but subjects were randomized to 6 arms receiving different treatments at 15 and 10 minutes before time 0. Data from Fabrizio Benedetti, Claudia Arduino, and Martina Amanzio, Somatotopic Activation of Opioid Systems by Target-Directed Expectations of Analgesia, *The Journal of Neuroscience*, 19 (9), pp. 3639–3648, figure 2, 1999.

Group 1 (n = 48) received a hidden injection of saline 15 minutes before the subcutaneous capsaicin. This arm represented the natural history of the capsaicin-induced pain.

Group 2 (n = 20) received a hidden injection of naloxone 15 minutes before the subcutaneous capsaicin. This arm was used to assess whether naloxone per se affected the burning pain sensation induced by capsaicin.

Group 3 (n = 25) received a placebo cream on the left hand before subcutaneous capsaicin along with the verbal suggestions that it was a powerful local anesthetic. A hidden saline injection was performed 15 minutes before subcutaneous capsaicin. In this arm, the effect of the placebo cream was assessed.

Group 4 (n = 27) received the same treatment as Group 3; however, a hidden injection of naloxone was performed 15 minutes before capsaicin. Therefore, this arm was used to see whether naloxone antagonized specifically the placebo effect on the left hand.

Groups 5 (n = 24) and *Group 6* (n = 29) were treated as Groups 3 and 4, however the placebo cream was applied to the right hand or left foot. These two arms were used to study the effects of naloxone on local placebo responses in two different parts of the body.

This experiment demonstrated local placebo analgesic responses that were specifically antagonized by naloxone, thus suggesting a somatotopic organization of the placebo-activated endogenous opioid systems (Benedetti et al., 1999; see also section 4.1.6).

12.2.4 The 4-arms experiment with nocebo, diazepam, and proglumide

The aim of this experiment (Benedetti et al., 2006a; see also section 4.2.3) was to investigate the role of anxiety as well as of CCK in nocebo hyperalgesia, by using an experimental ischemic pain model. It was performed in 49 healthy volunteers. Only those subjects within a predetermined range of hormonal plasma concentrations were included in the study, that is an adrenocorticotropic hormone (ACTH) plasma concentration of 14–30 pg/mL and a plasma cortisol concentration of 90–130 micrograms/L. The experiments were always performed at 9 o'clock in the morning in order to avoid variability in the basal activity of the hypothalamus–pituitary–adrenal axis, according to a randomized double-blind design. To do this, either the active drug or saline solution was given. To avoid a large number of subjects, two or three additional subjects per group received an infusion of saline in place of the active drug. These subjects were not included in the study because they were used only to allow the double-blind design.

The 49 subjects were randomly subdivided into four arms. The procedure is shown in Fig. 12.4.

Group 1 (n = 12) was tested twice (with an interval of 4 days) with the experimental ischemic pain without receiving any treatment. Therefore, this arm represents the natural history of the pain over the 2 days of the experiment.

Group 2 (n = 13) was tested twice, with an intertest interval of 4 days. In the first test these subjects did not receive any treatment, whereas in the second test they underwent a nocebo procedure. This consisted of an orally administered, inert talc pill 5 minutes before the induction of pain, along with the verbal suggestions that it was a powerful vasoconstrictor further increasing the experimentally induced ischemia. The subjects were further told that, due to the quick vasoconstriction, this would induce a faster and larger increase of pain intensity, so that a quite strong hyperalgesic effect should be expected. In order to further strengthen the nocebo verbal suggestions, the subjects were told that they could give up at any time. Therefore, this experimental paradigm represents a situation in which a stressor is anticipated.

	Pain induction in session 1	Pain induction in session 2
Group 1	No treatment	No treatment
Group 2	No treatment	Nocebo
Group 3	Diazepam	Nocebo + diazepam
Group 4	Proglumide	Nocebo + proglumide

Fig. 12.4 Four-arms experiment with nocebo, diazepam, and proglumide. Each group was tested twice with experimental ischemic pain, and the interval between sessions 1 and 2 was 4 days. In the "no treatment" condition, no drug was administered. In the nocebo condition, an inert talc pill was given along with verbal suggestions of hyperalgesia. Reproduced from Fabrizio Benedetti, Martina Amanzio, Sergio Vighetti, and Giovanni Asteggiano, The Biochemical and Neuroendocrine Bases of the Hyperalgesic Nocebo Effect, *The Journal of Neuroscience*, 26 (46), pp. 12014–12022, figure 6 Copyright 2006, The Society for Neuroscience, with permission. doi: 10.1523/JNEUROSCI.2947–06.2006.

Group 3 (n = 12) was tested twice (intertest interval 4 days), like Group 2, but these subjects received a pretreatment with the antianxiety drug diazepam 30 minutes before the induction of the pain.

Group 4 (n = 12) was tested with the experimental pain, like Groups 2 and 3, but 30 minutes after a pretreatment with the CCK-antagonist proglumide.

In all these arms, the plasma concentrations of ACTH and cortisol were assessed before the induction of pain and at 5 and 10 minutes during the pain challenge, according to standard clinical practice.

In this experiment, it was found that diazepam blocks both nocebo hyperalgesia and nocebo hormonal responses, whereas proglumide blocks nocebo hyperalgesia only, which indicates two independent mechanisms of drug action of diazepam and proglumide (Benedetti et al., 2006a; see also section 4.2.3 and Fig. 4.13).

12.3 Investigating sequence effects and learning

12.3.1 The design for expectation versus conditioning effects

This experiment (Benedetti et al., 2003; see also sections 4.1.3, 5.1.2, and 7.3.4) was aimed at assessing the contribution of expectation and conditioning in three different medical conditions: pain, Parkinson's disease, and hormone secretion (Fig. 12.5).

Pain

A total of 60 healthy volunteers participated in the study. The experiments were performed according to a randomized double-blind design. To do this, either ketorolac or saline solution was given. To avoid a large number of subjects, when the saline injection

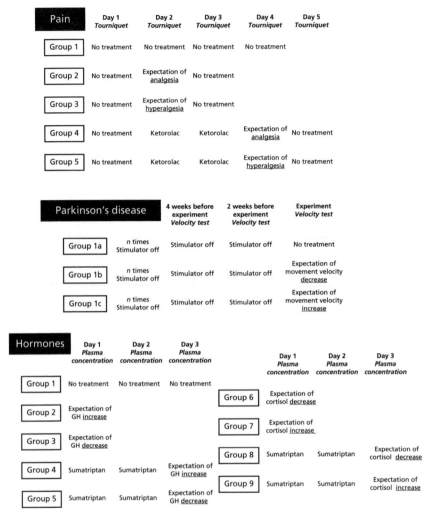

Fig. 12.5 Design used to test expectation versus conditioning effects in pain (5 arms), Parkinson's disease (repeated-measures design in the same patients) and hormone secretion (9 arms). Reproduced from Benedetti F, Pollo A, Lopiano L, Lanotte M, Vighetti S and Rainero I, Conscious expectation and unconscious conditioning in analgesic, motor and hormonal placebo/nocebo responses, *Journal of Neuroscience*, 23 (10), pp. 4315–23, figure 1 Copyright 2003, The Society for Neuroscience.

had to be performed, two or three subjects per group received ketorolac and were interspersed among those who received the saline injection. These subjects who received ketorolac in place of saline were not included in the study because they were used only to allow the double-blind design. All the injections were performed 10 minutes before the induction of the pain.

The subjects underwent experimental ischemic arm pain and were subdivided into five arms. The complete experimental procedure for pain is shown in Fig. 12.5.

Group 1 (n = 14) was tested for 4 days consecutively without receiving any treatment, and was used to assess the natural course of pain over a 4-day period.

Group 2 (n = 12) received an injection of saline solution on day 2 and was told that it was a powerful painkiller, a verbal suggestion aimed at inducing expectation of analgesia.

Group 3 (n = 12) received an injection of saline on day 2 and was told that it was a drug increasing pain. Thus, expectation of hyperalgesia was induced.

Group 4 (n = 11) was treated with the analgesic, ketorolac, on day 2 and 3 (conditioning) and received an injection of saline on day 4, with the verbal suggestion that it was ketorolac. Therefore, in this arm, expectation of analgesia was induced after pharmacological conditioning.

Group 5 (n = 11) was treated with ketorolac on days 2 and 3 (conditioning) and received an injection of saline on day 4, with the verbal suggestion that it was a drug increasing the pain. Therefore, expectation of hyperalgesia was induced after a pharmacological analgesic conditioning.

In this study, it was demonstrated that the expectation of hyperalgesia counteracted completely the pharmacological preconditioning with an analgesic drug, thus indicating that the placebo analgesic response was not attributable to conditioning but to expectation (Benedetti et al., 2003; see also section 4.1.3).

Parkinson's disease

Ten patients with idiopathic Parkinson's disease and with an implanted stimulator for deep-brain stimulation participated in the study. Each patient was tested for the velocity of movement of their right hand according to a double-blind experimental design. In order to check and set the stimulation parameters for clinical and therapeutic purposes, in all the patients the stimulator had been turned off many times, from the electrode implantation to the experimental procedure. Fig. 12.5 shows that movement velocity was tested 4 and 2 weeks before the experiment session. Three experimental conditions were analyzed in three different days, and their order was changed for each patient.

In *Condition a* the patients received no treatment, that is the stimulator was kept on and the patient did not receive any verbal instruction.

In *Condition b* patients were told that the stimulator was going to be turned off, but actually it was kept on. Therefore, expectation of worsening in motor performance was induced verbally.

In *Condition c* they were told that the stimulation intensity was going to be increased in order to improve motor performance, but actually no change in stimulus intensity was made. In this case, expectation of improvement of motor performance was induced verbally.

This study showed that that verbally induced expectations of motor improvement or worsening antagonized completely the effects of a conditioning procedure, which indicates that these placebo effects are mediated by expectation and not by conditioning (Benedetti et al., 2003; see also section 5.1.2 and Fig. 5.1C).

Hormones

A total of 95 healthy volunteers participated in this study and all the experiments were performed at 9 o'clock in the morning, after an indwelling intravenous catheter had been inserted into a forearm vein in order to take blood samples. All the experiments were performed according to a randomized double-blind design. To do this, either the antimigraine drug sumatriptan or saline solution was given. To avoid using a large number of subjects, when the saline injection had to be performed, two or three subjects per group received sumatriptan and were interspersed among those who received the saline injection. These subjects who received sumatriptan in place of saline were not included in the study because they were used only to allow the double-blind design. Fig. 12.5 shows the experimental design for hormones. The subjects were randomized to nine arms.

Group 1 (n = 15) received no treatment and was used to check for intraday and interday variations both in plasma growth hormone (GH) and plasma cortisol. To do this, a total of seven blood samples were taken at 15 minute intervals over 90 minutes. This procedure was repeated for 3 days in a row.

Groups 2, 3, 4 and 5 were tested for GH responses as follows:

Group 2 (n = 9) received a subcutaneous injection of saline solution in the lateral region of the thigh and subjects were told that GH was going to increase. Blood samples were taken 15 minutes before the injection, right after the injection (at 0 minutes) and 15, 30, 45, 60, and 75 minutes after the injection. This arm was used to assess the effects of expectation of GH increase on GH secretion.

Group 3 (n = 11) underwent the same procedure but subjects were told that GH was going to decrease. This arm was used to assess the effects of expectation of GH decrease on GH secretion.

Group 4 (n = 9) and *Group 5* (n = 11) were given the same saline injection with the same verbal instructions as Groups 2 and 3, respectively, but after preconditioning with sumatriptan, a selective agonist of serotonin type 1B/1D receptors that stimulates GH secretion and inhibits cortisol secretions. These arms were used to assess the effects of expectation of either a GH increase or decrease on GH secretion after pharmacological sumatriptan conditioning.

Groups 6, 7, 8, and 9 were tested for cortisol responses as follows:

Group 6 (n = 9) was given a subcutaneous injection of saline solution and told that cortisol was going to decrease. This arm was used to assess the effects of expectation of cortisol decrease on cortisol secretion.

Group 7 (n = 10) was told that cortisol was going to increase. This arm was used to assess the effects of expectation of cortisol increase on cortisol secretion.

Group 8 (n = 10) and *Group 9* (n = 11) were given the same saline injection and the same verbal instructions as Groups 6 and 7, respectively, but after preconditioning with sumatriptan. As described earlier, blood samples were taken 15 minutes before the injection, right after the injection (at 0 minutes), and 15, 30, 45, 60, and 75 minutes after the injection. These arms were used to assess the effects of expectation of either cortisol decrease or increase on cortisol secretion after pharmacological sumatriptan conditioning.

In this study, it was demonstrated that verbally induced expectations of increase or decrease of GH and cortisol did not have any effect on the secretion of these hormones. However, if preconditioning was performed with sumatriptan, which stimulates GH and inhibits cortisol secretion, a significant increase in GH and decrease in cortisol plasma concentrations were found after placebo administration, even though contrasting verbal suggestions were given. These findings indicate that placebo hormonal responses are mediated by conditioning and not by expectations (Benedetti et al., 2003; see also section 7.3.4 and Figs. 7.6 and 7.7).

12.3.2 The conditioning procedure for intraoperative recording

In this study (Benedetti et al., 2004; see also section 5.1.6), the purpose was to evoke large placebo responses intraoperatively in Parkinson patients during the implantation of electrodes for recording from single neurons in the subthalamic nucleus. Twenty-three patients participated in the study. They were randomly subdivided into two arms. The first received a placebo treatment (n = 11) whereas the second arm did not receive any treatment (n = 12).

In order to obtain powerful placebo responses, a preoperative conditioning procedure was performed, whereby repeated effective treatments for Parkinson's disease were given. The sequential steps of the entire procedure, both preoperative and intraoperative, are shown in Fig. 12.6. The Parkinson patients (in the medication-off state) were given a 2–3 mg dose of apomorphine subcutaneously 5 days, 2 days, and 1 day before surgery. In order to minimize nausea, they were treated with domperidone. Thus they received an effective antiparkinsonian treatment three times before surgical implantation of the electrodes. Each time a trained neurologist (not necessarily the same one who evaluated the patient intraoperatively) assessed symptom improvement using the Unified Parkinson's Disease Rating Scale (UPDRS), with particular regard to muscle rigidity at the wrist. Patients who developed dyskinesias after apomorphine injection were excluded.

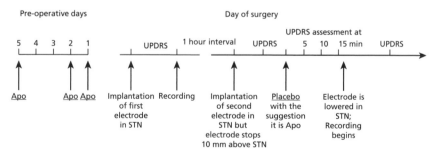

Fig. 12.6 The conditioning procedure for intraoperative recording. Both the preoperative and intraoperative steps are shown. Apo, apomorphine; STN, subthalamic nucleus; UPDRS, Unified Parkinson's Disease Rating Scale. Reproduced from Fabrizio Benedetti, Luana Colloca, Elena Torre, Michele Lanotte, Antonio Melcarne, Marina Pesare, Bruno Bergamasco, and Leonardo Lopiano, Placebo-responsive Parkinson patients show decreased activity in single neurons of subthalamic nucleus, *Nature Neuroscience*, 7 (6), pp. 587–588 Copyright 2004, Nature Publishing Group. doi: 10.1038/nn1250

On the day of surgery, during implantation of the first electrode, neuronal activity was recorded from the first subthalamic nucleus and the rigidity of both wrists was assessed several times.

After the first electrode was implanted, the surgical procedures for the implantation of the second electrode began. The time interval between the first and the second implantation was about 1 hour in all patients, and left and right implantation was randomized between subjects. During the second implantation, the tip of the electrode was stopped 10 mm above the subthalamic nucleus. This was done in order to avoid any possible microlesion-induced effects in the subthalamic nucleus produced by the passage of the microelectrode.

At this point, after rigidity assessment of the contralateral wrist, a subcutaneous injection of saline solution (placebo) was given with the suggestion that it was the same antiparkinsonian drug given on the previous days and that a motor improvement should be expected. More specifically, these patients were told that apomorphine was going to be injected and that a sensation of well-being should occur. Then wrist rigidity was assessed after 5, 10, and 15 minutes by a blinded neurologist, who did not know anything about the subcutaneous injection.

After 15 minutes the electrode was lowered into the subthalamic nucleus and neuronal recording began. An interval of 15 minutes between the placebo injection and the beginning of the recording was chosen on the basis of the action of apomorphine, as assessed the week before surgery. In fact, the effect of apomorphine begins after about this time lag.

At the end of the recording, arm rigidity was assessed again by the same blinded neurologist. After 15 minutes from placebo administration all the patients were asked to report any sensation of therapeutic benefit or, otherwise, of discomfort. In this way, it was possible to correlate the subjective report of the patient with the objective evaluation of the blinded neurologist. It is important to point out that the blinded neurologist did not know anything about the purpose of the study and that the arm rigidity assessment was done without knowing the subjective report of the patient. In fact, in order to avoid any influence of the patients' reports of well-being on the blinded neurologist, the patients described their subjective sensations when the neurologist was out of the operating room.

By comparing the pre-placebo neuronal activity in the subthalamic nucleus of one side with the post-placebo neuronal activity in the subthalamic nucleus of the other side, this study demonstrated that a placebo treatment caused reduced activity in single neurons in the subthalamic nucleus of placebo-responsive Parkinson patients (Benedetti et al., 2004; see also section 5.1.6).

12.3.3 The experiment on learning

This experiment (Colloca and Benedetti, 2006; see also sections 4.1.2 and 11.1.3) was aimed at investigating the role of prior experience in the magnitude of placebo analgesia following painful electrical stimulation. A total of 30 healthy volunteers participated in the study. After determination of pain threshold, each subject was randomly assigned to one of three experimental arms (Fig. 12.7).

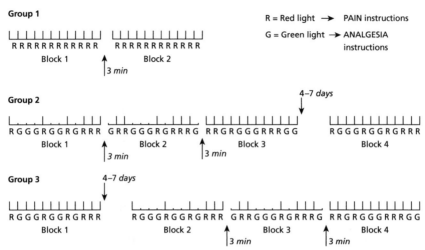

Fig. 12.7 Three-arms experimental paradigm to study learning. In all the conditions, a red light (R) means "pain" and is always associated with a painful stimulus (long vertical bar). Conversely, a green light (G) means "analgesia" and is associated either with a nonpainful tactile stimulus (short vertical bar) to train subjects, or with a painful stimulus (long vertical bar) to test placebo responses. Reproduced from Luana Colloca and Fabrizio Benedetti, How prior experience shapes placebo analgesia, *Pain*, 124 (1), pp. 126–33 Copyright 2006, The International Association for the Study of Pain, with permission. http://dx.doi.org/10.1016/j.pain.2006.04.005

In *Group 1* (n = 10), two blocks of 12 pain stimuli, each at twice the pain threshold (2T), were delivered. The interval between the two blocks was 3 minutes. Each stimulus was delivered at the end of a 12-second presentation of a red light (displayed on a computer screen). Subjects were told that the red light anticipated the delivery of a painful stimulus. Therefore, in this arm 24 associations (12 for each block) of red light and pain stimulus were performed. At the end of each association, subjects reported their perceived pain intensity according to an NRS that ranged from 0 (no pain) to 10 (unbearable pain). This arm was used as a control for possible sensitization and habituation effects. In other words, this arm represents the natural history group.

Group 2 (n = 10) underwent two experimental sessions on two different days. On the first day, three blocks of 12 stimuli each were delivered. The first block (block 1) consisted of six painful stimuli at 2T associated with the red light and six tactile stimuli (the intensity was surreptitiously lowered by 2 mA below pain threshold (T–2 mA)) associated with a green light. In the latter case, as done in previous studies, the subjects did not know that the intensity had been reduced. In fact, a sham electrode was applied to the middle finger of the hand that received the pain stimulus, and the subjects were told that the green light anticipated the activation of this electrode which, in turn, induced an analgesic effect. The second block (block 2) was the same as block 1. In block 3 the same random sequence of red and green lights was used, but all the 12 stimuli were painful (2T). Pain intensity was reported according to the NRS as in Group 1. It should be noted that this third block was actually an extinction trial, in that the green light was paired with the painful stimuli. Therefore, whether extinction occurred within a sequence as long as 12 stimuli was also tested. After 4–7 days, a further block (block 4) of 12 painful stimuli was delivered, which was exactly the same as the third block. This arm was used to assess both the short-lasting (minutes) and the long-lasting (days) effects of a conditioning procedure.

Group 3 (n = 10) underwent two experimental sessions on two different days. On day 1 one block of 12 stimuli was delivered, as per block 4 in Group 2. Subjects were told that a red light would anticipate a pain stimulus (six stimuli) while a green light anticipated a painful stimulus that was made analgesic by the stimulation of the middle finger (six stimuli). Actually, all 12 stimuli were painful, as they were set at 2T. After 4–7 days, three blocks each of 12 stimuli were delivered, as in the first session of Group 2. In other words, the two sessions of Group 3 were reversed compared to Group 2. Note that an extinction trial was run in this case also.

In this study it was shown that prior experience has a crucial influence on placebo analgesia, thus emphasizing the role of learning in the placebo effect (Colloca and Benedetti, 2006; see also sections 4.1.2 and 11.1.3 and Figs. 4.2C and 11.2).

12.4 **Comparing expected versus unexpected therapies**

12.4.1 **How to compare an open with a hidden treatment**

The experiment by Amanzio et al. (2001) (see also section 4.1.4) compared open (expected) versus hidden (unexpected) administration of four widely used painkillers in postoperative pain: buprenorphine, tramadol, ketorolac, and metamizole. A total of 278 patients who underwent different types of thoracic surgery were studied.

Straight after recovery from anesthesia, a single intravenous bolus of the painkiller was administered. Analgesia and respiratory depression, nausea, sedation and other side effects were assessed after 15 minutes. If adequate analgesia was not obtained, an equal bolus dose was given; this procedure was repeated until a satisfactory analgesic response occurred. We recorded the analgesic dose (AD) needed to obtain pain reduction of 50% (AD50) for each patient. Since it is not possible to observe a decrease of pain of exactly 50% in all patients, the AD_{50} was corrected according to the following formula:

$$AD_{50} = \frac{d(i/2)}{r}$$

where d represents the total dose administered, r is the decrease of pain according to an NRS ranging from 0 (no pain) to 10 (unbearable pain), and i is the initial pain intensity.

Open injections of the analgesic drug consisted of administration of the bolus by a doctor in full view of the patient. The patient was told that the medication was a powerful painkiller. In contrast, hidden injections were administered by a preprogrammed infusion machine without any doctor or nurse in the room so that the patient was totally unaware that a painkiller was being given. The NRS was assessed every 15 minutes.

Four drugs were studied: buprenorphine was given in boluses of 0.1 mg each, tramadol in boluses of 30 mg each, ketorolac in boluses of 10 mg each, and metamizole in boluses of 300 mg each. Both the open and hidden injections were performed with the same infusion time of 1 minute.

This study showed that in all cases the AD_{50} was larger with hidden injections, which indicates that the four analgesics were less effective when given covertly (Amanzio et al., 2001; see also section 4.1.4 and Fig. 4.3A).

In another study by Colloca and Benedetti (2005) (see also section 11.1.3 and Fig. 11.3) a different approach was used in order to better address some ethical problems that may occur with hidden administrations of drugs. In this study, the patients in the hidden condition knew that a painkiller was going to be given, but they did not know when. In fact, an infusion pump was preprogrammed to deliver the drug at the desired time, according to a double-blind design, in which neither the patient nor the doctor knew when the drug delivery was to begin.

12.4.2 The open–hidden paradigm in Alzheimer patients

This study (Benedetti et al., 2006b; see also sections 6.3.2 and 11.2.3, as well as Fig. 6.6) was aimed at correlating prefrontal executive control and functional connectivity with placebo responsiveness, as assessed by means of the open–hidden design. It was performed in 28 communicative patients with Alzheimer's disease. They were tested at the initial stage of the disease and after 1 year. All patients showed reduced connectivity among different brain regions after 1 year (see later). For comparison, the study included ten more Alzheimer patients who did not show a reduced connectivity.

Both the controls and the Alzheimer patients visited the hospital so that two blood samples could be taken on 2 days consecutively. Elderly people often complain of a painful burning sensation during and after insertion of a needle into the vein on the dorsal aspect of the hand. Usually a 1% solution of the local anesthetic lidocaine is applied to the cutaneous region where the needle had been inserted. Each patient and one of their relatives gave informed consent to receive either a lidocaine application or no application at all, depending on the situation. In fact, sometimes lidocaine is not applied because of the need to run a quantitative sensory test immediately after the blood sample. Thus, when a hidden application was performed, the patients believed that no lidocaine was applied.

In the open condition, the drug was applied in full view of the patients, telling them that their pain was going to subside in a few minutes. Then, according to routine clinical practice, the skin was covered with tape.

In the hidden condition, the drug was administered and the patient was completely unaware that a local anesthetic was being applied. In fact the same dose of lidocaine was contained within the tape that covered the skin. The tape was applied with no information about the treatment and the likely pain reduction in the following minutes. To justify the lack of lidocaine application, the patients were told that lidocaine would be applied or it would not, depending on the circumstances.

The patients rated their pain according to an NRS ranging from 0 (no pain) to 10 (unbearable pain) just before and 15 minutes after the application of lidocaine.

The open and hidden application of lidocaine was balanced on the left and right hand in different subjects.

Since the burning sensation after blood sampling also induces agitation and since heart rate (HR) is a good index of agitation and relaxation, an electrocardiogram was recorded using conventional techniques with two electrodes on the chest.

To study prefrontal functioning from a neurophysiological point of view, an electro-encephalogram was recorded and 'mutual information analysis' was used as a measure of functional connectivity, or coupling, among different intra- and interhemispheric brain regions. In this study, the mutual information among all pairs of electrodes (19×19) was calculated and plotted on a three-dimensional matrix.

By correlating the difference between open and hidden lidocaine with the electro-encephalogram functional connectivity, this study demonstrated reduced placebo responsiveness in those Alzheimer patients with disconnection of the prefrontal lobes from the rest of the brain (Benedetti et al., 2006b; see also sections 6.3.2 and 11.2.3, and Fig. 6.6).

12.4.3 The experiment with deep-brain stimulation

This experiment (Pollo et al., 2002; see also section 5.1.2 and Fig. 5.1B) used a somewhat different approach. It was performed in seven patients with Parkinson's disease who were implanted with electrodes for deep-brain stimulation.

Each patient was tested twice on different days, with an interval of 1 week, according to a double-blind design in which neither the patient nor the experimenter knew the intensity of the stimulation being delivered. In both the experimental conditions, "bad performance" and "good performance," stimulus intensity was changed in the same way and the movement velocity of the right hand was assessed.

After a first baseline test of movement velocity at 100% intensity (which represents optimal therapeutic stimulation) the stimulus was reduced to 80% of the initial stimulation and a second baseline test was run. Then the stimulus was reduced to 20% of the initial intensity and three velocity tests were run at 5, 15, and 30 minutes. The stimulus was then increased to 40% of the initial level and a test was run at 5 minutes. Finally the initial 100% stimulation was restored and a velocity test was run at 5 minutes.

Patients were tested in two different conditions in which opposite expectations were induced. The order of the two conditions was changed randomly in different patients. In "bad performance" they were told the truth about what was going to happen: when the stimulus reduction was from 80% to 20% (at 43 minutes from the beginning of the experiment) they were told that their motor performance was going to worsen; when the stimulus was increased from 20% to 40% (at 76 minutes) they were told that a small improvement in their motor performance was going to occur; and, finally, when the step was from 40% to initial stimulation (at 84 minutes) they were told their motor performance was going to return to normal values. In "good performance" they were told when the stimulus reduction was from 80% to 20% (at 43 minutes) that nothing was going to change in their motor performance, so no worsening was expected; when the stimulus was increased from 20% to 40% they were told that a big improvement in motor performance was going to occur because of a dramatic increase of subthalamic stimulation; they were told nothing when the stimulus was increased from 40% to initial stimulation.

This experiment demonstrated that the unexpected decrease in movement velocity induced a worsening in motor performance that was smaller than the expected decrease in velocity (Pollo et al., 2002; see also section 5.1.2 and Fig. 5.1B).

12.5 **Points for further discussion**

1   A 12-arms trial is conceivable with healthy volunteers but it is difficult to employ in real clinical settings. It can be used to answer specific questions about the action of drugs and biochemical mechanisms of the placebo effect.

2   A 4-arms trial is much simpler and might also be used in a real clinical setting to answer specific questions about mechanisms of placebo effects in specific diseases.

3   It would be interesting to use the designs about sequence effects and learning in different medical conditions and with different therapeutic interventions. In this way, both theoretical issues and practical implications could be addressed.

4   The open–hidden design is not easy to perform. As well as the technical problems relating to hidden administration per se, several ethical issues must always be taken into account.

References

Amanzio M and Benedetti F (1999). Neuropharmacological dissection of placebo analgesia: expectation-activated opioid systems versus conditioning-activated specific sub-systems. *Journal of Neuroscience*, **19**, 484–94.

Amanzio M, Pollo A, Maggi G and Benedetti F (2001). Response variability to analgesics: a role for non-specific activation of endogenous opioids. *Pain*, **90**, 205–15.

Benedetti F (1996). The opposite effects of the opiate antagonist naloxone and the cholecystokinin antagonist proglumide on placebo analgesia. *Pain*, **64**, 535–43.

Benedetti F, Amanzio M, Vighetti S and Asteggiano G (2006a). The biochemical and neuroendocrine bases of the hyperalgesic nocebo effect. *Journal of Neuroscience*, **26**, 12014–22.

Benedetti F, Arduino C and Amanzio M (1999). Somatotopic activation of opioid systems by target-directed expectations of analgesia. *Journal of Neuroscience*, **19**, 3639–48.

Benedetti F, Arduino C, Costa S et al. (2006b). Loss of expectation-related mechanisms in Alzheimer's disease makes analgesic therapies less effective. *Pain*, **121**, 133–44.

Benedetti F, Colloca L, Torre E et al. (2004). Placebo-responsive Parkinson patients show decreased activity in single neurons of subthalamic nucleus. *Nature Neuroscience*, **7**, 587–8.

Benedetti F, Pollo A, Lopiano L, Lanotte M, Vighetti S and Rainero I (2003). Conscious expectation and unconscious conditioning in analgesic, motor and hormonal placebo/nocebo responses. *Journal of Neuroscience*, **23**, 4315–23.

Colloca L and Benedetti F (2005). Placebos and painkillers: is mind as real as matter? *Nature Reviews Neuroscience*, **6**, 545–52.

Colloca L and Benedetti F (2006). How prior experience shapes placebo analgesia. *Pain*, **124**, 126–33.

Pollo A, Torre E, Lopiano L et al. (2002). Expectation modulates the response to subthalamic nucleus stimulation in Parkinsonian patients. *NeuroReport*, **13**, 1383–6.

Part 5

Beyond the healing context

Placebo effects are not limited to the pathological context, but extend to physiological situations in healthy individuals. These include physical performance in sport and cognitive performance. In addition, although the word placebo is used within the context of medical practice, both in pathological and physiological situations, it is worth pointing out that some similarities do exist with some effects within the domain of social psychology, for example, the effects of expectations on judgments, attitudes, and behaviors. Unfortunately, very little is known about the underlying mechanisms, particularly those related to biology and physiology. Therefore, in this part there are more questions than answers, but this will hopefully stimulate further debates and research.

Chapter 13

Physical and cognitive performance

Summary points

- In spite of the fact that very different experimental conditions have been investigated, all available data indicate athletes' expectations as important elements of physical performance.
- Although there is compelling evidence that physical performance in sport activities is boosted by placebos, the underlying mechanisms are not known.
- The use of placebo procedures in sport competition poses some important ethical questions about doping.
- Nocebo effects have been found to counteract good physical performance, and indeed they can interfere with training programs.
- Only a few studies have tried to investigate the effects of placebos on cognitive performance, and very little is known about either their effectiveness or their mechanisms.

13.1 **Physical performance**

13.1.1 **Placebos boost physical performance**

As for drug development, in the assessment of efficacy of the many substances revolving around the sport world, there is also a gray zone where placebos (and nocebos) can exert their influence. Here too, chemicals such as vitamins, ergogenic aids, or diet supplements are handed out, or physical treatments and manipulations of different kinds are delivered, and expectations about their effects are set in motion in the athlete's brain. And here too, care must be taken to distinguish between the psychobiological phenomenon and the overall improvement in the control arm of trials, which in spite of being called "placebo effect" is contaminated and amplified by other factors. Thus, only very recently and only few works have been published, focusing on placebo mechanisms in physical performance.

In general, all available data indicate athletes' expectations as important elements of physical performance, in spite of the fact that very different experimental conditions have been investigated (Beedie and Foad, 2009; Pollo et al., 2011). These range from short anaerobic sprints to long aerobic endurance cycling, and many different outcome

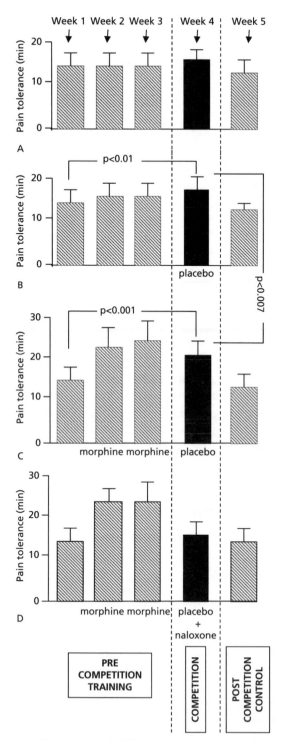

Fig. 13.1 Mean pain endurance times (±SD) in the precompetition training phase (weeks 1–3), on the day of competition (in week 4; black bars), and in the post-competition control (week 5) in four teams (A–D) that competed against each other in a competition

measures have been used, such as time, speed, and weight lifted. Indeed, many clinical trials of ergogenic and performance-boosting agents have been performed in a variety of sports. The most interesting trials have used untreated control groups, so allowing the identification of genuine placebo responses.

For example, Clark et al. (2000) investigated the placebo effect of a carbohydrate supplement on endurance performance in 43 cyclists in a simulated 40-kilometer timed trial. They were subdivided into three groups: the first received just water and was told nothing; the second ingested a drink containing 7.6 g per 100 mL of carbohydrate; and the third received a noncaloric placebo. The second and third groups were further subdivided into those who were told the drink contained nothing, those who were told it contained carbohydrate, and those who were told it contained placebo. The difference in mean power between the "told-carbohydrate" and the "told-placebo" group was 3.8%.

In a subsequent study, six cyclists in a laboratory 10-kilometer timed trial were told that they would receive either placebo or 4.5 mg/kg caffeine or 9 mg/kg caffeine, but actually they always received placebos (Beedie et al., 2006). A dose–response effect was found, whereby the cyclists who believed they had ingested placebo showed a decrease in power of 1.4%, those who believed they had ingested 4.5 mg/kg caffeine showed an increase in power of 1.3%, and those who believed they had received 9 mg/kg caffeine showed a 3.1% increase in power. Interestingly, some caffeine-related side effects were reported. By contrast, in a study on placebo responses associated with caffeine suggestions, only a limited effect of placebo was found (Flaten et al., 2003).

In a different study on the role of positive and negative expectations, Beedie et al. (2007) administered placebos to 42 athletes, along with opposite verbal instructions. In one group, athletes were told that the agent was ergogenic, thus they should expect an increase in performance. Athletes in a second group were provided with negative instructions about the possible negative effects of the substance. They were all tested by means of a sprint protocol before and 20 minutes after placebo administration. The first group showed a significant linear trend of greater speed with successive experimental trials, whereas the second group ran 1.57% slower than baseline.

In a simulation of sport competition in which subjects had to compete with each other in a competition of pain endurance, Benedetti et al. (2007) found that placebo administration on the day of competition induced longer pain tolerance compared to an untreated group (Fig. 13.1A, B). However, if pharmacological preconditioning was

---

Fig. 13.1 (continued) of pain endurance. On the day of the competition a significant increase in performance occurs after placebo administration compared to baseline in both groups B and C, whereas in groups A and D no increase in performance occurs. The performance of team C which was preconditioned with morphine is significantly better than that of group B, which receives the placebo without prior conditioning with morphine. Although team D receives the placebo on the competition day after morphine preconditioning, the beneficial effects are antagonized by the opioid antagonist naloxone. Reproduced from Fabrizio Benedetti, Antonella Pollo, and Luana Colloca, Opioid-Mediated Placebo Responses Boost Pain Endurance and Physical Performance: Is It Doping in Sport Competitions?, *The Journal of Neuroscience*, 24 (44), pp. 11934–11939, figure 2 Copyright 2007, The Society for Neuroscience. DOI: 10.1523/JNEUROSCI.3330–07.2007.

performed with morphine in the precompetition phase, the replacement of morphine with a placebo on the day of the competition induced an increase in pain endurance and physical performance that was significantly larger than placebo without prior morphine preconditioning (Fig. 13.1C). The placebo effect after morphine preconditioning could be prevented by administration of the opioid antagonist, naloxone, which suggests that this placebo response is opioid-mediated (Fig. 13.1D). These placebo analgesic responses were obtained after two morphine administrations that were separated as much as 1 week from each other.

Similar findings were obtained with a nonpharmacological conditioning procedure (Pollo et al., 2008) in which the effects of an ergogenic placebo on the quadriceps muscle, which is responsible for the extension of the leg relative to the thigh, were studied. A placebo, which the subjects believed to be caffeine at high doses, was administered twice in two different sessions. Each time the weight to be lifted with the quadriceps was reduced surreptitiously so as to make the subjects believe that the "ergogenic agent" was effective. After this conditioning procedure, the load was restored to the original weight, and both muscle work and fatigue were assessed after placebo administration. A robust placebo effect occurred, with a significant increase in muscle work and a decrease in muscle fatigue. These findings suggest a central mechanism of top-down modulation of muscle fatigue, which seems to be more important or as important as peripheral mechanisms arising from muscles.

Overall, by considering that these studies have used control groups, such as no-treatment groups, there is some compelling evidence that genuine placebo effects occur in sport. Within the context of recent theories of muscle fatigue, these placebo responses acquire a very important meaning. In fact, central mechanisms would play a role in muscle performance and fatigue, as postulated early in the 1910s by Krogh and Lindhard (1913) through the concept of central command. The notion of central command, or a central governor, implies that several physiological parameters like heart rate, arterial blood pressure, pulmonary ventilation, and muscle performance could be altered by manipulating the subject's perception of exercise. Indeed, we saw previously (section 5.2) that autonomic responses can be modulated by stimulation of several regions in the brain, like the subthalamic region in rats (Spencer et al., 1988; Van del Plas et al., 1995), in cats (Angyan and Angyan, 1996, 1999), and in humans (Priori et al., 2001; Thornton et al., 2002; Kaufmann et al., 2002; Benedetti et al., 2004; Lanotte et al., 2005). For example, stimulation of the subthalamic nucleus in freely moving cats induces a conspicuous increase in blood pressure, heart rate, and respiratory rate (Angyan and Angyan, 1999). In Parkinson patients, it has been found to induce heart rate increases and variable blood pressure responses (Kaufmann et al., 2002; Thornton et al., 2002) as well as autonomic responses according to the psychological context (Benedetti et al., 2004; Lanotte et al., 2005). In patients undergoing deep-brain stimulation, Green et al. (2007) found that anticipation of exercise resulted in increases in heart rate, blood pressure, and ventilation, which were accompanied by neural changes in the periaqueductal gray and subthalamic nucleus.

Muscle fatigue has also been found to be affected by a central governor (Box 13.1) (St Clair Gibson et al., 2003, 2006; Lambert et al., 2005). For example, St Clair Gibson et al.

Box 13.1 The central governor

At the end of 1800/beginning of 1900, the physiologist Angelo Mosso asserted that fatigue might appear at first sight as an imperfection of our bodies, but actually it is one of its most marvelous perfections, for it saves us from the injury produced by strenuous exercise. He also proposed that fatigue arises from the central nervous system, and that only a small contribution arises from the muscles. This idea was supplanted by that of Archibald Vivian Hill who believed that fatigue was the result of biochemical changes in the muscles (peripheral fatigue) to which the central nervous system makes no contribution. Today we witness a revival of Mosso's idea and model, whereby the brain uses the symptoms of fatigue as key regulators to ensure that the exercise is completed before harm develops. The existence of a central governor, or central command, in the central nervous system was suggested to explain fatigue after prolonged strenuous exercise in long-distance running and other endurance sports, emphasizing that subconscious and conscious mental decisions made by winners and losers are the ultimate determinants of both fatigue and athletic performance. The central governor model of exercise regulation and physical performance proposes that the central nervous system regulates exercise performance by continuously modifying the number of motor units that are recruited in the exercising muscles. This occurs in response to conscious and subconscious factors that are present before and during the exercise. The purpose of this control is to ensure that humans always exercise with reserve and terminate the exercise bout before there is a catastrophic failure of homeostasis. The brain uses the unpleasant sensations of fatigue to ensure that the exercise intensity and duration are always within the physiological capacity. The athletes who best control the progression of these subjective fatigue symptoms during exercise can reach the highest performances (Noakes, 2012).

(2001) found that, as fatigue increased in cycling, the electromyographic activity in leg muscles declined, even during sprint, thus indicating that fatigue is not due to muscle fibers hitting some limit. In many of these reported studies, athletes were asked to perform at their limit, in an all-out effort. Placebos apparently acted by pushing this limit forward. Therefore, it can be speculated that they could impact on a central governor of fatigue. The output of this center would continuously regulate exercise performance to avoid reaching maximal physiological capacity. This would provide protection against damage on one hand, and constant availability of a reserve capacity on the other (Hampson et al., 2001; Lambert et al., 2005). By altering expectations, placebos could then represent a psychological means to signal to the central governor to release the brake, allowing an increase in performance in a manner not dissimilar from that achieved by pharmacological means (for example, by amphetamines decreasing perceived fatigue).

13.1.2 **Should opioid-mediated placebo responses be considered doping?**

By taking all these studies into consideration, the increase in performance following placebo administration may have practical applications, but it also raises important questions as to how these effects should be exploited in sport competitions. The ethical issue is particularly significant when one wants to induce opioid-mediated placebo responses by means of pharmacological preconditioning with illegal drugs. In the study by Benedetti et al. (2007), described in the previous section, morphine was given twice in the precompetition training phase and was then replaced with a placebo which, in turn, mimicked the effect of morphine (Fig. 13.1). These morphine-like effects of placebos raise the important issue of whether opioid-mediated placebo responses are ethically acceptable in sports competitions or whether they have to be considered as doping procedures in all respects.

According to the Prohibited Drugs List 2014 of the WADA (World Anti-Doping Agency, 2014) drugs can be divided into those that are prohibited at all times and those that are prohibited only during competitions. For example, morphine is considered to be an illegal drug only during competitions, whereas its use out of competition is legal. Therefore, one could conceive of applying precompetition conditioning with morphine and then replacing it with a placebo on the day of competition. According to the Prohibited Drugs List 2014 of the WADA (World Anti-Doping Agency, 2014) the training procedures with morphine performed by Benedetti et al. (2007) should be considered legal because the athletes are allowed to consume narcotics out of competition. However, they could also be considered illegal because morphine administration is aimed at conditioning athletes for subsequent replacement with a placebo, which is supposed to have morphine-like effects during the competition.

Doping is a matter of great public concern. We should be aware that if a procedure like that of Benedetti et al. is carried out, whereby morphine is used as a preconditioning drug in the precompetition training phase, then illegal drugs in sport would not be discoverable and would not violate the antidoping rules.

13.1.3 **Nocebos can counteract good physical performance**

Nocebo effects are not limited to the pathological context, but extend to physiological situations in which intact individuals perform normal motor tasks. For example, Beedie et al. (2007) used a 30-meter repeat-sprint protocol, measuring speed in subjects receiving (placebo) starch capsules coupled with different instructions to elicit positive or negative expectations about the ensuing performance. While the positive belief group displayed increasing speed, the negative belief group worsened (Beedie et al. 2007) (see also section 13.1.1). Likewise, Pollo et al. (2012) showed that it is possible to negatively modulate the performance of subjects carrying out a muscle exercise to volitional maximum effort by employing discouraging suggestions and negative conditioning. In this study, the authors observed a significant decrease in the work performed under volitional maximal effort in the nocebo group compared to a significant increase of about 15% observed in the control group. In an attempt to evaluate whether a negative conditioning can strengthen the effect of expectation elicited by verbal suggestion, the authors coupled the application of a sham electrical stimulation of the quadriceps muscles with the surreptitious increase of the weight to lift (procedural conditioning). In this case also, a sharp group difference was found, with controls improving about 29% and nocebo subjects showing no changes in work performed. These findings may have profound implications for training strategies, because negative expectations may counteract the positive effects of training programs.

13.2 **Cognitive performance**

13.2.1 **Placebos boost performance within the cognitive domain**

A number of studies suggest that placebos and expectations enhance, at least in part and in some circumstances, cognitive performance (Green et al., 2001; Oken et al., 2008; Parker et al., 2011; Weger and Loughnan, 2013) and other cognition-related tasks, such as reaction times (Anderson and Horne, 2008; Colagiuri et al., 2011). For example, Green et al. (2001) used a balanced placebo design to investigate the extent of expectancy in the ability of glucose to affect cognitive performance. During two of the sessions, subjects were given a drink containing 50 g glucose and on the other two they were given a drink containing aspartame. For half the sessions subjects were accurately informed as to the content of the drink (glucose or aspartame), whereas in the other two sessions they were misinformed as to the content of the drink. The cognitive tests included a vigilance task, an immediate verbal free-recall task, an immediate verbal recognition memory task and a measure of motor speed (two-finger tapping). Interestingly, glucose administration was found to improve recognition memory times and performance on the vigilance task, but only in sessions where subjects were informed that they would receive glucose and not when they were told that they would receive aspartame. Therefore, expectation contributes to the positive effects of glucose on cognition. In another study, Oken et al. (2008) compared healthy seniors who took a 2-week supply of placebo pills, which they were told was an experimental cognitive enhancer, with seniors not taking any pills. The authors found a significant effect of pill taking on a wordlist delayed recall task and on a Stroop color word task. In an analysis of potential predictors of the expectancy effect, perceived stress and self-efficacy but not personality traits interacted with the pill-taking effect on cognitive function.

Colagiuri et al. (2011) tested whether an instructional manipulation could produce placebo effects on implicit learning, a nonconscious cognitive task. Students completed a visual search task while smelling an odor or no odor, in alternating blocks. Unknown to them, the task contained a contingency whereby on half the trials the target's location was cued by the pattern of distractors, which was achieved by repeating some configurations of targets and distractors. Prior to the task, participants received positive, negative, or no information about the odor's possible effects on performance. Those students who were given positive information showed faster reaction times on cued trials than the other students. Conversely, the students who received negative information showed slower reaction times on cued trials compared with students given no information. Similarly, Weger and Loughnan (2013) employed a placebo procedure which was told to unconsciously enhance the participants' knowledge, so that they should hence trust their skills in an upcoming knowledge test. It was found that performance was indeed enhanced, compared to a group that did not think the procedure would improve their knowledge. Placebo positive suggestions have also been found to decrease the cognitive conflict in a Stroop task, whereas negative suggestions have been found to increase the cognitive conflict (Magalhães De Saldanha da Gama et al., 2013).

Virtually nothing is known about the biological underpinnings of these possible cognition-enhancing effects by placebos. However, it is interesting to note that Stern et al. (2011) used the μ-opioid antagonist naloxone to test the role of endogenous opioids in the placebo response within the cognitive domain. Healthy men were required to perform a task-battery, including standardized and custom-designed memory tasks, to test short-term recall and delayed recognition. Tasks were performed twice, before and after intravenous injection of either saline or naloxone according to a double-blind paradigm. While the subjects of one group were given neutral information, the others were told that they might receive a drug with memory-boosting properties. Objective and subjective indexes of memory performance and salivary cortisol were recorded. Short-term memory recall, but not delayed recognition, was objectively increased after placebo-mediated suggestion in the saline group. Naloxone specifically blocked the suggestion effect without interfering with memory performance. These results were not affected when changes in salivary cortisol levels were considered, thus suggesting that stress was not involved. In addition, no reaction time changes were found, suggesting that there was no attentional impairment. Therefore, an opioid-mediated placebo effect seems to take place within a cognitive domain in healthy volunteers.

13.3 **Points for further discussion**

1　Physical performance includes a variety of factors, such as pain tolerance, fatigue endurance, muscle strength, motivation, and so forth. Therefore, several mechanisms are likely to be involved when placebos boost performance.

2　One of the main challenges of future research is to understand the biological underpinnings of all these factors and to integrate all the findings in order to identify possible practical implications and applications.

3　The ethical issue is one of the most important within this context. It entails discussion about the possible use of placebos to boost performance in athletes. The main question to answer is: Can the biological mechanisms triggered by placebo administration, such as endogenous opioids, be considered a form of doping?

4　We need to know whether illegal substances can produce conditioned placebo responses. For example, if an illegal substance is given for several days in a row and then replaced with a placebo on the competition day, can we obtain robust effects? This is an important ethical and legal issue, for a placebo can mimic the effect of a previously administered drug but an antidoping test could not detect it.

5　Virtually nothing is known about the real effects and the mechanisms of placebos on cognitive functions such as memory. A better understanding of the underlying neurobiology might lead to important implications. For example, placebo effects in memory might represent an interesting model to uncover some memory mechanisms.

References

Anderson C and Horne JA (2008). Placebo response to caffeine improves reaction time performance in sleepy people. *Human Psychopharmacology*, **23**, 333–6.

Angyàn L and Angyàn Z (1996). Cardiorespiratory effects of electrical stimulation of the globus pallidus in cats. *Physiology and Behavior*, **59**, 455–9.

Angyàn L and Angyàn, Z (1999). Subthalamic influences on the cardiorespiratory functions in the cat. *Brain Research*, **847**, 130–3.

Beedie CJ, Coleman DA and Foad AJ (2007). Positive and negative placebo effects resulting from the deceptive administration of an ergogenic aid. *International Journal of Sport Nutrition, Exercise and Metabolism*, **17**, 259–69.

Beedie CJ and Foad AJ (2009). The placebo effect in sports performance: a brief review. *Sports Medicine*, **39**, 313–29.

Beedie CJ, Stuart EM, Coleman DA and Foad AJ (2006). Placebo effects of caffeine on cycling performance. *Medical Sciences and Sports Exercise*, **38**, 2159–64.

Benedetti F, Colloca L, Lanotte M, Bergamasco B, Torre E and Lopiano L (2004). Autonomic and emotional responses to open and hidden stimulations of the human subthalamic region. *Brain Research Bulletin*, **63**, 203–1.

Benedetti F, Pollo A and Colloca L (2007). Opioid-mediated placebo responses boost pain endurance and physical performance: is it doping in sport competitions. *Journal of Neuroscience*, **27**, 11934–9.

Clark VR, Hopkins WG, Hawley JA and Burke LM (2000). Placebo effect of carbohydrate feeding during a 40-km cycling time trial. *Medical Sciences and Sports Exercise*, **32**, 1642–7.

Colagiuri B, Livesey EJ and Harris JA (2011). Can expectancies produce placebo effects for implicit learning? *Psychonomic Bulletin and Review*, **18**, 399–405.

Flaten MA, Aasli O and Blumenthal TD (2003). Expectations and placebo responses to caffeine-associated stimuli. *Psychopharmacology*, **169**, 198–204.

Green MW, Taylor MA, Elliman NA and Rhodes O (2001). Placebo expectancy effects in the relationship between glucose and cognition. *British Journal of Nutrition*, **86**, 173–9.

Green AL, Wang S, Purvis S *et al.* (2007). Identifying cardiorespiratory neurocircuitry involved in central command during exercise in humans. *Journal of Physiology*, **578**, 605–12.

Hampson DB, St Clair Gibson A, Lambert M I and Noakes TD (2001). The influence of sensory cues on the perception of exertion during exercise and central regulation of exercise performance. *Sports Medicine*, **31**, 935–52.

Kaufmann H, Bhattacharya KF, Voustianiouk A and Gracies JM (2002). Stimulation of the subthalamic nucleus increases heart rate in patients with Parkinson disease. *Neurology*, **59**, 1657–8.

Krogh A and Lindhard J (1913). The regulation of respiration and circulation during the initial stages of muscular work. *Journal of Physiology*, **47**, 112–36.

Lambert EV, St Clair Gibson A and Noakes TD (2005). Complex systems model of fatigue: integrative homoeostatic control of peripheral physiological systems during exercise in humans. *British Journal of Sports Medicine*, **39**, 52–62.

Lanotte M, Lopiano L, Torre E, Bergamasco B, Colloca L and Benedetti F (2005). Expectation enhances autonomic responses to stimulation of the human subthalamic limbic region. *Brain Behavior and Immunity*, **19**, 500–9.

Magalhães De Saldanha da Gama PA, Slama H, Caspar EA, Gevers W and Cleeremans A (2013). Placebo-suggestion modulates conflict resolution in the Stroop Task. *PLoS One*, **8**, e75701.

Noakes TD (2012). Fatigue is a brain-derived emotion that regulates the exercise behavior to ensure the protection of whole body homeostasis. *Frontiers in Physiology*, 3, 82.

Oken BS, Flegal K, Zajdel D, Kishiyama S, Haas M and Peters D (2008). Expectancy effect: impact of pill administration on cognitive performance in healthy seniors. *Journal of Clinical and Experimental Neuropsychology*, 30, 7–17.

Parker S, Garry M, Einstein GO and McDaniel MA (2011). A sham drug improves a demanding prospective memory task. *Memory*, 19, 606–12.

Pollo A, Carlino E and Benedetti F (2008). The top-down influence of ergogenic placebos on muscle work and fatigue. *European Journal of Neuroscience*, 28, 379–88.

Pollo A, Carlino E and Benedetti F (2011). Placebo mechanisms across different conditions: from the clinical setting to physical performance. *Philosophical Transactions of the Royal Society B*, 366, 1790–8.

Pollo A, Carlino E, Vase L and Benedetti F (2012). Preventing motor training through nocebo suggestions. *European Journal of Applied Physiology*, 112, 3893–903.

Priori A, Cinnante C, Genitrini S et al. (2001). Non-motor effects of deep brain stimulation of the subthalamic nucleus in Parkinson's disease: preliminary physiological results. *Neurological Sciences*, 22, 85–6.

Spencer SE, Sawyer WB and Loewy AD (1988). L-glutamate stimulation of the zona incerta in the rat decreases heart rate and blood pressure. *Brain Research*, 458, 72–81.

St Clair Gibson A, Baden DA, Lambert MI et al. (2003). The conscious perception of fatigue. *Sports Medicine*, 33, 167–76.

St Clair Gibson A, Lambert EV, Rauch LH et al. (2006). The role of information processing between the brain and peripheral physiological systems in pacing and perception of effort. *Sports Medicine*, 36, 705–22.

St Clair Gibson A, Schabort EJ and Noakes TD (2001). Reduced neuromuscular activity and force generation during prolonged cycling. *American Journal of Physiology: Regulatory Integrative Comparative Physiology*, 281, R187–96.

Stern J, Candia V, Porchet RI, Krummenacher P, Folkers G, Schedlowski M, Ettlin DA and Schönbächler G (2011). Placebo-mediated, Naloxone-sensitive suggestibility of short-term memory performance. *Neurobiology of Learning and Memory*, 95, 326–34.

Thornton JM, Aziz T, Schlugman D and Paterson DJ (2002). Electrical stimulation of the midbrain increases heart rate and arterial blood pressure in awake humans. *Journal of Physiology*, 539, 615–21.

Van del Plas J, Wiersinga-Post JE, Maes FW and Bohus B (1995). Cardiovascular effects and changes in midbrain periaqueductal gray neuronal activity induced by electrical stimulation of the hypothalamus in the rat. *Brain Research Bulletin*, 37, 645–56.

Weger UW and Loughnan S (2013). Mobilizing unused resources: using the placebo concept to enhance cognitive performance. *Quarterly Journal of Experimental Psychology*, 66, 23–8.

World Anti-Doping Agency (2014). *Prohibited drugs list 2014*. Available at: <http://www.wada-ama.org>.

Chapter 14

Halo effects

Summary points

- In this short chapter there are more questions than answers. It does not want to go into the complex domain of social psychology. It merely aims to stimulate further research on the effects of the context outside the healing setting.

- Halo effects can be considered, at least in part, similar to placebo effects because the context plays a crucial role in both.

- Whereas placebo effects have to do with the evaluation of symptoms, halo effects have to do with judgments of a person's quality and personality.

- The approach to placebo and halo effects is somehow related to expectations. If one expects pain reduction, one may experience a real analgesic effect. Likewise, if one expects either positive or negative qualities in a person, one may be misled to give either positive or negative judgments, respectively.

14.1 What they are

In the same way that the psychosocial context plays a crucial role in the placebo effect, the context is the key element in the halo effect. The term halo effect was coined by Thorndike (1920) while studying the personality traits of soldiers. He noted that two officers, who were asked to evaluate their soldiers for their physical, intellectual, leadership, and personal skills, tended to attribute positive qualities in all their judgments of a single individual. This holds true for negative qualities as well. In other words, there was a high correlation among both positive and negative judgments: if a soldier was judged to be intelligent, he was also judged to be loyal, cooperative, and a good leader. Likewise, if he was judged to be uncooperative, he was also judged to be nonintelligent and selfish. Therefore, the ratings about a soldier's quality by the two officers influenced the ratings of the other qualities.

A typical example of halo effect is a person's attractiveness. Someone who is perceived as attractive is likely to be perceived as intelligent and, similarly, people perceived as being more attractive are likely to be perceived as trustworthy and friendly. This, in turn, may affect perceptions tied to life success (Wade and Di Maria, 2003), which indicates that attractiveness may influence a variety of judgments. Different factors may take part in the halo effect, for example the emotional state. Forgas (2011) found that positive emotions affect the halo effect of a person's judgment about the philosophical attributes of an elderly man with a beard or a young woman. This approach to placebo and halo effects somehow overlaps with the expectation theory (Kirsch, 1999). If one expects either positive or negative qualities in a person, he/she may tend to give biased judgments.

Halo effects may pervade our daily life when judging persons, objects, and situations. For example, attractiveness is a strong predictor of decisions about leadership, especially in politics (Verhulst et al., 2010). Similarly, underestimation of caloric intake occurs when a restaurant is perceived as healthy (Chandon and Wansink, 2007).

This last chapter of the book does not want to go into the domain of social psychology, but rather it wants to pose some questions about some possible similarities between halo and placebo effects. In fact, whereas in the placebo effect the judgment is about a symptom like pain, in the halo effect the judgment is about a person's quality such as intelligence and skillfulness. But in both cases the judgments are influenced by the context. In future research, it will be interesting to replace the patient's evaluation of a symptom, as done in placebo research, with a person's evaluation of personality traits and qualities.

14.2 **Points for further discussion**

1 It will be interesting to understand similarities and differences between placebo and halo effects, and this will represent a bridge between medical sciences and social psychology.

2 We also need to understand the neurobiological underpinnings of halo effects in order to create a stronger bridge between neuroscience and social psychology.

References

Chandon P and Wansink B (2007). The biasing health halos of fast-food restaurant health claims: lower calorie estimates and higher side-dish consumption intentions. *Journal of Consumer Research*, **34**, 301–14.

Forgas JP (2011). She just doesn't look like a philosopher . . . ? Affective influences on the halo effect in impression formation. *European Journal of Social Psychology*, **41**, 812–17.

Kirsch I (1999). *How expectancies shape experience*. American Psychological Association, Washington, DC.

Thorndike EL (1920). A constant error in psychological ratings. *Journal of Applied Psychology*, **4**, 25–9.

Verhulst B, Lodge M and Lavine H (2010). The attractiveness halo: why some candidates are perceived more favorably than others. *Journal of Nonverbal Behavior*, **34**, 111–17

Wade TJ and Di Maria C (2003). Weight halo effects: individual differences in perceived life success as a function of women's race and weight. *Sex Roles*, **48**, 461–5.

Index